azing

Social Issues for Carers

Social Issues for Carers

TOWARDS POSITIVE PRACTICE

Second Edition

RICHARD WEBB BSc(Soc) MA CQSW PGCE
Lecturer in Social Care/Social Work, Castle Centre, Sheffield College

and

DAVID TOSSELL BSc(Soc) MSc CQSW PGCE
Lecturer in Health and Social Care/Social Work, College of North-East London;
Agency Social Worker and NVQ Assessor, Lewisham Social Services

ARNOLD

A member of the Hodder Headline Group
LONDON • NEW YORK • NEW DELHI

First published in Great Britain in 1991 by Edward Arnold

Sixth impression 1997

Second edition published in 1999

This impression reprinted in 2005 by

Hodder Arnold, a member of the Hodder Headline Group,

338 Euston Road, London NW1 3BH

http://www.hoddereducation.com

British Library Cataloguing in Publication Data
A catalogue record for this book is available from the British Library

ISBN-10: 0 340 70625 2
ISBN-13: 978 0 340 70625 1

5 6 7 8 9 10

Commissioning Editor: Nick Dunton
Production Editor: Wendy Rooke
Production Controller: Priya Gohil

Typeset in 10.5/14pt Janson by J&L Composition Ltd, Filey, North Yorkshire
Printed and bound by Replika Press Pvt. Ltd, India

What do you think about this book? Or any other Hodder Arnold title?
Please send your comments to www.hoddereducation.com

Every effort has been made to trace copyright holders of material. Any rights not
acknowledged here will be acknowledged in subsequent printings if notice is given to
the publisher.

To Emma, my daughter, with love
Richard Webb

To my mother, with love
David Tassell

Contents

Preface

This book is aimed at a wide range of people who are involved in the care of others, whether they are paid or unpaid. It draws on a number of study areas including health care, social care and social work practice, social policy and sociology.

We cannot claim that this book provides a comprehensive academic analysis of society. Instead, we have sought to focus on a range of social issues related to inequality, prejudice, discrimination, oppression, marginalization and social exclusion. Our aim has been to raise these issues for consideration, to stimulate discussion and to increase awareness of the effect of '*structural*' *disadvantage* on individuals.

The issues dealt with in this book are often complex and controversial, and invariably generate strong feelings and reactions whenever they are discussed. In a book of this size it would be impossible to explore fully all aspects of the issues raised. We have not sought to blame or accuse individuals of prejudiced views and behaviour; rather we have tried to shed some light on how discrimination has developed and why it occurs, and we have focused on the harmful effect of this process.

We are mindful of some of our own prejudices and limitations, which stem in part from the fact that we are two white, middle-class, middle-aged men who have been born into, and exposed to, the conditioning of British society. In order to present a fuller discussion of social issues, we have sought the assistance of a number of different people including women, disabled people, people from ethnic minorities, and people with different life-styles and sexual orientation. Along with others, we are engaged in the lengthy process of discovering and challenging our own behaviour. We hope that this book makes a contribution to a fuller appreciation of social issues and their significance for positive practice.

Richard Webb and David Tossell 1998

Acknowledgements

We should like to thank the following people for their advice, assistance and time:

Cath Baldock, Helen Barrett, Heidi Caldwell, Susan Cawthorne, Andy Dick, Ken Douglas, Mike Fowler, Ruth Hendry, Eileen Hendry, Keith Hendry, Richard Johnstone, Sue Ledger, Hector Medora, Alison Millerman, Linda Moore, Johnnie Murphy, Sue Myatt, Robin Parker, Laura Timms, Phil Timms, Umut Ugur, Ian Warwick, Pam Warwick, John Wilkinson, Leslie Wilson and Linsey Wilson.

In addition, we should like to thank the helpful library staff and publicity officers from the following organizations:

- Campaign for Racial Equality (CRE)
- Equal Opportunities Commission (EOC)
- Joint Council for the Welfare of Immigrants (JCWI)
- MIND
- National Children's Bureau (NCB)
- National Institute for Social Work (NISW)
- Race Equality Unit (REU)
- Terrence Higgins Trust
- Age Concern
- Stonewall

and the staff and students of the College of North-East London, for their ideas and support.

Finally, we are indebted to Joyce Tossell for her grammatical insight.

Introduction

AIMS OF THIS BOOK

This book aims both to inform and to stimulate carers into thinking about the influence of society by examining the important social issues that affect both the lives of those we care for and ourselves as carers. Caring takes place within a social setting and is carried out by a range of different people, including health and social work professionals, health and social carers, volunteers, and those caring for a friend or relative at home. It is necessary that the service-users' social context is understood in order that we, as carers, are able to appreciate the impact of the wider society on the individual and so obtain a more rounded perspective. Otherwise it is far too easy to observe an individual – for example, a person who has mental health problems or someone who is physically abusive to members of his or her family – and blame that person and say that they are entirely responsible for their situation. Categorizing individuals in this way may make the person making the judgements feel better, even superior, but it does not lead to a helpful understanding of the situation, nor does it point towards a resolution of the difficulties. Whilst it is fair to say that we are all in some way responsible for what we do, we are not always able to control our circumstances. An appreciation of the effect of external factors enables us to develop a more balanced and less judgemental view of the person we care for.

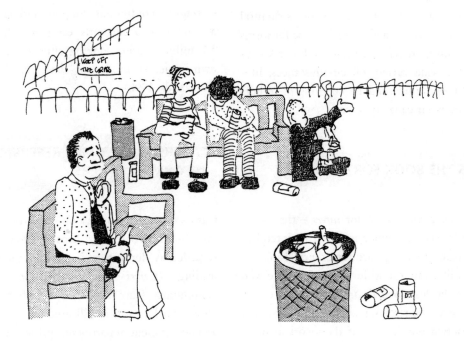

To what extent is society responsible?

THE FOCUS AND RELATED THEMES

The central focus of the book is *structural inequality*, by which we mean the systematic, uneven distribution of life-chances and how this affects each individual from the moment he or she is born. The different forms that structural inequality takes are explained alongside a number of interrelated themes, including: *prejudice, stereotypes, discrimination, oppression, powerlessness, marginalization* and *social exclusion.*

The main forms of structural inequality are social class, gender and race. However, social divisions are prevalent in other important respects, including disability, sexual orientation, age, life-style, health, citizenship and political status. Of course, individuals may experience structural inequality in a number of different forms simultaneously. For instance, an 80-year-old black woman may be said to be structurally disadvantaged in three main ways, owing to her age, gender and race. Likewise, a disabled young man who is gay will experience discrimination on at least two grounds, namely his impairment and his sexual orientation.

An appreciation of the effects of structural inequality on ourselves and those we care for forms a basis for our approach to caring – a fuller knowledge of the wide variety of circumstances, lifestyles, cultures, values and perceptions of others can strengthen our capacity to care.

WHO IS THE BOOK FOR?

This book has been written for *carers* – that is, all those people who are either involved or intend to be involved in providing care for others. Table 0.1 attempts to illustrate the wide range of people who can properly be described as *carers*, whether they are paid or unpaid. Their roles, positions and duties are all very different, but the core of their work involves a responsibility towards others. This responsibility is

to ensure that wherever care is provided, it is of a high quality, that it is offered with compassion, and that it is respectfully administered so that the independence, dignity and individuality of the person being cared for are upheld and maintained.

WHO ARE THE CARERS?

Most care takes place in the home. Only a relatively small number of adults are permanently cared for in institutional or residential accommodation. For instance, the proportion of people under 65 years of age who are cared for in a long-stay hospital, residential home or nursing home is less than 0.05 per cent of the population. For the 65–74 years age group the proportion is only 1 per cent, rising to 5.5 per cent for the 75–84 years age group, and over 25 per cent for people who are over 85 years of age (Age Concern, 1996).

Greatly outnumbering those who are receiving hospital, residential or nursing-home care are the many people, who – owing to disability, frailty, learning difficulties or challenging behaviour patterns – require continuous support and are cared for at home. It is currently estimated that there are 5.7 million carers looking after someone in their own home; 3.4 million of these carers are women (Rowlands, 1998).

CARERS, SOMETIMES REFERRED TO AS 'INFORMAL' CARERS

Carers themselves have long since rejected the epithet 'informal', mainly because it was variously regarded as 'derogatory, inaccurate, unclear or misleading' (*Carers' National Association Newsletter*, Community Care Project, November 1989, p. 1). However, the word is still used by some academics and government departments, primarily in order 'to make a distinction between those who are employed

Table 0.1 Who are the carers and where are they based?

Carer	Home/ domiciliary	Day/resource centre	Field/outreach and community	Residential care/nursing home	Hostel	Hospital unit/ hospice	Schools, nurseries and creches/child guidance clinics	Specialist settings prisons, therapeutic communities, young offender institutions
Care assistant/officer	0	✓	0	✓	0	0	✓	0
Health care assistant/worker	0	0	✓	0	0	✓	✓	0
Home carer/home support worker	✓	0	✓	0	0	0	0	0
Home help	✓	0	✓	0	0	0	0	0
Hospital support worker	0	0	0	0	0	✓	0	0
Assistant/one-to-one worker	✓	0	✓	✓	0	0	✓	✓
Carer of a friend or relative	✓	0	0	0	0	0	0	0
Adult carer/(foster carer for children)	✓	0	0	0	0	0	0	0
Residential social worker	0	0	0	✓	0	0	0	✓
Field social worker/care manager	0	0	✓	0	0	✓	✓	✓
Approved social worker (ASW)	0	0	✓	0	0	✓	✓	0
Probation officer	0	✓	✓	0	✓	0	0	✓
Education welfare officer (EWO)	0	0	✓	0	0	0	✓	0
Youth worker	0	✓	✓	0	✓	0	0	0
Community worker	0	✓	✓	0	0	0	0	0
Community psychiatric nurse (CPN)	0	0	✓	✓	0	✓	✓	✓
District Nurse (DN)/Health Visitor	0	0	✓	0	0	0	0	0
Occupational therapist (OT)	0	✓	✓	✓	0	✓	0	✓
Speech therapist	0	0	✓	0	0	✓	0	0

Table 0.1 Who are the carers and where are they based? (*cont.*)

Carer	Setting							
	Home/ domiciliary	Day/resource centre	Field/outreach and community	Residential care/nursing home	Hostel	Hospital unit/ hospice	Schools, nurseries and creches/child guidance clinics	Specialist settings prisons, therapeutic communities, young offender institutions
Art, drama and music therapist	O	O	✓	O	O	✓	O	O
Chiropodist	O	O	✓	O	O	✓	O	O
Physiotherapist	O	O	✓	O	O	✓	O	O
GP	O	O	✓	O	O	O	O	O
Junior doctor	O	O	O	O	O	✓	O	O
Consultant	O	O	✓	O	O	✓	O	✓
Psychiatrist	O	O	✓	O	O	✓	O	✓
Clinical psychologist	O	O	✓	O	O	✓	O	✓
Educational psychologist	O	O	✓	O	O	O	✓	O
Counsellor	O	O	✓	O	O	✓	O	✓
Speaker, signer advocate	O	O	✓	O	O	O	O	O
Housing tenancy support worker	O	O	✓	O	O	O	O	O
Police	O	O	✓	O	O	O	O	O
Creche-worker	O	✓	O	O	O	✓	✓	O
Nanny	✓	O	O	O	O	O	O	O
Officer/nursery nurse	O	✓	O	O	O	✓	✓	O

The above table shows where carers are *based*. However, although home-carers, home-helps and support workers are, strictly speaking, based in offices within the community, they have also been included as being based in a person's home, because this is where they carry out the bulk of their care work. Other carers, notably psychiatrists, CPNs and OTs, are not based in a person's home but visit people there as part of their regular practice. Similarly, carers such as social workers, probation officers and GPs who are based in the community may also periodically be called upon to carry out practice in a residential, nursing, hospital or specialized setting. Consultants, junior doctors and GPs have been included as carers so that the full spectrum of carers may be seen (some people would not categorize qualified doctors as carers, but they do spend much of their time talking to people and attempting to help them with problems or difficulties they may be facing, so are included within the broad definition of carer).

by an organization, authority or company to care and those who are not employed' (*Carers' National Association Newsletter*, Community Care Project, November 1989, p. 1).

Until relatively recently their circumstances were unknown, but the work of carers' organizations such as the Carers' National Association and the Alzheimer's Disease Society have done much to highlight the plight of people caring at home, to such an extent that specific legislation was introduced on their behalf in April 1995. The Carer's Recognition and Services Act 1995 entitled all carers to an independent assessment of their needs, separate from the needs of the person they were looking after.

It would be wrong to assume that carers always freely choose to undertake this role. Many of them have little or no option because of the lack of a satisfactory, realistic alternative. Either the dependent relative's condition is not severe enough to warrant residential care or hospitalization, or community services are inadequate or not sufficiently developed. Consequently, the burden of care falls mainly on families and, more particularly, on women. In fact, more women stay at home to care for elderly or disabled relatives than stay at home to look after young children.

VOLUNTEERS

Many organizations in our society depend for their successful functioning on the unpaid efforts and dedication of volunteers. Some voluntary and self-help organizations rely almost exclusively on voluntary help. Other larger voluntary and statutory bodies depend to a lesser extent on volunteers, who will often complement the work of paid employees. The motivation to volunteer is varied. For example, some people may not have satisfactory human contact in their daily lives, and have a need to help others, unemployed people may find that voluntary work provides a source of fulfilment, while others

may use the opportunity to gain experience and knowledge in the field of social care or social work. Some people, of course, have a committed spiritual or humanitarian motivation, while others simply have a strong moral conscience.

HEALTH AND SOCIAL CARERS

So far we have discussed people who are not paid for their caring. We shall now turn to those who are paid to care for others. In the UK there has traditionally been a somewhat artificial distinction between social carers and social workers, and between that which is considered to be *social care* and that which is regarded as *social work*.

In the field of health there is much less blurring of the roles and responsibilities of carers, including professionally qualified workers and basic-grade health carers. The distinction between roles is usually more clearly demarcated, owing to health cares more rigid and defined occupational structure. Health care may be said to include medical, surgical or psychiatric intervention, and this inevitably contains elements of both social work and social care.

Social care has come to be understood to mean only the direct physical care of clients, i.e. the washing, dressing, feeding and toileting of the client. Social work, on the other hand, still stands for purposeful enabling intervention on behalf of the whole person. This has arisen mainly as a result of historical factors. Although there have been social workers and social work training since the beginning of the century, social work practice as it is known today did not become established until the late 1950s, when it began to incorporate the prevalent psychoanalytical theories of the time. Since then there has been the establishment, in 1971, of the Social Services Departments in England and Wales and the Social Work Departments in Scotland; the latter were created following the Social Work (Scotland) Act 1968. Training has become established within higher education for both social workers and probation officers, and social work has used such developments to press its claim for professional status. Partly as a consequence of this, social work has been at pains to distance itself from the more pragmatic, routine element of its function, which has in turn been seen to be the province of social care.

A difference in status developed between field social workers and their contemporaries who worked in residential, domiciliary and day-care settings. This was compounded by the tendency for field workers to be provided with Certificate of Qualification in Social Work (CQSW) training, which was full-time and was offered almost exclusively in institutions of higher education, while residential and other workers were mainly expected to undertake Certificate in Social Services (CSS) training, which was provided on a day-release basis and required the student to remain at work. When the CSS was first introduced in 1975, it was not regarded as a professional qualification. It was only after it became recognized that the work carried out on the CSS was as thorough and comprehensive as that undertaken on CQSW courses that they were, in November 1987, officially deemed to be equivalent by the Central Council for Education and Training in Social Work (CCETSW) and social work trade unions and professional organizations. In 1994, the Diploma in Social Work replaced both the CSS and the CQSW, which was phased out over a period of 4 years. Whereas the majority of field social workers have received professional training, only a minority of residential social workers have had the opportunity to qualify.

The distinction between social care and social work is misleading for two main reasons. First, physical care is not carried out in isolation – it is an integral part of what has been traditionally regarded as social work. When, for example, a care-plan is designed for an older person, that person's physical needs, such as the planned visit to the chiropodist, the required changing of dressings, dietary needs and toileting arrangements, are taken into consideration, and so too are the client's social needs, such as the need to maintain links with loved ones and to attend gatherings wherever possible. Similarly, the client's intellectual need to be stimulated and to be engaged as much as possible in their surroundings is taken into account, together with their emotional and psychological need to be able to take risks and make decisions, to express themselves and to feel valued. The client's cultural requirements are also acknowledged and arrangements made to accommodate them. Physical care, essential as it may be, is neither more nor less important than any of the other elements of the social work task.

Secondly, if it is to be carried out properly, physical care cannot be performed without an understanding of the whole person, including the need for privacy, the need for time and space, and a person's right to have his or her cultural expectations met. In other words, that which is commonly regarded as social care is informed by social work principles.

Although, in practice, those people who are employed primarily as social care workers are predominantly concerned with the immediate, practical caring tasks of clients, their actions form part of a process of social work intervention. In this way social care can be seen to be part of social work.

Social work and social care are part of the same continuum – they overlap in practice. The field social worker may well be called upon to attend to the personal needs of his or her disabled clients; medical social workers may well have cause to deal with their clients' incontinence on home visits in the community. In the same way, residential social workers, particularly key-workers, are in a position to offer sustained emotional support and case-work intervention equivalent to that provided by their field-work colleagues. Care assistants or care officers and other residential staff, by the very nature of their situation, are often well placed to form meaningful relationships with clients and so contribute to the social work process. As Joan Beck, President of the Social Care Association, says, 'Living with your clients day in and day out provides the ideal situation to carry out social work. Even doing something like washing up together provides a natural environment in which to talk, unlike the artificial "home visit" situation' (*Social Work Today*, 19 October 1989, p.12).

The relationship that is formed between residential workers and residents can be stronger and more meaningful than that which exists between fieldworkers and their clients.

Among practitioners and academics alike there is no universal agreement about what constitutes social care and what constitutes social work. Consider the following definition. In your opinion does it relate to social care or social work?

> the term used to describe the activities and processes undertaken by all sectors/agencies (statutory, voluntary and independent) which seek to enable individuals, families and groups who are disadvantaged, or deprived in some way, to achieve a higher, self-determined level of functioning and quality of life. It is about the planned meeting of clients' needs. It concerns the physical, intellectual, emotional, cultural and social aspects of the client's development and well-being. It involves mutual trust and respect; it involves a sense of purpose and change; it recognizes the interaction between people and their environments.
>
> (Mallinson, 1988)

In fact the author was defining social care. However, it can be seen from the content that this definition is very similar to a description of conventional social work.

According to the British Association of Social Workers, 'social work' is said 'to be the purposeful and ethical application of personal skills in interpersonal relationships directed towards enhancing the personal and social functioning of an individual' in order 'to help create a social environment conducive to the well-being of all' (Bamford, 1990, p.30). Surely much of this, too, pertains to social care?

One way of clarifying the confusion that exists between social care and social work is not to focus on the separate tasks carried out by different workers, or on the authority and responsibility invested in particular roles. Instead, we need to consider the whole activity which is defined either as social care or social work.

As we have already stated, social care and social work can be seen to be part of the same continuum. Figure 0.1 shows the range of personal needs which can be met by the activity of social care and social work. As we move from social care on the left along the continuum towards social work on the right, we pass from more basic, physiological needs, through emotional and cultural needs, to less tangible and more general psychological and social needs. Social care informs social work, just as social work informs social care.

ORGANIZATIONS PROVIDING HEALTH AND SOCIAL CARE

Health and social care services are provided by a range of different types of organizations that are collectively referred to as the *mixed economy of care* (Fig. 0.2). This is composed of the statutory sector and the independent sector, which consists of voluntary organizations, not-for-profit organizations, private companies and individuals. The National Health Service and Community Care Act 1990 required local authorities to encourage the development of a mixed economy of care.

Paid carers may be employed by *statutory* or *non-statutory* organizations.

Statutory sector

Statutory organizations, as the name suggests, are those which have been set up by law. They operate at either national, regional or local level. The two main statutory care organizations in the UK are the National Health Service and Local Authority Social Services Departments (Social Work Departments in Scotland). (In Northern Ireland both Health and Social Services are administered by the National Health Boards.)

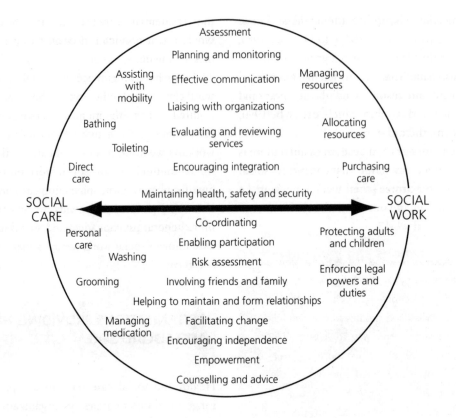

Fig. 0.1 The relationship between social care and social work.

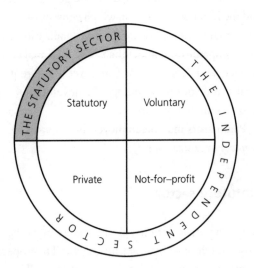

Fig. 0.2 Types of organization that make up the 'mixed economy of care'.

Other statutory agencies include Housing Departments, Education Departments, the Probation Service, the Prison Service and the Police.

Non-statutory sector

Non-statutory organizations together make up the *independent sector*. They are independent of the state and are not legally obliged to provide a service. The exception is the NSPCC, which is voluntary by status, but has statutory rights relating to intervention with children.

Voluntary organizations are self-governing and non-profit-making. Less than half of them are registered as charities, but all are run by their own committees. Some of the principal health and social care national organizations include the British Council of Organizations of Disabled People (BCODP), the Sickle Cell Society, Age Concern, MIND, the Terrence Higgins Trust, Women's Aid, the National Association for the Care and Resettlement of Offenders (NACRO), Stonewall, Values into Action (VIA), the National Gypsy Council, the Joint Council for the Welfare of Immigrants (JCWI),

Shelter, and the Carers' National Association (CNA).

Not-for-profit 'Trusts' form a growing number of bodies that have been set up to manage former local authority provision. Under the National Health Service and Community Care Act 1990, Local Authorities were required to reduce their provider role in favour of their assessment and purchasing function. The Act also required local authorities to encourage the development of a mixed economy of care.

Private organizations and individuals

Private health and social care organizations are profit-making concerns. They are increasingly to be found in nearly all areas of health and social care provision. Private health care has been provided within the National Health Service (NHS) since its inception, and independent private hospitals and private nursing homes have been with us for some time. Social care, too, has a long history of being supplied by private companies, particularly within

the residential care sector. In the 1980s the Government provided incentives to private companies to encourage them to extend their activities. This policy, strengthened by the requirements of the NHS and Community Care Act 1990, has resulted in a proliferation of private care, chiefly at the expense of local authority provision.

Individuals and private companies initially established themselves within the residential care and nursing home sector, and mainly provided care for older people. They have since become involved in providing residential care for all service users, including children and young adults. In addition, private companies now offer day-care and domiciliary-care services.

HEALTH AND SOCIAL CARE SETTINGS

Health and social care has always taken place in a variety of settings, ranging from large-scale institutions to an individual's own home. Today the philosophy of community care dominates both health

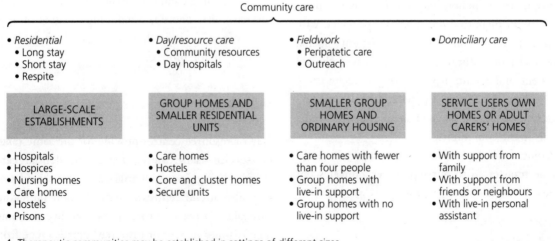

1. Therapeutic communities may be established in settings of different sizes.

2. Care may be seen as taking place within settings along a continuum where there is considerable overlap. For example, someone living in their own home may also spend periods of time in residential care, attend a resource centre and receive visits from fieldwork health and social care staff as well as domiciliary service support. Similarly, someone living in residential care may also attend a day centre, receive visits and support from social work or peripatetic health care staff, and make use of community resources.

Fig. 0.3 Continuum of community care settings.

care and social care strategies, so the emphasis is now on maintaining a person in her or his own home or within the community for as long as possible.

Hospital care

People are admitted and treated in hospital when they are either physically or mentally unwell. The provision of care in large-scale institutional settings has tended to give way to smaller, more specialized units. A patient's stay in hospital is now kept to a minimum, and treatment may be continued at home or elsewhere in the community as soon as the patient is well enough to cope away from the hospital.

The 'community-care' process originated in this country with the decanting of people from large psychiatric hospitals in the 1960s and early 1970s. The continuation of this policy has resulted in the closure of some hospitals and the partial closure of others. Most major hospitals remain large-scale settings, although they are often divided into individually specialized units. In addition, smaller cottage or community hospitals may operate as satellites of the main hospital.

People remain in hospital while there is a medical necessity for them to do so. The care provided will, as far as possible, aim to meet the patient's social, emotional and cultural needs, but – when clinical treatment and attention is no longer necessary – they will be discharged. Peripatetic health professionals may continue the medical treatment of individuals in the community.

People defined as having 'continuing care needs' may be transferred to nursing homes, convalescent homes or hospices as appropriate.

Residential care

Residential care homes are provided for a range of service users:

- homes for older people, including physically frail people with various forms of dementia;
- homes for people with physical disabilities, including degenerative diseases, head injuries, sensory impairment and those with continuing care needs (including individuals who are HIV-positive);
- homes for people with learning disabilities, including those with autism and severe physical and behavioural disabilities;
- homes for people with a range of mental health problems or conditions (excluding acute psychiatric facilities);
- homes for people with problems related to substance misuse;
- homes or hostels for offenders, including unconvicted people on bail or ex-offenders;
- homes for families;
- homes for children and young people.

(based on information from Des Kelly, cited in National Institute for Social Work, 1996).

Care homes vary in size. Some may cater for up to 40 residents, while others may be established in ordinary housing, accommodating only two or three residents who may live independently or semi-independently, with or without live-in support.

Therapeutic communities also exist for a range of service-users. There is often a high degree of self-determination within these settings, which is part of the daily living process.

Day-care

Day or resource centres provide for the same range of service-users catered for by residential care. People living in residential-care accommodation may also attend centres as part of their individual care-plan. Other day-care users may live at home. The regimes of day or resource centres range from those that offer drop-in facilities for service-users to make use of when they wish, through to the more structured programmes. The ethos of day-care provision has changed recently, and an increasing number of individuals and organizations now use the day or resource centre as a base from which to exploit the resources available in the wider community as part of a policy of integration.

Domiciliary care

As the name implies, domiciliary services are provided within a person's own home. They may include health services, such as those provided by general practitioners (GPs), occupational therapists (OTs), physiotherapists, community nurses, community psychiatric nurses (CPNs), health visitors, district nurses and community health-care workers.

Social care may be provided by social workers, social work assistants, home carers and home-helps, night-sitters and family aides. Other services provided for people in their own homes include laundry services, structural adaptations and the provision of daily living aids for the home, and meals on wheels.

Fieldwork

Fieldwork refers to work carried out in the community by office-based social workers and probation officers. They are mostly engaged in assessment, counselling, care management, support and supervision. Social workers are increasingly likely to specialize in working with service-users from one client group.

Community care

Day-hospital services and residential, field, day-care and domiciliary services make up what is known as community care. Traditionally, hospitals, nursing homes and residential-care homes have been regarded as separate from the community. This, in part, reflects their institutional policies and practices. Many establishments are now attempting to integrate more fully into the communities in which they are situated. The level of integration that they achieve will determine the extent to which they are regarded as a community resource.

Care at home

The largest proportion of community care is carried out by unpaid family members, relatives, friends or neighbours. The time involved in caring for a dependent friend or relative can range widely, from a few hours a day to prepare a meal, or to do washing or shopping, to virtually 24-hour support. The tasks undertaken will also vary from simple help with dressing and feeding to more complex or arduous ones, which may include bathing, lifting, toileting and having to apply paramedical skills, such as changing dressings and administering medication. Caring for a friend or relative invariably involves the carer in having to make sacrifices in terms of time, energy and money. Often they are isolated in their activity, since essentially it ties them to the home, and carers forsake their own involvement in the outside world. Opportunities for paid work and career progression may have to be sacrificed, and carers' social and leisure time is often severely curtailed.

To sum up

As we have already mentioned, carers may be paid or unpaid, qualified or unqualified, and employed by statutory or non-statutory organizations. Care may take place in a variety of settings, and carers may be full-time or part-time. Some carers are not employed, and work as volunteers or carers in the home.

THE UNDERVALUING OF CARING

There can be no doubt that caring – whether 'informal', voluntary or paid – is seriously undervalued in our society. It is chiefly carried out by women, and is largely taken for granted. Furthermore, much of it is unpaid. This undervaluing results in a generally low status for all those involved in caring. It is manifested in the absence of resources and support available for 'informal' carers, and it is reflected in the relatively-

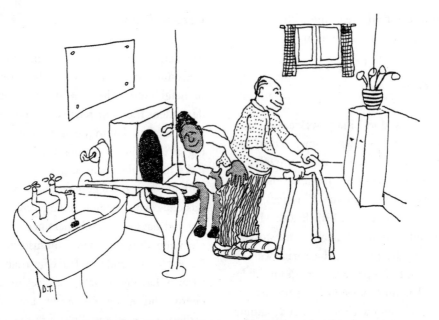

Social care is generally undervalued by society and is mainly undertaken by women.
Care is seen as an extension of the traditional woman's role.

low salaries of qualified nurses and social workers compared to other professions, and the poor remuneration that residential, domiciliary, day-care and health-care workers receive.

Social carers, domiciliary workers and health-care workers are, as we have said, predominantly female. They are also disproportionately often from working-class backgrounds, and many of them are from ethnic minorities. This contrasts sharply with the make-up of senior and managerial personnel, who are mainly white and male. The very name 'care assistant' trivializes the work that is done by social carers and fails to convey accurately the responsibilities that they undertake. This is now recognized by some authorities, who are rejecting the title of 'care assistants' in favour of 'care officers'. Similarly, the range of work and responsibilities carried out by 'home-helps' has been acknowledged, and they are now increasingly being referred to more broadly as 'home carers'.

There are other encouraging signs of the revaluing of both social care and health care.

- The aim of the National Vocational Qualifications (NVQ) in England, Wales and Northern

Ireland (or Scottish Vocational Qualification (SVQ) in Scotland), namely to achieve a better qualified work-force, provides carers with an opportunity to demonstrate good practice and to receive official recognition of their daily work. The rationalization of the care standards in early 1998 simplified the qualification process and made the awards more flexible' to cover a wide range of different care roles.

- The Carers' National Association was founded in 1988 in order to 'address the needs of all (informal) carers to support them and to enable them to speak in a stronger voice.' It has helped to bring the needs of carers to the attention of policy-makers, and has been instrumental in the passing of the Carers Recognition and Services Act 1995.

- At the end of 1997, it was announced that the CCETSW is to be subsumed within a new General Social Care Council (GSCC) which will regulate social workers and home-helps and other unqualified staff. The new body promises to improve and co-ordinate training for care staff, and has been generally welcomed by social care organizations.

HOW TO USE THIS BOOK

This book is designed to be read sequentially or to be dipped into selectively according to the reader's interests. Whichever way you decide to use the book, we would stress the importance of initially familiarizing yourself with the material contained in Chapter 1.

In addition to the text, the book contains a number of diagrams, illustrations and quotations from literary sources, and at the end of each chapter there are exercises, questions for essays or discussion and suggestions for further reading. The further reading includes both academic references and literary sources. In some instances we have recommended one specific work by an author, although several of her or his publications could equally well have been recommended, as they cover similar or closely related themes.

EXERCISES

These are designed to broaden the reader's understanding of the issues and to help her or him to think through the practical implications, particularly in relation to caring. Directions are given on how these exercises may be carried out, although these may be modified to suit the needs of particular groups or settings. All case-study material is based on real situations, but the names are fictitious for reasons of confidentiality.

QUESTIONS FOR ESSAYS OR DISCUSSION

Again these are designed to broaden the reader's understanding of the issues. Most of them build on the text, while others introduce new material.

FURTHER READING

Academic sources

In this section we have recommended academic texts which we consider to be both accessible and up to date.

Other literary sources

Here we have selected works of fiction and poetry which comment on or allude to the material in the text. Social care and social work are as much an expression of art as they are theoretical and practical disciplines. Among other things, they draw on intuition, feelings, spontaneity, insight, imagination, compassion and spirituality.

Films or plays

We have selected a small number of films or plays which in some way explore ideas and viewpoints contained in the text (except in Chapters 6 and 7). The film director's name is given before the title of the film.

I

An unequal society

Today inequality is not only widespread, it is also widely accepted. Those who advocate equality are going against the social tide.

(From *Towards equality: a Christian manifesto*, Bob Holman, 1997)

We live in an unequal society, and this is apparent from observation of everyday living. Not everybody has the same life-chances. Some people, owing to differences in social class, gender, skin colour or physical and mental health, are more likely to enjoy and participate in a fuller range of society's benefits than others. Inequality in society manifests itself in different ways, and we might usefully break equality down into three different forms, namely *formal* equality, equality of *opportunity* and equality of *outcomes*.

Formal equality refers to the principle that everyone in society is equal. They are born equal and will receive equal treatment at the hands of society's political, administrative and legal institutions. Examples of this are that all adult citizens have the right to vote in democratic elections, that they have a number of common civil rights and liberties, and that they are all entitled to the same treatment under the law.

Equality of opportunity refers to the principle that everyone has an equal chance to achieve their potential in society. According to this principle society provides equal access to health, education and job opportunities. In other words, society endeavours to mitigate against any disadvantages individuals may experience with regard to their social class, gender, race, age, culture, disability, sexual orientation, lifestyle or religion.

Equality of outcomes refers to the principle which ensures that, as far as possible, all individuals obtain an equal share of society's benefits. Outcomes would include income, wealth, life-style, influence, power and status, as well as equal health treatment and quality of education, housing and employment.

It is important to stress that these forms of equality are principles, and that in reality no society has translated them entirely into practice (or could do so). For example, in our society formal equality under the law is adversely affected by power, wealth, prejudice and discrimination. Statistics indicate that black people have a greater chance of being arrested, charged, remanded in custody and imprisoned than white people. Similarly, most men who apply for care and control of their children in divorce proceedings are unsuccessful.

True equality of opportunity would mean that society would have to control all political, economic and social influences on all individuals from birth. This is clearly impossible to achieve. For example, in our society a child born into a wealthy family that can afford to provide greater stimulation can have an enormous advantage over other children, even before he or she attends school. According to statistics, the child is already likely to be healthier and more educationally advanced than a child from the working class. Thus, although it is declared that we have a free and open education system, in reality this is not so, because some children start with socially bestowed advantages.

Likewise, equality of outcome is impossible to implement absolutely, since so many variables would need to be controlled. Intervention would constantly be required to restore the imbalances that would continually develop. Income is linked to status and power, and as individuals will always use it differently, so inequalities will always be arising. In addition to individual differences, there are also social structures which prevent the achievement of full equality.

There have been attempts within our society to create various equal opportunities policies – for example, those aimed at enabling more black and Asian people to enter social care and social work. It has been recognized that black and Asian people are under-represented within the profession, and that this is caused in part by the existence of structural racism within our society. Equal opportunities policies have aimed to redress this imbalance. However, equality of opportunity can only really be effective if equality of outcome is also established. The two principles are inextricably linked.

For example, the policy of providing access to the Diploma in Social Work courses to black and Asian students can only be successful as an equal opportunities policy if those students go on to complete the course successfully and obtain appropriate jobs within social work. If black access students still face discrimination during training, at the job recruitment stage, or later, then equality of outcome will not be achieved.

Similarly, equal opportunities policies aimed at attracting women back into employment will only ultimately be successful if they are accompanied by other social changes. Employers' expectations would need to change, and hours of attendance, leave arrangements, working conditions, child-care arrangements and facilities would have to be altered to accommodate women's specific needs. Obviously outcomes would ultimately determine the effectiveness of equal opportunities.

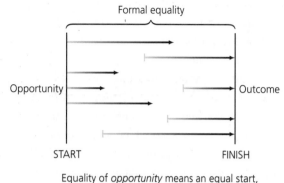

Equality of *opportunity* means an equal start, but not necessarily an equal *outcome*.

Fig. 1.1 Forms of equality.

INDIVIDUAL AND STRUCTURAL INEQUALITIES

During the depression years of the 1930s, cookery classes were organised for women in poor communities in an attempt to help them to provide nutritious meals for their families despite their low incomes. One particular evening, a group of women were being taught how to make cod's head soup – a cheap and nourishing dish. At the end of the lesson the women were asked if they had any questions. 'Just one,' said a member of the group. 'Whilst we're eating the cod's head soup, who's eating the cod?'

(Langan and Lee, 1989, p.140)

Inequalities exist both among individuals and within the structure of our society. There are differences between people at birth, including differences in physical and mental capacity. Whether or not these potential abilities develop will depend to a large extent on the person's social circumstances. No social structure can eliminate essential innate differences between people. However, it can help to determine the distribution of power, influence and life-chances.

There is plenty of evidence of structural inequality in our society. Consider, for example, the composition of the House of Commons. In this democratically elected chamber, of the 659 members only a small proportion are from working-class backgrounds, 120 members are women, nine are from ethnic minorities, four are 'out' gay MPs, including one lesbian, and only two members are disabled. This is a reflection of the structural imbalance of power, influence and prestige within society. Similar observations could be made of many of society's major institutions, for example, the Civil Service, legal and professional organizations, the media, and social and welfare services.

Society can be said to be divided in three major ways – by social class, gender and race. It is also structured according to other factors, such as age, disability and sexual orientation. In our society, non-disabled, white, middle-class, heterosexual males are more likely to achieve social success, obtain power and derive more of society's benefits and rewards. All other groups will to a certain extent experience a corresponding lack of power and influence. In this way they can be said to be *marginalized* within society. A factor that contributes towards the process of marginalization or oppression is the extent to which people experience *prejudice*.

Prejudice

Prejudice is not easy to define, and it can take many different forms. It is usually a strongly held attitude towards individuals or, more commonly, towards groups, which is to a greater or lesser extent unreasonable or irrational. It is irrational because it is *not* based on reasonable, factual evidence. To some extent prejudice is expressed in a person's behaviour, but much of it may remain secret or unconscious and may, as a result, be very hard to recognize or admit to. Usually it is very deep-seated and powerful, and can affect what a person thinks, feels and does.

Prejudice is based on either fear or a lack of knowledge, or both. It is most often applied by the more powerful – those with authority and influence – to the less powerful. When used in education or in

work, its application can profoundly affect the prospects and feelings of those to whom it is directed. Again, it tends to be working-class people, women and black people who most often suffer from the harmful effects of prejudice. Those in authority who can affect our lives and life-chances may express prejudice through fear, because they feel threatened in some way, or because they feel they will lose out. Whatever its cause, an ignorance of those to whom it is directed is nearly always present.

Discrimination

The expression of prejudice leads to *discrimination* – that is, to a situation where people are treated unequally, some being favoured and others not. Discrimination may appear to be arbitrary, since it is subject to the whims of those expressing it.

Stereotyping

Prejudice is commonly based on, or justified by, a *stereotype*. The two are closely related. A stereotype 'lumps together' all members of a particular group as if they *all* possess the *same* characteristics. Examples of negative stereotypes used in our society are that 'all Scotsmen are mean', 'all Jewish people are wealthy' or 'all men are uncaring'. Thus a person might say 'I do not mix with a certain kind of person, because they are. . .', so his or her action has been governed by a stereotype.

Most stereotypes are negative. They may describe a group as 'lazy' or 'dirty', 'mean' or 'criminal'. Whatever the epithet used, they fail to see a person as a whole individual. Instead, particular traits or characteristics are isolated, and from this a generalization is made which denies a person's uniqueness.

The actual process of stereotyping is simple and follows this pattern:

> This person is an 'X'
> All 'Xs' are selfish.
> Therefore, this person is selfish!

It is difficult to say from where stereotypes originate. There is almost certainly a range of sources – for example, parents, our socialization, our friends or peers, teachers, literature, the mass media and advertising. Stereotypes are certainly contained in the very language we use, and many of them take the form of clichés. There are, for example, more derogatory terms for marginalized groups, including minorities and women, than there are for more established members of society. This is because stereotyping is so deep-seated that it is extremely difficult to modify, let alone eliminate completely.

It is important to point out at this stage that we also use stereotypes in a good and positive way. We do this in order to make 'short cuts', so that living is made easier and more manageable. Huge amounts of information continually bombard our senses, and we have to continually select or 'stereotype' in order to make sense of the world. For example, the 400 or more recognized shades of green become a single 'green' for the purpose of conversation and making sense quickly to one another. Again, we refer to 'a drug', whereas in reality there are thousands of different drugs doing very different things to different people. Using stereotypes as a form of 'shorthand' saves us time when we have no opportunity for prolonged thought or speech.

LABELLING AND STIGMATIZATING

If we use a different phraseology, stereotyping may be described as *labelling* or *stigmatizing*. When a person is said to have been 'labelled', then frequently a stereotype with negative associations is being used. It is common for those in a powerful position to employ a label in order to 'put people down'. Thus someone in work might 'label' an unemployed person as 'work-shy'.

It is extremely difficult for people who are labelled to attempt to modify the label and its associated stigma, let alone rid themselves of its taint

completely. They act from an inferior position and lack the power and influence with which to do so.

OPPRESSION, MARGINALIZATION AND SOCIAL EXCLUSION

The overall effect of the interrelated processes of stereotyping, prejudice and stigmatizing is to *marginalize* the victim. This means that they are prevented from taking a full part in the life of our society; instead, they live as it were 'on the edge' or 'margin' of society. They do not share full citizenship with regard to the social, economic and political life of the community, and they may be said to be *socially excluded*.

Many marginalized individuals will be without paid work and will be dependent on state benefits, as will many older and disabled people. Others may be among the one million single-parent families in the UK, or they may be among those experiencing mental health problems or those who have a learning disability. Many people who are marginalized lack a satisfactory income which would enable them to take a full part in economic life. Such groups are likely to be over-represented in the so-called '*underclass*'.

Marginalization needs to be distinguished from the closely related but stronger word *oppression*. Oppression relates to the systematic putting down of people or their opinions, behaviour and life-styles. Essentially the process subjugates the expression of less powerful people by denying aspects of their identity and a chance for them to flourish.

Oppression consists of a combination of elements, which can operate at both an individual and an institutional level. For instance, single parents, asylum-seekers and gay people may be abused by other individuals, as well as being structurally oppressed by financial limitations and absence of available child care, bureaucratic constraints and punitive welfare policies, and the denial of rights that are open to other citizens and a free expressive social life.

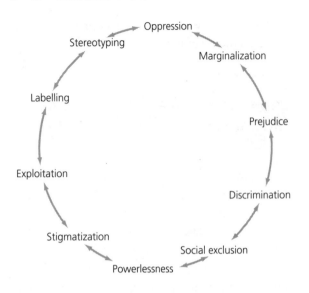

Fig. 1.2 Processes that adversely affect less powerful groups and individuals (all of the processes are interrelated).

POVERTY

One in ten children is 'poor' on the basis that their family cannot afford at least three of the things most families take for granted – such as three meals a day, a bed of their own and shoes bought new and properly fitted. One in 30 children is 'severely poor' as they lack at least five of these things.

(extract from the Joseph Roundtree Foundation Report; *Guardian*, 10 July 1997, p.5)

Poverty is directly related to oppression, because people who are poor do not have the same extent of choice or control over their lives as other members of society. For example, they have a greater reliance on public utilities and services, and they are less able to afford to buy labour- and time-saving appliances for the home. The goods within their purchasing range are often of inferior quality and not cost-effective, and may need to be replaced sooner than more expensive items.

Poor people undergo a great deal of inconvenience because they are forced to depend on public transport, which is often unreliable. This makes tasks such as shopping more difficult, and it means that many poor people have to shop in more expensive and smaller local stores. They are not able to take advantage of a monthly trip to the supermarket in order to stock up their food cupboards and freezers with lower-priced goods.

Reliance on public telephones and the nearest launderette add to their inconvenience. More affluent families will not only have all the required appliances within their homes, but they will also often buy in domestic help for cleaning, child care, decorating and gardening.

The consequences of poverty are felt just as deeply in rural areas as they are in an urban environment. A church report entitled *Faith in the Countryside* (Archbishops' Commission on Rural Areas, 1990) highlighted the significance of rural poverty: 'the weak, the poor and vulnerable and the elderly have their choices further curtailed, since without readily available personal transport, access to basic facilities is restricted' (p.311).

TIME POVERTY

The extent to which money buys time in our society is often overlooked. As Sue Ward has pointed out, 'being poor takes up an enormous amount of time and energy' (Ward, 1986, p. 37). She adds, 'Money also buys better housing and working conditions. These also affect the amount of time you have. Keeping clean, warm and fed – even just keeping going – in a damp council flat on the 14th floor, where the lifts don't work and the nearest supermarket is a mile away, is going to be a struggle anyway' (Ward, 1986, p.38).

Money buys time. People in highly paid occupations are able to pay others to undertake their domestic tasks for them. A Mintel survey published in January 1997 showed that families in the UK spend '£4 billion in one year on nannies, cooks, cleaners and gardeners – four times as much as they spent ten years ago' (*Observer*, 19 January 1997, p.14).

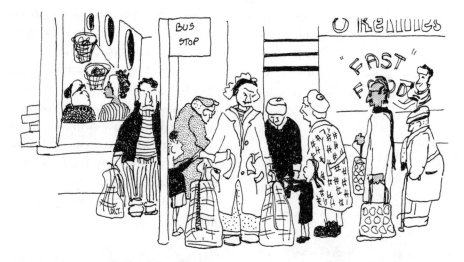

Poor people are affected by 'time poverty' – they do not have facilities and modern appliances in their own homes, and are dependent on public utilities and transport.

The survey revealed that the people undertaking this work 'come from families lower down the social scale, where part-time work is the only option, because they have their own children to look after. In effect the rich are buying leisure time from the poor' (*Observer*, 19 January 1997, p.14).

As a reaction to their deprivation many people turn inwards to their homes and families, and rely exclusively on the privatized entertainment of television and video. Lack of money effectively prohibits poor people from having the chance to engage fully in local activities. Thus the possibility of corporate, communal life becomes ever more remote.

It is not surprising that many oppressed or marginalized people, families and groups feel 'trapped' in their situation. It is extremely hard to work one's way out of this predicament. For those who have committed offences, the existence of a criminal record will make it harder still. We may consider it small wonder that in the 1980s many large cities saw extensive unrest, and that there were increasing numbers of instances of antisocial activities directed at wider society. Such unrest had many complex interrelated causes, and it would appear that anger and frustration were certainly among them.

In addition to those who experience marginalization as a result of their material deprivation and the associated prejudice of the more privileged sections of society, there are others who suffer similarly as a result of their so-called 'unconventional' life-styles, or their involvement in grass-roots political activity. These include groups that are sometimes referred to as 'alternative', such as the 'eco-warriors', some feminist groups, and other alternative life-style groups such as the so-called 'New Age Travellers'. To a large extent such people choose to be unconventional and therefore anticipate a marginalized identity. Whether individuals are passive victims because of their class, gender or race, or whether they have made a more conscious decision to live a 'marginalized' life-style, the result is the same. A substantial proportion of the population does not play a full part in the life of our community.

To be structurally oppressed or marginalized is not automatically an entirely negative experience. Some individuals and groups draw strength from their social exclusion, and rise above it despite the adversity. Some people have chosen to exist on the edge or margin of society, while others have no choice. Social exclusion and material deprivation have been the elected province of many great writers, artists and spiritual thinkers throughout history. Similarly, many creative women and men have expressed themselves eloquently despite the existence of unwanted discrimination and/or poverty. Many influential social movements had, and still have, their roots in the experience of marginalization and subjugation, and were established on the collective strength of those who were commonly oppressed.

> If my life as a priest and religious leader in the inner city has done anything to me personally, it has above all things led me to a profound respect for, and wonder at, the depth of power in the lives of the powerless.
>
> (Fr Austin Smith, quoted in Joint Council for the Welfare of Immigrants, 1997a, p.4)

This is not to romanticize exclusion, poverty or suffering. Indeed, there is plenty of evidence – as the rest of this book shows – that people's life-chances are permanently adversely affected by the existence of structural inequality, and that individual potential for development is systematically thwarted. However, the very experience of oppression may lead to an understanding of its general effect and deepen one's understanding of a fellow person's suffering. For instance, black people may identify with the powerlessness felt by disabled people, and in the same way, women may recognize the struggle that gay men have in their fight for basic rights. Experience of exclusion, discrimination and hardship may extend a person's empathy and ultimately increase their resourcefulness and ability to stand by and enable both themselves and others.

> If I hadn't grown up queer and Jewish – and being as I had gone to such an ordinary, you know, absolutely classic public school and then to Cambridge – then I might have been someone with much less sympathy or interest in other people's lives. I might have believed myself to be better than others.
>
> (Stephen Fry, actor and writer, *Gay Time TV* 3rd series, 6 August 1997)

EXERCISES

1. Living on benefits

Obtain from your local DSS office information concerning the exact financial benefits to which any of the following people are entitled:

- a family of two adults, neither of whom is in paid work, and two children under the age of 10 years;
- a single parent, who is not in paid work, with one child under 10 years old;
- a single person who is not in paid work;
- an older male, post-retirement age, living on his own.

Find out the average rent and council tax contribution typical of your area. Then make an estimate of essential everyday expenses, including a proportion of standard bills such as electricity, gas and water. In the light of this, calculate as accurately as possible how much disposable income remains to meet the cost of other essentials.

2. Pejorative words and terms

Either individually or in pairs, make a list of 20 derogatory terms/swear-words and consider at which group of people they are targeted. Share these with the whole group. Now, in discussion as a whole group, consider the following question. What does this say about general social attitudes towards those groups which you have identified?

3. Examining prejudice

On the opposite page are 10 photographs. Study each face carefully while considering the following questions.

(a) Who would you be most likely to share a personal problem with? Rank order the remainder.

(b) What occupation (if any) do you think each of them has?

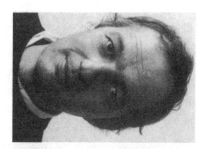
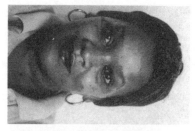
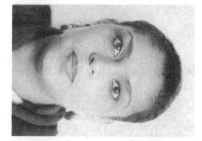
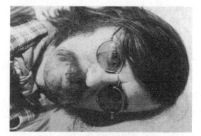
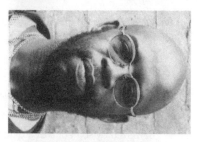
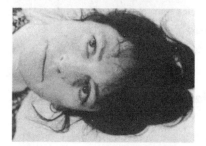
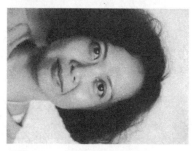
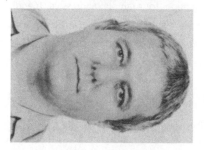
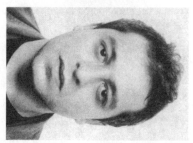
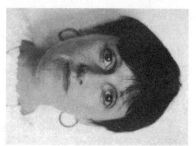

(c) What social class grouping does each individual belong to?

(d) Which of them might have a drink- or drug-related problem?

(e) Which of them might live alone?

(f) Which of them would most readily resort to violence?

Note that this list is not exhaustive, so you can add other suggestions of your own.

As a whole group discuss your answers to the following questions.

(a) Are you aware of the roots of your own prejudice?

(b) What steps can you take to eradicate your own prejudice? Note that this exercise is designed to elicit personal prejudice in a spontaneous way. It should be undertaken in a spirit of trust, and no criticisms or blame should be levelled at or attached to any individual contribution.

4. The effects of labelling

The trainer needs to produce a different label for each member of the group – for example, aggressive, friendly, depressive, assertive, withdrawn, etc. These labels should be randomly allocated to each group member and fixed to his or her forehead so that other participants can immediately see the label. Participants will react towards others in accordance with the label they are displaying.

The setting is a social services day centre (for any client group) in which a group of service users are planning a range of future social events. This task should take about 20 minutes. The purpose of the exercise is to focus on the labelling process. It is important for participants to refrain from using the specific word or words which make up the label. The discussion following the exercise should explore the varied responses to the label, as well as the different feelings evoked as a result of being labelled.

5. How we think others see us

In pairs, each person takes it in turn to explain to their partner how others will see them in terms of the following criteria.

(a) *Class*. Having established their own class position, the participant proceeds to describe in detail how someone from a different social class will see them.

(b) *Gender*. The participant relates to their partner how someone of the opposite sex will see them.

(c) *Race*. The participant imagines how they will be perceived by someone of a different race or culture, and relates this to their partner.

When this process is complete, the whole group should examine what they have learned from the experience.

QUESTIONS FOR ESSAYS OR DISCUSSION

1. A.H. Halsey has said 'Society means a shared life. If some and not others are poor then the principles on which life is shared are at issue; society itself is in question'. In what ways does inequality put shared or corporate social life in jeopardy?

2. Which of the following do you consider to be the most significant structural disadvantage – social class, gender or race? Explain your reasons.

3. Often in our society the rich are made richer and the poor are made poorer as a way of encouraging their respective efforts and initiatives. Why should society's approach to the two groups differ in this way?

4. Describe the practical ways in which 'time-poverty' affects the lives of individuals and families.

5. Explore the ways in which equal opportunities policies can work towards eliminating discrimination and inequality in our society.

6. With regard to a group of your own choosing, e.g. women, black people, working-class people, homeless people, unemployed people, gay people or disabled people, describe what form their social exclusion takes.

FURTHER READING

Academic sources

Bishops' Advisory Group on Urban Priority Areas 1995: *Staying in the city – faith in the city ten years on.* London: Church House Publishing. Published 10 years after the *Faith in the City* Report which examined inequality, environmental decay and social disintegration, this report provides an update on what has happened in our major cities during the intervening years.

Goffman, E. 1968: *Stigma.* Harmondsworth: Penguin. Subtitled *Notes on the management of spoiled identity*, this classic sociological study examines the close relationship between stigma and stereotypes, and looks at the strategies open to the stigmatized with which they could minimalize what we would now refer to as their 'marginalization' or their social exclusion.

Lister, R. 1990: *The exclusive society – citizenship and the poor.* London: Child Poverty Action Group. A short text which examines both the responsibilities and the rights of citizenship in the UK. The author goes on to study how poverty threatens full citizenship, especially in relation to black people, women and children. Along the way she attacks the concept of an 'underclass'.

Taking Liberties Collective 1989: *Learning the hard way.* London: Macmillan. This book is a compilation of working-class and black women's experiences of oppression and discrimination, and their struggles in everyday living.

Oppenheim, C. and Harker, L. 1996: *Poverty: the facts*, 3rd edn. London: Child Poverty Action Group. This book provides statistical information on poverty in the UK and comparative figures for the European Union. It reveals income and regional inequalities and devotes two separate chapters to how women and black people, respectively, experience poverty.

Townsend, P. 1996: *A poor future.* London: Lemos & Crane. The UK's foremost authority on poverty provides a short, succinct account of inequality and social polarization in Britain. The book contrasts poverty levels in this country with those in European countries and other places in the world.

Other literary sources

Crisp, Q. 1985: *The naked Civil Servant.* London: Fontana.

Greenwood, W. 1993: *Love on the dole.* London: Vintage.

Hesse, H. 1965: *Steppenwolf.* Harmondsworth: Penguin.

Healy, J. 1991: *Streets above us.* London: Paladin.

Morris, J. 1997: *Conundrum.* Harmondsworth: Penguin.

Michael, L. 1994: *Under a thin moon.* London: Minerva.

Films and plays

Huston, J. 1972: *Fat City.* USA.

Lynch, D. 1980: *The Elephant Man.* USA.

Pollack, S. 1969: *They Shoot Horses Don't They?* USA.

Schlesinger, J. 1969: *Midnight Cowboy.* USA.

2

Social class and the creation of an 'underclass'

. . . class, that peculiarly British hang-up.

(Ros Wynne-Jones, *Sunday Mirror*, 9 February 1997)

The class war is over – and the middle class have won . . . the working class have been made strangers in their own land. The old certainties have gone forever. The working class is a divided class. The future is middle class.

(Tony Parsons, from *Parsons on Class*, BBC2, April 1996)

Increasingly, and accelerated by the great push of Thatcherism, Britain has become, like the rest of Europe, a middle-class society.

(Ralf Dahrendorf, *Observer*, 9 March 1997)

INTRODUCTION – THE CUTTESLOWE WALLS

In 1934, in the Cutteslowe area of North Oxford, it was proposed to re-house some 28 'slum-clearance' families in public housing adjacent to a new private housing development. In December of that year, the company that had erected the private housing responded by building large brick walls topped by metal spikes across the two roads which connected the separate developments. An outcry from many sections of the local community followed, but it was not until March 1959 (following protests, court injunctions, partial demolition and rebuilding of the walls) that the walls were finally removed.

For 25 years the 'Cutteslowe walls', or 'snob walls' as they became known locally, had remained *in situ*. Edmund Gibbs, a city councillor whose father had campaigned vigorously to have the walls removed, ceremoniously knocked out the first bricks with a pickaxe in 1959. He said later, 'I was delighted to be there when those dreadful walls came down at last, but it is depressing that class prejudice is still around, and even getting stronger' (*Limited Edition*, October 1988, p.12). This was an extreme and unique example of class prejudice, and it indicates the depth of feeling that can sometimes occur around the issue of social class.

The Cutteslowe walls may be unique, but the sentiments which led to them resurfaced in another case more recently. In September 1995 the *Daily Mail* reported that 'Homeowners on a private estate are demanding a "Berlin Wall" to hide poorer families they fear could devalue their properties' (*Daily Mail*, 22 September 1995, p.5). This occurred in Coleford, Gloucestershire, and the report continued '... they want the local council to build a wall across their street and lay a new road to provide independent access to 17 rented homes'. One of the home owners was quoted as saying: 'I wanted the council to protect the value of my property or pay us compensation'.

WHAT IS SOCIAL CLASS?

Class is a good thing for the country, because I think successful people are always respected. I was born in Watford by the football ground, my dad was a builder – he worked his way up. I was born in a bed-sit . . . I can mix with millionaires . . . and I *do* enjoy their company and they enjoy my company because they think I'm different.

(Vinnie Jones, footballer, from *World in Action*, ITV, 2 December 1996) [his emphasis]

Most of us have some concept of class, and of our own place within a 'class system'. We might rank ourselves or others as 'working class', 'middle class' or 'upper class'. We will do this according to various factors, including the way we speak or dress, what we or members of our family do for a living, where we live, what kind of car we drive, what we spend our leisure time doing, and so on.

People generally think of social class hierarchically, implying that being 'upper class' is somehow better than being 'middle class', which in turn is better than being 'working class'. Many object to the generalized use of the term 'social class' on the grounds that it emphasizes differences and inequalities between people who are essentially the same, and creates an unfounded snobbery.

We begin to see that social class is an extremely complex concept which, in common usage, has almost as many meanings as there are people prepared to make generalizations about it! However, a technical and generally accepted use of the term 'social class' is extremely important for people who study society. Above all, it is a useful *analytical tool*. It enables researchers to make observations about social need and the effectiveness of social policy. Most importantly, it can highlight the plight of particular groups of people, defined by their social class, and consider whether their needs are being met. In this way the effects of policies concerning education, housing, health, social care or income maintenance can be examined.

SOME POSSIBLE MISCONCEPTIONS ABOUT CLASS

We need to remember that there is nothing 'natural' about social class. Rather, it is an artificial concept designed for the benefit of social analysis. Social class is not *fixed* – there is movement between classes, both within and between generations. If we perceive class as a hierarchy, this movement can be either up or down the social scale. A child born into a particular social class may change his or her position as he or she grows older and enters the worlds of education and work. We refer to this movement as 'social mobility'. It usually takes place between adjacent groupings, rather than between extremes of 'top' and 'bottom'.

As we shall see later, the concept of social class alters over time. It has to be updated in response to changes in society, particularly those concerning the people who make up the work-force.

The concept of social class applied in the UK will not necessarily be transferable to other countries or cultures. It has evolved from the analysis of our own particular society. All nations are unique, having a different history, culture and traditions. The work-force will be organized in different ways and patterns of income and wealth will not be the same. We must treat each nation state in ways that are sensitive to its own particular qualities. One of these qualities will be its own unique pattern of social class.

We should always attempt to make the concept of social class an objective analytical tool. Therefore no moral judgements should be implied or intended when using class analysis. For example, if we discover that working-class children do less well at school, the implication is that the education system is failing to deliver effectively to such children, not that they are less able or intelligent than children from other social classes.

> It's a thing of being discreet and just being well behaved and well mannered – that's class.
>
> (Tara Palmer-Tomkinson, *Class*, ITV, 10 June 1997)

> What we have today is an entirely middle-class world. What we've seen since the turn of the century is the hands-down victory of all the middle-class values.
>
> (A. A. Gill, journalist, *Class*, ITV, 24 June 1997)

> There's not enough class war in Great Britain. The British working classes take what's coming to them, they accept their inferior position in society . . . they take it without a moment's resentment.
>
> (Roy Hattersley, *Class*, ITV, 17 June 1997)

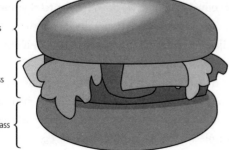

Fig. 2.1 Social class has been likened to a sandwich. The middle class form the filling, and without that filling there is no sandwich. Each layer has its own distinct perspective.

SOCIAL STRATIFICATION

Outside of an ideal society, it is hard to imagine a society that is not divided in some way between those who are less well off and those who are better off. In reality, all societies – past and present – have been and are divided into a range of groups associated with varying material resources (wealth, income, property, land, etc.). All societies are therefore said to be stratified, i.e. divided into different *strata*, a concept which social scientists have borrowed from geology which refers to the various layers found in the structure of the earth.

Social stratification is a neutral term which simply refers to the different divisions or groups within society. *Social class* is simply *one* of the ways in which societies can be divided.

Not all previous societies have been divided along *class lines*. For example, they may have been divided (or 'stratified') by *age* – with older people occupying the most powerful positions of authority and having more status than others. Societies can also be stratified by *gender* – they can be *patriarchal* or *matriarchal*, where those in powerful positions are either male or female, respectively.

Race or ethnicity (or colour) may be the crucial stratifying factor, for example in the late *apartheid* system in South Africa. This was based on the supposed superiority of a minority white group who, by dominating the major economic and political institutions of society, were able to treat the black majority as subservient and keep them under repressive control.

Some societies have been divided on *status* lines. This has taken many forms. *Slavery* was one example where masters literally *owned* their slaves and treated them as their property.

In some countries, e.g. India, the *caste* system is another example. This fixes a person's social position at birth, and strict rules govern what relationships there will be between castes. At the lowest end of the caste system, the 'untouchables' are barred from social interaction with all higher groups and lack the civil rights enjoyed by others. This is illustrated in the novel *The God of Small Things*, when the author refers to the application of the caste system at the beginning of this century:

> Paravans, like other Untouchables, were not allowed to walk on public roads, not allowed to cover their upper bodies, not allowed to carry umbrellas. They had to put their hands over their mouths when they spoke, to divert their polluted breath away from those whom they addressed.
>
> (Arundhati Roy, 1997, p.74)

This system has lately undergone change, and a 'loosening up' of rigid divisions has occurred.

It is important to point out that such stratification systems are not mutually exclusive, i.e. more than one system can operate in a society at any one time. For example, gender and age could be the prevalent factors, with older women in positions of authority, or gender and status could be prevalent, with male masters holding power.

To sum up, social stratification refers to the structural inequalities in society – that is, inequalities between different groupings of people which are determined by the way in which society is organized. Ruling groups may have a vested interest in preserving inequalities in order to continue deriving benefits and privileges.

SOCIAL CLASS – A DEFINITION

Most modern societies are today stratified by what we call *social class*. Unfortunately, there is no general agreement about the definition of class and there are a large number of competing definitions, theories and explanations. Broadly speaking, class refers to *socio-economic* differences between groups of people. These differences will affect people's lifestyles, life-chances and future prospects.

Explanations of social class tend to include both *objective* factors (e.g. those tangible material factors

that can be more easily measured, such as *income* or *wealth*) and *subjective* factors (e.g. a person's *attitudes* and *values*, including perhaps how they view their own class position). Whereas it is reasonably straightforward to assess the former, it is far more difficult to assess the latter.

We shall now turn to three of the most prominent explanations of social class which have been applied to the British class system, in order to consider their usefulness in helping us to understand our present society.

KARL MARX (1818–1883)

Marx, a German economist and political scientist who lived and wrote for most of his life in London, has to be included in any discussion of social class. His work is still extremely important for social scientists today, despite being over 100 years old. Marx was the first to make social class central to an analysis of society and to a theory of social change.

For Marx, 'the history of all hitherto existing society is the history of class struggles' (Marx and Engels, 1975, p.32). In other words, he felt that social class characterized all previous forms of society. In ancient societies the division was between masters and slaves, and in feudal times society was fundamentally divided between landlord and serf (although there were intermediary groupings). In each case the former group dominated the numerically larger latter group. The social-class system changed once more when society was transformed from being basically agrarian to a society based on industry and commerce.

According to Marx's theory, a person's social class is determined by her or his relationship to what he called the *'means of production'* – the means by which material goods are actually produced, that is, the technology, situated in workshops and factories. Within this system, *capitalists* (or industrialists) *own* the means of production, while *workers* (or the *working class*) earn their living by selling their labour to capitalists. Marx used his own terms to refer to these social classes:

- the *bourgeoisie* referred to the owners of the means of production;
- the *proletariat* referred to the workers.

These two social classes were engaged in the class struggle, but Marx also referred to a third class:

- the *lumpenproletariat* Marx referred to in derisory terms because it included the idle or 'work-shy' – as they did not work, they took no part in the class struggle.

Capitalists derived their wealth by exploiting workers, who were never paid a wage which reflected the true value of their labour. This wealth, 'creamed off' by the capitalist class, was referred to by Marx as 'surplus value'. In this way profits were made by the capitalist class, while workers had to continue working day after day, week after week, simply in order to survive.

As the capitalist class gained in wealth, they also grew in power and influence, although a small, landed aristocracy remained. They were therefore able to control and dominate all of the institutions in society, namely the law, the education system, religion, politics and the media. Their ideas, attitudes and values (or *ideology*) became dominant, and contrary views had to struggle to find a voice and be heard.

Thus Marx viewed social classes as real, objective entities. The class system required inequalities to exist in society. We could describe these inequalities as *structural*.

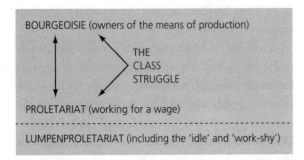

Fig. 2.2 Marx's three social classes.

Criticisms of Marx's concept of class

We must not be unfairly critical of Marx, and we should appreciate that our society has changed a great deal since his death in 1883. Society today is far more complex. It has become less easy to place certain groups of people in one or other of Marx's two great opposing classes.

With the development of our modern, industrial society, a large state apparatus has grown, including the Civil Service and other large bureaucratic organizations operating at both national and local levels. These include, for example, the Department of Social Security (DSS), the National Health Service (NHS) and the local authority Housing Departments, and Social Services Departments (or Social Work Departments in Scotland). Marx did not foresee these developments in the public sector, so his class analysis is unable to accommodate the personnel working for such government organizations. They are clearly not capitalists in Marx's sense of the word, and neither are they working directly for the capitalist class. They perform their duties for the good of the community, or society as a whole. Such people we would now refer to as 'middle class' because, in a sense, they fit between Marx's two classes, but they cannot be accepted into his scheme of things on his terms.

Another fundamental criticism of Marx is that by focusing exclusively on class he ignored other ways in which society is stratified, e.g. race, gender and age. In his day, most waged workers working outside the home were male. Consequently, women appear to be largely *invisible* in his work. Yet today women represent over 45 per cent of the work-force, and this proportion is increasing. Despite this, however, most top jobs are held by men. We might conclude from this that in terms of employment, *gender* is as important a factor as *class*.

Thirdly, some of Marx's historical predictions have not been borne out. He believed that the two major classes would become more clearly demarcated, but in fact they have become more fragmented and, as we have seen, the divisions between them have become blurred. The working class has shrunk in size rather than growing as he predicted, and its revolutionary potential has not been realized in this country. So much then for Marx's referring to the working class as the 'gravediggers of capitalism' (Giddens, 1982, p.63).

THE REGISTRAR-GENERAL'S 'SOCIAL CLASS BASED ON OCCUPATION'

There are at present two official socio-economic classifications used in the UK. Both are used to analyse data gathered by the national census and other surveys. In this century, the census (introduced in 1801) has taken place every 10 years since 1901, with the exception of 1941, when it was abandoned because of the Second World War.

1. Socio-economic groups

Introduced in the 1951 census, this is a non-hierarchical classification which groups together people who have jobs of similar social and economic status. In total there are 20 different groups, ranging from 'employers and managers in central and local government, industry, commerce, etc.' through to 'skilled manual workers', 'agricultural workers' and 'members of the armed forces'. For our purposes, this is not as useful as the second form of classification.

2. Social class based on occupation

This was first used by the then 'General Register Office' in relation to the 1911 census. Frequently known as the 'Registrar General's' classification, after the person who heads up the 'Office for National Statistics', a central government body formed in April 1996 from the merger of the 'Central Statistics Office' (founded in 1941) and the 'Office of Population Censuses and Surveys' (OPCS) (founded in 1970). It recognizes five social classes, one of which (Class III) is further sub-divided (see Table 2.1).

Table 2.1 Social class based on occupation

Class	Category of occupation
I	Professional occupations
II	Managerial and technical occupations
IIIN	Skilled occupations (non-manual)
IIIM	Skilled occupations (manual)
IV	Partly skilled occupations
V	Unskilled occupations

NB: People of 'foreman' status whose basic social class is IV or V are allocated to social Class III. People of 'manager' status are allocated to Social Class II, with certain exceptions.

In total, there are over 20 000 different occupational titles used by the Registrar-General, but below we shall give only a handful of examples of occupations in the various class categories.

- *Social Class I*: accountant, architect, barrister, chemist, doctor, judge, member of parliament, optician, solicitor, university lecturer.
- *Social Class II*: chiropodist, college lecturer, farmer, nurse, pilot, police officer, probation officer, schoolteacher, social worker.
- *Social Class III (non-manual)*: clerical worker, estate agent, sales representative, secretary, shop assistant, typist.
- *Social Class III (manual)*: bricklayer, bus driver, carpenter, cook, hairdresser, miner, police constable, train driver.
- *Social Class IV*: agricultural worker, bar person, bus conductor, hospital orderly, postman, street vendor.
- *Social Class V*: chimney sweep, kitchen hand, labourer, office cleaner, railway porter, window cleaner.

For the purposes of the 1991 census, people were assigned to one of the social classes depending on their occupation in the week preceding the census, or where they were not in paid employment, on the basis of their most recent paid job within the previous 10 years. The person who filled in column 1 of the household census form, whether male or female, is taken as a reference person in the household, and the socio-economic position of the whole house-hold is inferred from that person's occupation.

Current developments

The data derived from the census and from other government surveys such as the 'General Household Survey' are analysed and subsequently used as a basis for making changes in social policy. The data may be utilized when measuring poverty or monitoring health, when assessing need, or when evaluating the effectiveness of welfare services.

The Economic and Social Research Council (ESRC) has reviewed the two government socio-economic classifications and considered their relative shortcomings. It concluded that there should be just one, revised, occupationally based socio-economic classification, incorporating the most useful qualities of both. The new classification system will include a category for people who are not in paid employment. This applies to 40 per cent of the UK population, and includes some people who have never had a paid job. The new classification will be used to analyse material produced by the 2001 census.

Criticisms of the Registrar-General's 'Social Class Based on Occupations'

Many academics and commentators have long been calling for the kind of changes now being explored by the ESRC. Clearly, a classification which only involves the 60 per cent of the UK population who are in paid work is limited. It ignores, in addition to unemployed people, students, carers remaining at home to care for their children, retired people, and those who are unable to work owing to a physical or learning disability. As women outnumber men in the second and third of these categories, far fewer of them than men are included in the classification. The effect, therefore, has been to marginalize women.

Leaving out unemployed people also means leaving out the very rich, who have great wealth and/or

private incomes. They do not have an occupational title and so are excluded. This group has been referred to as the 'upper class' or 'aristocracy' and, more recently, as the 'super-class' or 'over-class', to contrast it with the recently designated 'underclass'.

We shall now turn to a third explanation of social class – a more useful and sophisticated one that is well respected by a wide range of academics and commentators who have a special interest in this subject.

JOHN GOLDTHORPE'S CLASS MODEL

In the course of many years' work on class and social mobility (how people move up and down the class system), John Goldthorpe (working largely from the 1960s onwards) has devised a sophisticated model of class in Britain (Goldthorpe, 1980). His work is highly respected by other social scientists who have also studied class. For example, a major study of class in this country in the late 1980s, which was part of a larger, world-wide study involving some 19 countries, found Goldthorpe's analysis to be the most useful. This study, based at the University of Essex, involved a national sample survey of men and women aged 18–65 years. Almost 2000 responses were received, and the survey included a one and a half hour interview with each respondent (Marshall *et al.*, 1988).

At its most elaborate, the Goldthorpe model of class identifies 11 social classes. These can be reduced to seven, five and even three major classes depending on their use. These are entitled *service*, *intermediate* and *working* classes (see Table 2.2).

Goldthorpe has reviewed his class categories at times in order to stay up to date with changes in the work-force and other social developments. His classes are determined by two major factors fused together, namely a person's occupational title (including their source and level of income, financial security and financial prospects) and their employment status (how much autonomy they have,

Table 2.2 John Goldthorpe's three major social classes (adapted from Goldthorpe, J. 1980: *Social mobility and class structure in modern Britain*. Oxford: Oxford University Press)

- **Service class** – professionals, administrators and managers, including the supervisors of non-manual workers
- **Intermediate class** – routine non-manual workers (e.g. clerical and sales personnel), less senior technicians, the supervisors of manual workers and the self-employed
- **Working class** – All skilled, semi-skilled and unskilled manual labourers, including agricultural workers

or what control they exercise over their roles and tasks at work).

Criticisms of Goldthorpe's class model

Although Goldthorpe's class analysis is an improvement on the Registrar General's classification because it involves employment *status* as well as occupation and occupational skills, it is still inadequate in some respects.

First, social class positions are still too much determined by a person's occupation – the kind of job they do. Therefore, as with the Registrar General's classification, those who are very rich, those with other sources of income and those who do not need to work are not included. Again, those who are not classified as working, including unemployed people, pensioners, housewives and students, are also 'invisible' to the analysis.

Secondly, women generally tend to have many more part-time, less well paid and less secure jobs than men. The relationship between women and work and men and work is thus very different. Goldthorpe's class analysis does not do full justice to this situation, because the nature of much of women's paid work leads to their being over-represented in the 'working class'. This is a distortion, since it ignores other social class determinants, such as life-style, leisure pursuits and cultural interests. In fact, this particular issue has led some writers on class to suggest that we should seek to devise a completely different class analysis for women as opposed to men. This may therefore be a future development.

A SUMMARY OF CLASS ANALYSES

So far, by focusing on three important contributions to an understanding of social class, we have seen that the concept remains far from simple. So many different variables need to be taken into account, depending on our definition of social class – occupation, income, wealth, status, skill, autonomy in work, values, attitudes, life-style, leisure interests – that the task is a daunting one! A major problem is that these complex variables frequently contradict each other, making classification difficult. Consider, for example, where a high-earning manual worker, who lives in a leafy middle-class suburb, and whose friends and leisure activities are middle class, should be placed. Furthermore, where would you place his wife, who does not have paid employment?

Each explanation of class that social scientists have put forward appears to be incomplete or inadequate in some way. In particular, two issues of key importance, namely *gender* and *race*, appear to be largely ignored in class analyses.

Writing on class still tends to be very *male-oriented* and to use outdated concepts such as 'head of household'. Many households in the UK today do not comprise the traditional 'nuclear family', i.e. two parents and the average number of children – somewhere between two and three. There are now over 1 million single-parent families, and many of these parents will not be able to take any kind of work because of their child-care responsibilities. Most of them are women, and they are not represented in our 'gender-blind' class theories and analyses.

Analyses of class also ignore the fact that there are racial issues of importance. For example, a large proportion of black people are to be found in poorer-paid, less secure, and in the case of black women, part-time jobs. Black people, along with people with physical disabilities and those with learning difficulties, are not evenly represented in all occupations, and a social class analysis fails to portray this. British society is stratified by gender and race in ways that are too important to be ignored or rendered 'invisible'.

WHY USE THE CONCEPT OF SOCIAL CLASS AT ALL?

In the past few years, some academics have talked about the *death of social class*. They feel that it is indistinct and no longer a useful sociological concept, and so should be abandoned. Some politicians have also argued that the UK is no longer divided along class lines. Most famously, John Major, in referring back to what he had said in the run-up to the 1992 general election, commented, 'I said that I believed in a nation at ease with itself – the development of a truly classless society – with opportunities for all from wherever they came, to do whatever they can with their own life'.

When this comment was repeated on ITV's *World in Action* programme in December 1996, the Labour MP Tony Benn responded by saying, 'when the Prime Minister said he wanted a "classless society", what he really meant was he didn't want class discussed anymore'. He added, 'The pretence that there's a common interest between the guy working on £3.00 an hour or £2.00 an hour and the man who employs him is nonsense. But if you take class out of politics, which was the Prime Minister's intention, then, of course, the sense of class solidarity disappears and that gives him and the government the power to tell everybody that life is natural; it's:

> *God bless the Squire and his relations*
> *and keep us in our proper stations.*

That was the Victorian poem and that's what he'd like to go back to.' Here, Tony Benn was refuting the claim that we are now living in a classless society. For him the divisions are effective and remain.

However, for all its inadequacies, inconsistencies and incompleteness, and for all that it is a crude measure involving generalizations and the grouping of individuals into wide categories, the nomenclature of social class *does* continue to have some value. It can still inform us about the quality of life for some groups of people. Let us look at its application when examining two important areas of social policy.

Social class and health

One guaranteed way to live longer, grow taller, avoid chronic illness, have healthier children, increase your quality of life and minimize your risk of premature death. The secret is BE RICH – because all the major health indicators are directly related to income.

(Dr John Collee, *Observer,* 27 September 1992)
[his emphasis]

Of the factors contributing to structured variations (or patterns) in life and death, SOCIAL CLASS is the most significant.

(Perry, 1996, p.212)

Social scientists have demonstrated that people from class positions higher in the social scale tend on average to be healthier and taller, and to live longer than those in lower-class positions. Class differences are greatest with regard to infant mortality and the death of children. In addition, people from lower-class positions are more likely to die at any age in life than people from higher-class positions. There are a number of reasons for this, but the main one is the lack of financial resources of those in lower-class positions. This nearly always leads to a poorer diet. A report from the Health Education Authority written by a National Health Service dietitian, Issy Cole-Hamilton, stated that people on low incomes could not afford to eat healthily. Lack of money, rather than lack of knowledge of what healthy foods to eat, led to this situation (*Observer*, 15 October 1989, p.4).

More recently, in 1994, two further reports shed light on the link between poverty and diet. A National Childrens' Home report based on research conducted by the Food Commission stated that social security benefits did not provide enough money for a basic, healthy diet. Secondly, an international research group, Mintel, produced research which was published in *British Lifestyles, 1994* (Mintel, 1995). It found that people living on benefits were least likely, of all social groupings, to eat vegetables or fresh fruit regularly. Healthier food is more expensive, but the research found that poor people are also affected by a lack of good cooking facilities, the cost of fuel for cooking, and a reluctance to experiment with new, healthier recipes which their children might not like – thus causing food to be wasted.

In April 1997, the National Food Alliance published a report entitled *If They Don't Eat a Healthy Diet, It's Their Own Fault! – Myths About Food And Low Income* (Lobstein, 1997). The report asserted that ignorance or fecklessness are not the main problems, as is often claimed in connection with a poor diet, but rather lack of money, inadequate shopping facilities and poor transport. In referring to what it called 'food poverty', it said that some low-income families eat as little as 95 grams of fresh green vegetables per week – the equivalent of barely one brussel sprout per person per day. The report also showed that about 40 per cent of women on low incomes were seriously lacking in iron, potassium and vitamin B_6 (necessary for healthy blood, teeth and gums and a healthy nervous system).

The report calculated that the money available for food for a family on benefit amounts to about 63 pence a day for children of primary-school age, 93 pence for older children and £2.73 for adults. The same report estimates that a 'modest but adequate' diet for a family of two adults and two children aged 16 and 10 years would cost £69.20 pence per week.

Finally, the report points out that most good bargains are for bulk buys, which is not much use for someone who cannot afford them, does not have a car to take them home and does not have the space and facilities to store them.

In addition to diet, a number of other factors are involved in the relationship between health and class. Those lower down the class scale tend to live in poorer housing and environmental conditions. Those with jobs tend to suffer from poorer working conditions (i.e. dirtier, noisier and more dangerous) and those lower in the class structure generally are less able to afford holidays or breaks, which are an important part of a healthier life-style.

Such findings were aired in a major report called *Inequalities in Health,* written by a working group set up in 1977 and chaired by Sir Douglas Black (the Black Report). The report was published by the DHSS (as it then was) in 1980, and generated a great deal of controversy because of its disturbing findings. Its most important conclusion was clear – that *material deprivation* played the most important part in poor health for those in lower social classes. Other contributory factors were biological and cultural, and those centred around life-style.

The report indicated that people in higher social classes also tend to benefit more from medical care. They have more access to such care, being able to draw on private as well as public (NHS) services. Such people are statistically more likely to self-refer to such services. They also spend longer on average in sessions with their general practitioner.

In 1986, the Health Education Council commissioned research which updated the evidence of the Black Report. The report, entitled *The Health Divide: Inequalities in Health in the 1980s,* stated:

> In some respects the health of the lower occupational classes [Registrar-General's] has actually deteriorated against the background of a general improvement in the population as a whole. While death rates have been declining, rates of chronic illness seem to have been increasing, and the gap in the illness rates

> between manual and non-manual groups has been widening too, particularly in the over-65 age group.
>
> (Health Education Council, p.266)

One of the report's conclusions was that 'the weight of evidence continues to point to explanations which suggest that socio-economic circumstances play the major part in subsequent health differences' (p.304). Another conclusion indicated that, 'disappointingly, in the intervening eight years [since the publication of the Black Report] there seems to have been little progress on the basic problems underlying inequality in health' (p.350). Among these underlying problems are mentioned 'poverty', 'poor nutrition' and poor 'housing and working conditions' (p.350).

There appears to be no firm evidence that class differentials in health are narrowing in the 1990s. Two influential reports published in 1995 confirmed that poor people suffer ill health more than rich people. First, the King's Fund, an independent health charity, produced *Tackling Inequalities in Health: An Agenda for Action* (King's Fund, 1995), which concluded that poorer people experience more illness and disability, and that people in impoverished circumstances are likely to die 8 years earlier than those who are more affluent. At the public launch of the report, Sir Donald Acheson, former Chief Medical Officer for England, was quoted as saying, 'The existence of health inequalities in Britain is indisputable'. He went on to state: 'Any successful effort to reduce inequalities in health must look beyond the NHS and encompass a broad range of actions involving every aspect of society.'

Secondly, in October 1995 the Department of Health published a report which stated that life expectancy was 7 years longer for someone born into social class I than for someone born into social class V. Furthermore, children born into the former class were four times less likely to suffer accidental death than those born into the latter (Department of Health, 1995).

So concerned was the new 1997 Labour Government with inequalities in health that it created a new post – a Minister of Public Health. Tessa Jowell, the first person to occupy the post, confirmed that the government would be updating the findings of the Black Report (*Inequalities In Health*) of 1980, and said, 'We want to attack the underlying causes of ill health and break the cycle of social and economic deprivation and social exclusion' (*Guardian*, 8 July 1997, p.7).

Social class and education

> Clearly there is a relationship between how much one earns and how good an education one's child gets.
>
> (Paul Haddock, parent of public schoolboy *Class*, ITV, 24 June 1997)

The education which our society provides for our children and young adults tends to reaffirm class inequalities, rather than change them. The tripartite system of state (or public) education introduced by the Butler Education Act 1944, i.e. grammar, technical and secondary modern schools, enshrined the principle of 'equality of opportunity'. It aimed to offer children of all classes the chance to win a grammar school place. Grammar schools were more committed to academic achievements than the other two types of school, and young people leaving them tended to have gained better qualifications and thus were more likely to go on to higher education and better paid jobs with better prospects.

The 1944 Act also introduced the '11-plus' examination, and success in this secured a grammar school place. What has been discovered since is that home environment was the dominant feature in a child's educational success or failure. Those children from higher social classes whose homes were more comfortable and conducive to study performed better. It was also felt that the 11-plus examination contained an inbuilt cultural bias which favoured children from higher social classes (the style of language used is a key feature here, it being more 'foreign' to children from lower social classes). There also tended to be too few grammar schools in working-class areas of our towns and cities, so there was a dearth of places for less privileged children.

A University of Oxford social mobility study (Goldthorpe, 1980) surveyed 10 000 men, asking them what their own occupation was and what their father's had been. Using John Goldthorpe's three major class divisions – service, intermediate and working class – the movement between them over a generation was studied. What was discovered was a 1:2:4 rule, whereby whatever chance a working-class boy had of moving into the service class, a boy from the intermediate class had twice the chance, and a service-class boy had four times the chance.

Working-class children are far more likely to drop out of education earlier than others. In the Oxford survey, the service-class child was four times more likely to be still at school at 16 years of age, eight times more likely at 17 years, and 11 times more likely to enter university. Less than one in 40 boys from working-class families gained 'O' levels (now GCSEs), compared to one in four service-class boys. Writing in a collection of essays published in 1996, John Goldthorpe (with Gordon Marshall) reviewed research conducted to date on class and education. Rather pessimistically, he had to conclude that the situation had not significantly improved.

Of course, not being so successful in educational terms has a 'knock-on' effect for lower-class children. It means that their prospects of higher education, better paid jobs and promising careers are severely curtailed. Add to this the fact that more privileged people in the top social classes can also afford to take advantage of the growing sector of private education, and the result is considerable inequality.

> If you wanted the one defining attribute of the middle classes it is a reverence for education.
>
> (A.A. Gill, journalist, *Class*, ITV, 24 June 1997)

THE EMERGENCE OF AN 'UNDERCLASS' IN BRITAIN

> Two nations, between whom there is no intercourse and no sympathy, who are as ignorant of each other's habits, thoughts and feelings as if they were dwellers in different zones or inhabitants of different planets.
>
> (Benjamin Disraeli, Conservative Prime Minister, in *Sybil, or the Two Nations*, 1980, originally published in 1845) [His description of the rich and the poor might well apply to the situation today between a more comfortable majority and a marginalized 'underclass']

In the past few years some commentators on social class have begun to talk of a new phenomenon in the UK, particularly in our class structure. This is the emergence of a so-called 'underclass'. For many social scientists and those concerned with the future of our welfare services, this recent development should be of deep concern to us all.

The first use of the term 'underclass' has been attributed to an American sociologist, Gunnar Myrdal, who wrote of the concept as far back as 1962 in a book entitled *Challenge to Affluence* (Myrdal, 1962). He used the term to refer to people who are marginalized and excluded from the labour market as a result of structural economic change. Later in the 1980s, and again in America, the term was popularized by a journalist called Ken Auletta. Today, however, use of the word and concept is most closely associated with the name of a third American, Charles Murray, a social policy analyst. He developed his own meaning of the 'underclass' in an American setting, in a book called *Losing Ground: American Social Policy 1950–1980* (Murray, 1984). Later he came to the UK, and in November 1989 *The Sunday Times* magazine published an article by him, headed 'The emerging British underclass'.

Debate about the concept of the 'underclass' has intensified. The term has been used by both those on the 'right' and those on the 'left' of the political continuum. When used by those on the right it tends to have a morally judgemental element, in that members of the 'underclass' are depicted negatively as 'fickle' or 'immoral', 'criminal' or 'work-shy'. For writers such as Murray or Ralf Dahrendorf, the concept appears to be a resurrection of the Victorian idea of the 'undeserving' as compared to the 'deserving' poor, who they would now refer to merely as 'the poor'. We can refer to this approach as a *behavioural* or *cultural* explanation.

Murray's description of those he would define as being members of the 'underclass' appeared early in his *Sunday Times* article, where he described a 'handful' of people in the small Iowa town in which he grew up:

> Then there was another set of poor people. These poor people didn't lack just money. They were defined by their behaviour. Their homes were littered and unkempt. The men in the family were unable to hold a job for more than a few weeks at a time. Drunkenness was common. The children grew up ill-schooled and ill-behaved and contributed a disproportionate share of the local juvenile delinquents.
>
> (*The Sunday Times* magazine, November 1989, p.23)

For those on the left, there has been disagreement about the use of the concept, and it is recognized that the word itself has negative connotations. Ruth Lister believes that it is imprecise, emotive and value-laden. Bob Holman agrees, rejects the term completely, and prefers simply to refer to those who experience 'social deprivation' (*Social Work Today*, 16 August 1990). Both authors believe that the very use of the term is likely to worsen the plight of those to whom it refers, and to increase the social stigma which they face.

Others – such as Frank Field, whose definition of the term is discussed more fully below, and Bill Jordan – use the concept, but in doing so they concentrate on the economic, political and social *forces* or *structures* which exclude certain poor people from full citizenship. They focus on what Miller has

referred to as 'the insufficiencies of current economic and social policies to bring a subsection of the poor out of poverty conditions' (cited in Bulmer, 1989). Bill Jordan considers that we have 'a social structure in which the most important division in society is between the relatively comfortable majority and an underclass' (Jordan, 1989, p.18). We can refer to this approach as a *structural* or *structuralist* explanation.

Despite the disagreement surrounding the term 'underclass', it does still have its uses. We use the concept throughout this book in a non-judgemental way as a means of drawing attention to the economic, political and social elements which have conspired together to exclude a section of our society from full citizenship. Perhaps a more satisfactory term will soon be discovered. For now we have placed the word in inverted commas in order to emphasize its imprecise nature.

What do we mean by an 'underclass'?

> Throughout this century people have defined themselves by their work. They were miners, engineers, printers, draymen, tanners. And they were predominantly male. But as the manufacturing industries collapsed, more jobs were taken by women and millions of badly educated men could no longer define themselves. 'I'm a printer' could be said with pride; 'I'm on benefit' is a mark of exclusion.'
>
> (Barry Hugill, *Observer*, 13 April 1997, p.29)

Perhaps the description of the 'underclass' which appears to be most useful for the UK is that spelt out by Frank Field (1989), a Member of Parliament and former Director of The Child Poverty Action Group (CPAG). He believes that the 'underclass' has been recruited from three groups of people, namely the long-term unemployed, single-parent families and elderly pensioners. All of these groups are on fixed incomes, i.e. they receive state benefits of one kind or another.

It is important not to think of these groups as being homogenous - in fact their situations, ages, gender and race are various. For example, the long-term unemployed will include young people who have not had paid work since leaving school, and older workers who have lost their jobs and, owing to the ageism prevalent in society, have found it difficult to obtain new employment. A large proportion of unemployed people are to be found in, or near, inner-city areas owing to the above-mentioned decline in heavy manufacturing industries. There is also a higher than average proportion of ethnic minority members among them (given their numbers in society), whose families had originally moved to inner-city areas for the available work in traditional industries. Again, because of racism, people from ethnic minorities have found it extremely difficult to obtain work. There are now over 1 million single-parent families in the UK, and the vast majority of parents in these families are women. Child-care responsibilities are most frequently taken on by mothers, and the plight of those who have been on welfare benefit for a long time is particularly harsh. Their child-care responsibilities mean that they cannot work, especially in full-time jobs.

Those elderly pensioners who are completely dependent on their old-age pension and income support are also particularly deprived. They do not have an additional occupational pension, they often live in very poor housing, and they also have to contend with the increasing ill health and disability which the ageing process can bring.

A final group that we should include are disabled people. An official report from the Office of Population Censuses and Surveys (1988) estimated that there are just over 6 million disabled people in this country, i.e. about 1 in 10 of the total population. Another report from the same source that was published soon afterwards noted that two-thirds of disabled people were living at or below the poverty line.

Around the same time, a report from the Disability Alliance (1988), which represents about 100 voluntary organizations that champion the interests of disabled people, showed that disabled people of working age are twice as likely to be living on or below the poverty line than are their non-disabled counterparts. Those particularly hard hit were disabled people who had never been able to work, and who had therefore never made any national insurance contributions. Such people only received basic state benefit for disabled people. Older disabled people were particularly badly affected because of this situation.

The 'underclass' – permanently marginalized

> Yes – there is an underclass that cannot take physical necessities for granted.
>
> (T. Kaczynski, *Unabomber's Manifesto, Washington Post* and *New York Times*, 19 September 1995)

The most depressing and distressing aspect of the social position of members of the 'underclass' is the *fixedness* of their situation. They are *trapped*, and their situation is almost certainly permanent. If they earn a little money on a part-time or casual job, their benefit is cut. It would appear that their only escape is well-paid, secure employment, and this is extremely unlikely given their multiple deprivation.

Blaming the victim

As they are no longer needed by our economy as workers, it is easy for our society to ignore and lose interest in them. It is possible to make the mistake of treating the deprivation from which members of the 'underclass' suffer (poverty, poor housing, etc.) as the 'cause' of their plight. If this mistake is made, it becomes dangerously easy to unfairly 'blame' the 'victim' for her or his predicament.

Bob Holman has pointed out that the behaviour of the rich is less vulnerable to public censure.

Cabinet ministers who beget children outside marriage, Oxbridge students who use drugs, stock-brokers who commit fraud, the London Docklands' affluent who . . . build security fences to make themselves a separate group, do not lead [commentators] to write an attack on the 'overclass'. By just blaming the poor [they make] them victims.

(*Social Work Today*, 16 August 1990, p.38)

How large is the 'underclass'?

It is probably impossible to come up with an accurate figure for the number of people in the 'underclass'. We must be clear that this is not equal to the number of people living in poverty, of whom there are far more.

In 1987, Dahrendorf estimated that the 'underclass' he defined represented around 5 per cent of the UK population – that is, nearly 3 million people. John Vincent, as a supporter of Church Action on Poverty (an organization representing a number of different church denominations), calculated the size of the 'underclass' at the end of 1989 to be between 1 and 2 million people (*Today*, Radio 4, 11 December 1989). Will Hutton's '30-30-40 model' of society (see Fig. 2.3) substantially increases the proportion of the population who are described as 'absolutely disadvantaged', to nearly one-third of society. Some would equate this to an 'underclass'.

Not only is it extremely difficult to measure the size of the 'underclass' with any accuracy, but the situation is of course changing all the time, as social and economic factors and conditions alter.

Deprived of full citizenship

Society means a shared life. If some and not others are poor then the principles on which life is shared are at issue; society itself is in question.

(A.H. Halsey, in Foreword to Mack and Lansley, 1985, p.xxiii)

The top 40 per cent

The privileged full-time employed or self-employed who have held their jobs for over 2 years. Hutton also includes part-time workers who have held their jobs for over 5 years.

The intermediate 30 per cent

Those in insecure and poorly protected jobs, including the growing number of part-time and casual workers.

The bottom 30 per cent

Hutton refers to this group as the 'disadvantaged'. They are unemployed, and do not even find 'scraps' of part-time work.

Fig. 2.3 Will Hutton's model of a 30-30-40 society. (Will Hutton is an economist and ex-stockbroker who works as a journalist. He is currently editor of the *Observer* newspaper. His 30-30-40 model appeared in his 1995 book, *The State We're In*, (published by Jonathan Cape). Reproduced with permission.

The material deprivation which members of the 'underclass' suffer also deprives them of a number of other things. Their children's education, which will be impoverished by poor living conditions, and diet – the direct result of poverty – will be further harmed by a lack of financial resources. Parents are not able to send or take their children on educational visits, trips or 'exchange holidays'.

The mobility of those same families is severely restricted because they will not have access to a car, and they have to rely on an often limited public transport service (especially in rural areas). This also means they will have to rely on local shops, where prices are often higher than in larger stores in city or town centres, or in superstores on the edge of urban areas.

Entertainment, hobbies, leisure pursuits and sport all cost money to a greater or lesser extent, and therefore members of the 'underclass' will have severely limited access to all of them. This means they will be confined to their homes with little to break up the daily tedium except radio or television.

Poverty is much more than simply a lack of finance. It is also a poverty of experiences. Life in the 'underclass' will be dispiriting and depressing, and how many feel they will ever escape from such an existence?

Members of the 'underclass' are deprived of being able to take a full part in social, political and economic life. They are *socially excluded*. As we have said earlier, their marginalization appears to be *fixed*. The majority of them may be said to be *trapped* in a condition that is likely to last for the rest of their lives.

> The existence of an underclass casts doubt on the social contract itself. It means that citizenship has become an exclusive rather than an inclusive status. Some are full citizens, some are not. If some have no stake in the society, the society puts itself at risk. It becomes defensive and, in the end, closed. Extending full citizenship rights to all is therefore the main task of social policy.
>
> (R. Dahrendorf, *New Statesman*, 12 June 1987, p.14)

For the sake of the well-being of every member of our society, the existence of the 'underclass' – of a sector of the population that is cut off in many different ways from mainstream social life – should not be allowed to continue. The new Labour Government revealed plans in August 1997 to re-integrate the 'underclass' into mainstream society. Ministers felt that this could be achieved over a 10-year period.

As Tony Blair observed, 'After several years of economic growth, 5 million people of working age live in homes where nobody works. Over 1 million have never worked since leaving school' (*Independent*, 3 June 1997, p.1). The Prime Minister went on to say:

> There is a case not just in moral terms but in enlightened self-interest to act, to tackle what we all know exists – an underclass of people cut off from society's mainstream, without any sense of shared purpose. . . . Our task is to reconnect that workless class

> – to bring jobs, skills, opportunities and ambition to all those people who have been left behind by the Conservative years and to restore the will to win where it has been lost.
>
> (*Yorkshire Post*, 3 June 1997, p.1)

The government has set up a 'Social Exclusion Unit' to operate in the Cabinet Office which reports directly to the Prime Minister. Announcing this new initiative, the Minister without Portfolio, Peter Mandelson, said 'We must tackle the root causes of social exclusion' and the Prime Minister, Tony Blair, pledged that 'there would be no forgotten people in the Britain I want to build' (*Independent*, 14 August 1997, p.1).

In practical terms, 1300 inner-city housing estates were initially targeted, which contained 3 million of Britain's poorest people. The Unit aims to focus on the following issues: young people excluded from school; those drifting into criminality or substance misuse; and those under 25 years of age who have not worked since leaving school. More money has also been allocated to the 'Rough Sleepers Initiative', introduced by the previous government, in order to extend it beyond London. The unit also has a racial dimension in acknowledgement of the fact that black people figure disproportionately frequently among lone parents, those excluded from school, and people who are long-term unemployed.

CLASS, CARERS AND CLIENTS

> The majority of social workers are white middle class and the majority of clients are working class.
>
> (C. Jones, *State Social Work and the Working Class*, 1983, p.9)

No substantial research has been conducted on the social class position of the clients of the personal social services. From our own working experience and the testimony of others in social welfare, we know that the majority of clients are working class and poor. We know that material deprivation will be the root cause of many problems which people, as clients, will take to a social worker. Saul Becker, who conducted research into the extent of poverty among social-work clients in the mid 1980s, wrote, 'This showed that nine out of ten users of social services were claimants of social security benefits' (*Community Care*, 26 June 1997, p.19). Bob Holman has referred to research which reported that '88 per cent of child-care referrals to the Strathclyde Social Work Department (in Scotland) [came] from low-income families' (Holman, 1992, p.7).

In 1969, Frederick Seebohm (Chair of the Seebohm Committee which reported in 1968) considered that poverty and bad housing 'probably caused something like 60 per cent of the work that is now carried on by social workers'. Poverty and poor-quality housing (the two are closely linked) will be experienced disproportionately by members of lower social classes.

The class position of the clients of the personal social services will, of course, vary depending on the need. For example, residential care for elders and day-care for disabled people or those with learning disabilities will tend to be provided to a wider cross-section of social classes in the UK. We *all* get old, and disability or learning difficulties occur in all kinds of families from all kinds of social class background. However, those individuals or families who approach a social worker and whose problem has its root in deprivation will be more exclusively drawn from a lower social class.

It is also important to look at the other side of this question. Why are members of the higher social classes able to *avoid* becoming the clients of the personal social services? There are three possible answers. First, their general level of affluence means that they do not suffer, either directly or at second hand, from poverty, poor housing or a poor environment with few facilities. Secondly, they are able to purchase care from the private sector and to employ carers in their own home for themselves or their children. Thirdly, research such as the Black Report

and *The Health Divide* shows clear signs that the better off actually derive more benefit from public services such as education or the National Health Service than do lower-class people. Middle-class people tend to be more assertive and better able to seek out what is available to them.

Material deprivation, such as poverty, low income and poor housing, makes a contribution to a client's difficulties. These are often inextricably linked with emotional, relationship, or psychological problems that clients may experience. For carers and clients it is frequently unclear precisely where the origins of difficulties lie.

As the quote at the start of this section highlighted, most social carers and social workers are middle class. We have become accustomed to seeing advertisements for jobs in social care which state that the employer is an 'equal opportunities employer'. These adverts usually state that the employer will take on people regardless of their *gender* and *race*. Less often *disability* is mentioned, and still less frequently *sexual orientation*. *Social class* is never mentioned at all. Employers do not have equal opportunities policies which state that members of the 'working class' are welcome to apply, let alone members of the 'underclass'!

Why should this be? It is difficult to come up with a clear answer to this question. Social class does not appear to be treated with the same importance or urgency as the other factors we have mentioned. Perhaps one key to the answer is to be found in a general awkwardness or embarrassment in British society towards class. Although we know that our society is deeply divided along class lines, many people do not like to acknowledge this. They choose to ignore it, as if this will diminish its significance. Others might find the mere mention of class in a job advertisement actually offensive. Many people like to render class invisible – to push it into the background.

What should our reaction, as social carers, be to social class? First, we should acknowledge that our own social class position will frequently differ from that of our clients, no matter what our specific field may be. The quality of life we enjoy, our life-style and material well-being will usually be more privileged than that of our clients. Many field social workers and probation officers will have completed a professional training course in higher education, and will therefore have benefited from a vocational education course at a higher level than the average person in our country.

Secondly, such privileged life experience may well have implications for how well we can empathize with, and have knowledge and understanding of, those who become our clients. The trapped position of a member of the 'underclass' will not usually accord with our own more flexible situation. We are not subject to the particular stress and depression that being in such a position can engender.

Thirdly, an awareness and knowledge of social class are imperative if we are to be effective social carers. We must attempt to understand the client in her or his social class and cultural context. This will inform our practice and ensure that we do not fall into the trap of *blaming the victim(s)* of the social class system – the victim(s) of *structural inequality*. Thus our understanding, awareness and empathy will be enhanced.

In increasing our awareness of social class, we shall be better placed to see *communalities* of experience between clients who share a common social class position. We can attempt to raise our clients' own awareness of this situation, and thereby help them not to be defeatist or blame themselves over-much for their own predicament where this situation is a direct cause of structural inequalities or other social factors that are beyond their control.

Sometimes this is summed up as a way of empowering the client – helping them to take more initiative with regard to their situation, and to become more pro-active. This is of great importance if we believe that it is their very lack of power over their own lives and situations which is the main effect of our clients' frequent marginalization. It is also important that this empowerment (which will be dealt with more fully in the final

chapter of this book) is real, and that it leads to definite, progressive change, rather than being merely fine-sounding rhetoric.

Turning from the individual social carer to the agencies for which they work, it would be encouraging to see social class, along with other factors such as gender and race, included in their equal opportunities policies and recruitment advertising. As we indicated earlier, the issue has been ignored or conveniently avoided. It is extremely important for a balanced social-care work-force that members of social classes lower in the scale are recruited, along with more people from minority groups in our society. A predominantly middle-class social-care work-force dealing with a largely deprived clientele leads to an unhealthy situation which reflects the 'powerful-powerless' divide in our society. Social care should be at the forefront of moves to change this situation radically for the better.

THE FUTURE OF SOCIAL CLASS

Society is never static – change is constant. In particular, the nature of work and the constituency of the work-force has changed dramatically during the last few years. Although the work that people perform is only one of several factors influencing which social class they belong to, it is extremely important. Changes in work and the nature of the work-force must therefore be considered in any discussion of social class. Some of the important changes in the work-force are indicated below.

A decline has taken place throughout the UK, but particularly in South Wales, Scotland and northern areas of England, in the traditional 'heavy' industries such as shipbuilding, steel and coal-mining, and also in general manufacturing industries. These industries had always employed a large number of people belonging to the working class – workers (virtually all men) of a skilled, semi-skilled and unskilled *manual* nature. This has led to a corresponding decline in the communities in which they

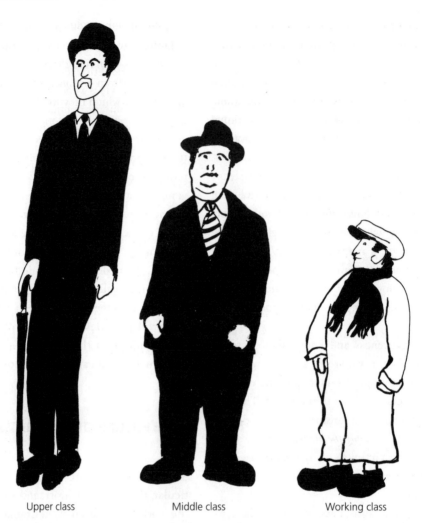

Upper class   Middle class   Working class

Are these traditional images of social class outmoded?

lived in large numbers. Particular areas that were hit by unemployment in these types of work were the shipbuilding industry in the north-east of England and on the River Clyde in Scotland, steel manufacture in the 'steel city' of Sheffield and in the surrounding districts in the English north-Midlands, and coal-mining, which has been reduced nationally to a handful of pits.

The decline in other types of work affected different parts of the country. For example, the complete closure of the London docks in the east of the City and the Isle of Dogs occurred within only a few years. Many thousands of dockers lost their employment in these areas.

Whilst the 'heavy' and manufacturing industries have seen dramatic decline, the service sector and white-collar work have enjoyed tremendous growth. As old technologies are phased out, so new technologies have shown rapid growth. Automation, computerization and the massive increase in the use of microchip technology have brought about what might be referred to as a 'revolution' in working practice. New areas of work, such as information systems, have blossomed, while more established areas of work have completely changed their working practices. The newspaper industry is one such example. The move of all major national newspapers out of Fleet Street has been accompanied by investment in new plant and new technological ways of communicating news and producing the finished article.

All of these changes have had two important effects. First, they have led to an expanded middle (or 'intermediate') class and a declining working class. Secondly, they have increasingly fragmented the middle class into new divisions as the nature of work has changed.

During the last few years a fatalism has developed in this country concerning the future of work. The main aspects of this fatalism are as follows:

- that we are now living in a time of post-full employment;
- that full employment will never return;
- that full-time, well-paid, secure *jobs for life* in large numbers are a thing of the past;
- that we can do little, if anything, about these developments because economic necessity and efficiency have taken precedence over the political will;
- that we have no alternative but to accept long-term, mass unemployment;

- that a socially excluded 'underclass' has become a permanent feature of our society.

It is important that those of us who are involved in the caring services vehemently resist such fatalism. We must encourage politicians to do the same, and to search for practical measures which will eradicate social exclusion. The setting up by the government of the Social Exclusion Unit is a positive sign that fatalism is being replaced by optimism and positive action.

Class explanations, theories and analyses must 'sharpen up' in response to all of the changes discussed in this chapter. They need to develop in a more flexible way in order to take increased account of gender, race, age and unemployment. Far from 'withering away', research shows that social class is actually growing in importance for people in the UK. The opinion poll company Gallup has asked research participants in this country since 1961 whether they think there is a class struggle in this country? Of the sample asked, in 1961 56 per cent believed that there was. In 1996, 6 years after the then Prime Minister John Major had promised to aim for a classless society, this figure had risen to 81 per cent.

EXERCISES

1. Which class are you?

Advertisers (along with opinion pollsters) have used a six-point social class classification in recent years which they hope will help them to market their wares more effectively.

- A – the so-called 'upper middle class', who have top professional or managerial jobs. It represents only about 3 per cent of the population.
- B – the so-called 'middle class', who are middle-managers and professionals. It represents 14 per cent of the population.
- Cl – might be called the 'lower middle class' – consists of junior managers or professionals or those

that own small businesses with premises and staff. It respresents 26 per cent of the population.
- C2 – the 'skilled working class'.
- D – semi-skilled or unskilled workers.
- E – the poorest in society, mostly consisting of unemployed people and retired elderly people relying on the state pension.

(a) Place yourself in what you believe is your own or your family's category. Give your reasons for your decision.

(b) Now place yourself in your relevant class position using the three major class analyses discussed in this chapter. Again, give your reasons for your decision.

2. Social mobility

Go back three generations (to your great-grandparents) and place each adult from the different generations in what you believe to be their relevant social class positions. Again use the three major class analyses discussed in this chapter (Marx, the Registrar-General and Goldthorpe). Now trace the pattern of social mobility – whether it has been upward, downward, or remained unchanged. Account for the changes in this pattern.

3. Identifying social class

Where in the social class structure would you place the following personnel in the caring services?

- Nursery nurse/nursery officer
- Home help (home carer)
- Receptionist
- Care manager
- Ward sister
- Officer-in-charge, residential home for children
- Occupational therapist
- Home help/care organizer
- Education welfare officer
- Senior social worker
- Probation officer
- Care assistant/officer, residential home for older people
- Registered general nurse
- Chief probation officer/assistant chief probation officer

4. The middle class

Read the following poem:

> Another thing about the English middle classes
> Is how they hate their children.
> Those under fifty, and more still, those under forty
> They instinctively hate their own children
> Once they've got them.
>
> At the same time, they take the greatest possible care
>   of them -
> Nurses, doctors, proper food,

> hygiene, schools, all that –
> The greatest possible care
> And they hate them.
>
> They seem to feel the children a ghastly limitation –
> But for these children I should be free –
> Free what for, nobody knows. But free! –
> Awfully sorry, dear, but I can't come because of the
>   children.
>
> The children, of course, know that they are cared for
> And disliked.
> There is no means of really deceiving a child.
>
> So they accept covered dislike as the normal feeling
>   between people
> And superficial attention and care and fulfilment of
>   duty
> As normal activity
> They may even, one day, discover simple affection as
>   a great discovery.
>
> (*Middle-Class Children*, from *The Complete Poems of D.H. Lawrence* (1964, 1971) reproduced with permission from Laurence Pollinger Limited and the Estate of Frieda Lawrence Ravagli)

(a) Is the poet's message based entirely on prejudice, or is there some truth contained within it?

(b) Is disadvantage experienced by people from *all* social classes? If so, what forms does it take?

5. Media study

Make a selection of national daily and Sunday newspapers, e.g. two tabloids and two more 'serious' papers. Read them carefully and try to ascertain which social class they might appeal to most. Give your reasons for your judgements.

QUESTIONS FOR ESSAYS OR DISCUSSION

1. We are all middle class now.
2. Britain is increasingly becoming a classless society.
3. Regardless of income, wealth, home- and share-ownership, social class is largely determined by a person's life-style.
4. Social class is a more important factor than a person's race or gender status.

5. Poverty is only one deprivation affecting members of Britain's 'underclass'. What other forms of deprivation do they suffer?
6. In order to be an effective social carer, should you be from the same social class background as your client(s)? Give your reasons for your answer.

FURTHER READING

Academic sources

Crompton, R. 1993: *Class and stratification: an introduction to current debates.* Cambridge: Polity Press. Includes discussion of what she calls the 'pseudo-debate' between sociologists of different 'schools', who often do not understand each other's views.

Goldthorpe, J. 1987: *Social mobility and class structure in modern Britain.* Oxford: Clarendon Press. An academic account of a very large research project on the modern development of social class in Britain. Covers social mobility and the ways in which it has occurred.

Lee, D. and Turner, B. (eds) 1996: *Conflicts about class: debating inequality in late industrialism.* Harlow: Longman. A selection of up-to-date readings on social class, including a section which focuses on British sociology and class analysis.

Lister, R. (ed.) 1996: *Charles Murray and the underclass: the developing debate.* London: Institute of Economic Affairs. Brings together in one book Murray's two major articles on a British 'underclass', with several commentaries from writers who are generally hostile to his views.

Marx, K. and Engels, F. 1996: *The Manifesto of the Communist party.* London: Pluto Press. Originally commissioned by the Communist League, an international workers' organization, in 1847. A readable introduction to some of Marx's key concepts in his analysis of capitalist society.

Saunders, P. 1990: *Social class and stratification.* London: Routledge. An analysis of social class in modern Britain, unusually sympathetic to a variety of 'New Right' perspectives.

Other literary sources

Bleasdale, A. 1985: *Boys from the blackstuff.* London: Hutchinson.

Grossmith, G. and Grossmith, W. 1993: *The diary of a nobody.* London: J.M. Dent.

Lawrence, D.H. 1994: *Lady Chatterley's lover.* Harmondsworth: Penguin.

Orwell, G. 1989: *The road to Wigan Pier.* Harmondsworth: Penguin.

Sillitoe, A. 1990: *Saturday night and Sunday morning.* London: Paladin.

Tressell, R. 1991: *The ragged-trousered philanthropists.* London: Paladin.

Films or plays

Gilbert, L. 1983: *Educating Rita.* UK.

Ivory, J. 1991: *Howards End.* UK.

Loach, K. 1969: *Kes.* UK.

Ivory, J. 1993: *The Remains of the Day.* UK.

3

Gender, inequality and sexism

Women are an oppressed majority. They represent 51 per cent of the UK population, yet they do not have the same access to society's resources as do men. Women are less likely to obtain positions of power, own wealth, achieve job satisfaction, develop leisure pursuits, or fulfil creative interests, due to the existence of visible and invisible barriers to their development.

The discriminatory process known as structural *sexism* begins at birth and is maintained through childhood and reinforced during adulthood by society's expectations and practices. While society is constantly changing and inroads towards equality are continually being made, its structure and institutions are so deeply rooted that change, somewhat inevitably, is often only gradual.

The sexist nature of society is abundantly manifest, and it is just as apparent in the continued under-representation of women in positions of power, authority and influence as it is in the over-representation of women in service-related occupations and their role as caregivers. Women disproportionately bear society's responsibility to provide care for children and dependent adults. Furthermore, women are more likely than men to experience poverty, be the victim of violence within a relationship, and receive treatment for mental ill-

ness. This chapter will look at the nature of this imbalance.

Men, too, may be adversely affected by sexism, particularly in relation to the care of children. Less than 2 per cent of child-care workers are men. Furthermore:

Society – as represented by judges, court welfare-officers and other family care workers – regards fathers as second-class citizens. In most cases, unless a father can prove that his ex-partner is seriously unfit, he will never again live with his children. The most he can hope for, if his case ends up in court, is a sleep-over every other weekend, and tea during the week.

(Burgess, 1997b, p.22)

THE DIFFERENCE BETWEEN WOMEN AND MEN

At the beginning of a mixed student seminar discussion group the tutor posed the question 'What is the difference between women and men?' For a long while there was silence among the 20 or so sociology degree students, until one brave young woman eventually spoke up. 'Er ... I know the difference but I can't quite put my finger on it!' The tension was broken and laughter ensued.

But what was it that this student was trying to articulate? And why did her colleagues have such difficulty in answering such a seemingly straight-forward question? The answer is, of course, that it was not an easy question. Defining the differences between women and men is not easy because of the confusion surrounding that which is 'natural' and that which is socially defined as being appropriate for females and males – in other words, the difference between *sex* and *gender.*

The age-old debate about how much human behaviour is derived from innate factors and how much is a result of social conditioning cannot be settled in these pages. Suffice it to say that there are distinct biological differences between women and men, and there are observable differences in the way they live their lives.

The biological differences are determined at conception. *Sex* is the word used for the classification of the species into either female or male. Females alone can give birth and suckle children, and males have a different hormonal and genital structure to females. *Gender* is the word used to describe social and personality differences between women and men. It refers to that which society defines as masculine and feminine.

Although it is normally assumed to be so, gender need not necessarily be related to sex. For example, in our society usually only women are seen wearing skirts, which are considered a 'feminine' mode of dress. Yet in other societies – Sri Lanka, for example – both men and women wear wrap-around sarongs in everyday life and there is no notion of masculinity or femininity associated with this form of dress. However, the kilt is a symbol of masculinity when worn by men in Scotland or Ireland, because of its connotations with honour and bravery.

Unlike 'sex', which is a relatively stable character-istic, 'gender' is a more variable concept that is defined differently between societies and within the same society over time. For instance, in some tribal

societies it is deemed masculine to wear ornaments, whilst the women are shaven-headed and unadorned. In other societies women do all of the agricultural and other heavy work, and thus these heavy duties are considered to be feminine tasks.

In modern industrial society it is claimed that the basic differences between women and men have been greatly exaggerated. It is argued that a woman's biological capacity to reproduce and pro-vide nourishment for her offspring has restricted women's role generally to the care and social-ization of children. Because only women can give birth and naturally feed children, the care and upbringing of young children has been defined as feminine.

Social roles are defined by society but, because they appear to stem from biological differences between women and men, they are also claimed to be 'natural' and therefore appropriate. Con-sequently, childbirth and child care have been in-exorably linked. The essential biological differences between women and men have tended to divide society unequally in terms of women's and men's labour, power roles and expectations.

GENDER ROLE STEREOTYPING

CHILDREN'S WRITER
John in the garden
Playing goodies and baddies

Janet in the bedroom
Playing mummies and daddies

Mummy in the kitchen
Washing and wiping

Daddy in the study
Stereotyping.

(From *Defying Gravity,* by Roger McGough (1992), reproduced by permission of Peters, Fraser & Dunlop Ltd on behalf of Roger McGough)

Consider the following variation on an old riddle. A father takes his son for a ride in the family car. Unfortunately the car becomes involved in a crash and the boy is injured. He is immediately taken to hospital, whereupon he is rushed to the operating theatre. On looking down and seeing the boy's face the surgeon cries, 'Oh my goodness! My own son!' What relation is the surgeon to the boy?

The solution will be quite straightforward for some of you, notwithstanding its context within this chapter. Others of you may be forgiven for not establishing immediately that the surgeon is in fact the boy's mother. Society's stereotyped image of a surgeon is not female (it is more likely to be a white, middle-aged male). This is not to say that women are incapable of performing the work of a surgeon, but because the work is associated with high status, scientific precision, responsibility and the world outside the home, it is firmly entrenched within the male domain.

Various attributes are commonly associated with women and men; they are considered to be either *feminine* or *masculine*. Look at the following list of adjectives and see if you think they can be applied exclusively to women, exclusively to men, or equally to either sex.

---

tender, artistic, sporty, sensitive, handsome, secretive, mean, vicious, pretty, emotional, submissive, strong, flirty, feminine, neurotic, creative, practical, dominant, ambitious, self-confident, home-orientated, masculine, entertaining, hilarious, tearful, sexy, flatterable, egotistical, nagging, caring, aggressive, warm, promiscuous, boastful, appearance-oriented, independent

---

In fact, all of the above qualities may be applied equally to either women or men, although traditionally most are associated more firmly with one or other of the sexes. The crudest stereotype portrays men as being strong, aggressive, logical and confident, while women are portrayed as sensitive, caring and timid. These are harmful images of both women and men because they limit individual growth and development. Stereotypes restrict the fulfilment of our human potential. Unfortunately, however, they are powerful images which often affect people from the moment they are born.

GENDER-PROCESSING

Gender-processing begins from the moment of birth when baby girls are traditionally covered in pink blankets and boys in pale blue ones. Initially the parents and immediate family are the child's primary socializing influence, but as the child grows and interacts with the wider social world, other people – such as relatives, neighbours, nursery or other day-care staff, siblings, peers and the media – contribute to the child's understanding of his or her social role. At every stage the child is subject to beliefs about how females and males ought to behave based on society's prejudicial notions of femininity and masculinity. Eventually, by the time the child has reached his or her mid-teens, he or she has a good idea of what is expected by society.

Studies have shown that babies are treated differently according to their sex. For example, it has been established that there is a tendency for mothers to breastfeed boys for longer periods than girls. Even this action, whether it is done unconsciously or not, tends to reflect an inclination to foster independence and responsibility in girls (who are later to be the principal caregivers) whilst tolerating dependency in boys.

That children internalize society's expectations of them is apparent in subtle behavioural differences which can be observed between girls and boys at a very young age. An observation of a nursery class of children getting ready to go into the playground, where it was raining, indicated differences displayed by girls and boys in carrying out the simple task of putting their coats on. Whilst the girls were generally seen to attempt to get their coats on, struggling with awkward buttons in the process, the boys more often than not sought assistance.

It is hardly surprising that boys act in this way. For example, consider the world through the eyes of a young boy who is receiving a rather stereotyped traditional upbringing. He develops a primary dependency relationship with his mother, who feeds and cares for him for most of the day. He sees very little of his father, who is out for much of the time. Even when his father is not at work he may still be unavailable – he may be absent, tired or 'recuperating' from his work outside the home. The child will be used to having his needs attended to largely by his mother. If the boy attends a nursery or play-group setting he will observe that it is predominantly women who care for the children. When he ventures outside to the doctor, the shops or hospital he will again see mainly women in the role of receptionist, assistants and carers. His picture of men is likely to be very different because he sees them in the more 'interesting' and 'exciting' social roles of builder, transport driver and policeman.

Susie Orbach (1978), in her book *Fat is a Feminist Issue*, claims that within the family girls are instilled with an inferior sense of self. She argues that mothers tend to hold back their daughters' desires to be autonomous and self-directed. Instead, from an early age, a young girl is guided to put her energy into taking care of others. At the same time, boys are taught to accept emotional support without learning how to give this kind of loving in return. She suggests further that, in some cases, this imbalance in a girl's upbringing may later manifest itself in the development of depression or, in extreme cases, one of the various eating disorders such as bulimia or anorexia nervosa. As women struggle with their need to be themselves conflicting with the pressure to create and maintain a body shape that is desired by the male-dominated outside world, they are particularly prone to such disorders.

> Between 1940 and 1985 Miss America got taller and thinner, reflecting a changing ideal woman. Her bust size fluctuated. Meanwhile, the number of American women with anorexia and those undergoing breast augmentation soared.
>
> (*Nursing Times*, 14 February, 1996, p.23)

The consequence for boys who, as Susie Orbach states, do not learn to return the emotional support they are given, is that as men they are less able to give emotionally. This inability to relate on an emotional level inevitably becomes a major factor contributing to marital and partnership breakdown. According to NSPCC worker John Roberts, 'social workers are often confronted with the inherent sadness men convey in not being able to reach out to other men (or women) with their own feelings and in not being able to share their insecurity and vulnerability' (*Community Care*, 25 August 1990, p.22).

Many more women than men suffer depression, and whereas single men are more prone to depression than married men, married women are more likely to become depressed than their single counterparts. One explanation for this is that the traditional housekeeping role is so poorly regarded by society that it represents an insufficient challenge to a woman's intellectual capacity. Consequently, those women who are confined to the home are more likely to break down than those who have paid jobs or are engaged in stimulating experiences.

Brown *et al.* (1975), in their classic study on women and depression which was conducted in Camberwell, highlighted the contribution made to women's depression by the absence of emotional support from their partner. They point out that many women fail to receive the closeness, mutual trust and opportunity for expression of feeling that they need from a relationship. They identified four main factors contributing to depression in women:

- the loss of one's mother in childhood;
- having three or more children under 14 years old living at home;
- the absence of paid work;
- the lack of a close, confiding relationship.

Apart from outside employment, all of these vulnerability factors are class related. For example:

> 43 per cent of working-class women had three or more children living at home ... 9 per cent of working-class women had experienced the loss of their own mother in childhood compared to 3 per cent of middle-class women, and only 37 per cent of younger working-class women enjoyed a relationship of high intimacy, compared to 75 per cent of middle-class women. ... Social structural factors are certainly at the root of some of the events that we call severe ... they partly explain their greater incidence amongst working-class women.
>
> (Brown *et al.*, 1975, p.276)

Shere Hite confirms the frustration felt by women towards men regarding their unwillingness to share their feelings. In her study *Women and Love* (Hite, 1988) she canvassed the views of 4500 women on love and sex. She found that 98 per cent of the women in her study 'wanted more verbal closeness with the men they loved; they wanted the men in their lives to talk more about their own personal thoughts, feelings and plans and to ask them about theirs' (Hite, 1988, p.5). For most women their best friends were women; these were the people with whom they chose to share their intimate secrets. Men, too, turned to women when they needed to be close to someone.

MEN AND SOCIALIZATION

There is much in the socialization of men that discourages them from expressing their feelings. Pressure on them always to appear strong and in control in front of others means that they learn from an early age to hide their true feelings. 'Big boys don't cry' is a clear message throughout childhood which is reinforced in books and other forms of popular culture. The lyrics of the 1980s song *Boys Don't Cry* by The Cure is just one example. Another can be found in the earlier sentimental classic by Elvis Presley, *Old Shep*, in which tears finally come to a small boy who is forced to shoot his dying dog, only after a great struggle.

Formaini discusses the narrow definition of masculinity to which society expects boys to conform. One of the 160 men on which her study was based explained what this definition of masculinity entailed. 'If I am a little boy, I have to cut off everything that means being a little girl. I don't cry any more, I keep a stiff upper lip and I pretend to like games even if I am terrible at them and I am stoic and all that sort of stuff' (Formaini, 1990, p.9).

She comments, 'Giving up feelings is a very heavy price to pay for one's masculinity. Without feelings, it is very difficult to make the kind of decisions that men need to make, whether the decision concerns personal relationships or something else' (Formaini, 1990, p.11).

In her 1997 report, Esther Rantzen, chairwoman of Childline, stated that, 'Stereotyping seems to reach its height in adolescence when boys feel under great pressure to show they are tough'. She added, 'But the 71 per cent increase in suicide by young men in the past 10 years shows how dangerous it can be to bottle up distress' (*Guardian*, 17 April 1996, p.12).

Signs of emotion and expressions of tenderness are often interpreted as weakness, and men rarely admit to them to other men, except perhaps obliquely through jokes. Consequently, many men find themselves locked in an image-conscious macho world built on bravado, banter and outward signs of success – a world in which they compete more easily than they relate.

Men are less guarded in other cultures. Ros Coward points out that the British are still peculiarly repressed about touching in order to comfort or express closeness. 'Grown male relatives and friends never kiss or hold each other; adolescent boys are exiled from physical tenderness; and we find it difficult to hug dying people' (*Guardian*, 23 April 1996, p.14). She compares this view with those of people from other countries, notably Eugene Skeef, a South African musician living with his children in this country, 'In my culture we touch all the time. We are

Men are increasingly being depicted in films and television programmes as being distressed or expressing grief, there are more instances of male politicians allowing themselves to show visible signs of emotion at the scene of national tragedies, and more men are giving themselves permission to express closeness.

In the radio programme *Pucker Up: The 60-Minute Kiss*, one contributor explained:

> I went out with a girlfriend who was very tactile; she was very kissy and very affectionate. She was always horrified with me because I never hugged or kissed my parents. And I remember when I was about 22, she said, 'Well try it.' And I probably hadn't had a hug or a kiss from my Mum and Dad since I was about six, because I was from Yorkshire and you didn't do that kind of thing! Anyway I went home and I tried it on my Mother and she loved it. Then I tried hugging my father and he loved it. And now, now I'm 30, I go home and I hug and kiss them both and it's funny because I had to start kissing my Dad because he felt so left out because my Mother was getting it and it's really funny now. But I really like it because it makes me feel so much closer to them.
>
> (*Pucker Up: The 60-Minute Kiss*, Radio 2, July 1997)

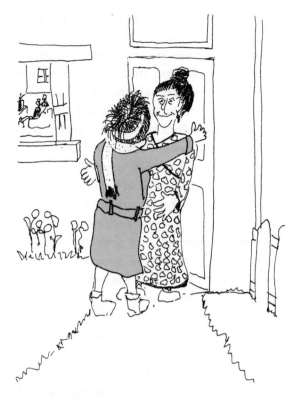

Women tend to be more spontaneous than men in the way in which they touch each other.

not ashamed of our bodies. Much of my music reflects that pleasure and reverence to the body. This is difficult to express in England' (*Guardian*, 23 April 1996, p.14).

For most heterosexual men the physical expression of feelings is restricted to acts of aggression or acts of horseplay, or it is ritualized in social situations (for example, at football and rugby matches). The typical male greeting involves the formal handshake or the slapping of palms – rarely do men freely wrap their arms around one another. In contrast, women are more spontaneous. They touch each other more readily and kiss or hug one another when they meet. Gay men are generally more able to express their emotions than other men. They, too, touch and kiss more easily, and have done much to break down the rigidity of the unfeeling male stereotype.

There are signs within our society of slow change occurring as greater awareness develops.

The fact that many men are unable either to acknowledge or express their feelings and to communicate at a more intimate level has detrimental consequences both for their partners and for their children. By avoiding a deeper expression of what they feel, they also do themselves great harm by denying an essential aspect of their lives.

As Ros Coward claims: 'That inability to comfort either by touch or words amounts to a disability' (*Guardian*, 23 April 1996, p.14).

PATRIARCHY

We live in a patriarchal society. The word patriarch means 'male head of family' or 'father', but when it is applied to society it is used to imply male domination. Men hold a disproportionate amount of power in society, and consequently many of the rules, institutions and values of society support the notion of male superiority and reinforce the corresponding subjugation of women.

Consider the overwhelming presence of men in official positions of power in this country. They currently represent 75 per cent of the House of Commons, and dominate more completely the House of Lords. They predominate in the higher echelons of the Civil Service, the armed forces, the police, the judiciary and the legal and financial institutions. Not only is this the position now, but it has been established for as long as those organizations have existed. Men's power in the past helps them to maintain notions of superiority today.

Women hold very few senior positions in political, public, industrial and commercial life. For example, 'women make up less than 18 per cent of MEPs, less than 3 per cent of senior managers and directors, 10 per cent of the top three grades of the Civil Service, 25 per cent of local authority councillors and around one-third of public appointments' (Equal Opportunities Commission, 1995a, p.1).

In some areas of the UK the figures are considerably worse. In Northern Ireland, for instance, there are no women MPs or MEPs.

Academic institutions are male dominated, and much of what is studied relates to male activity. History has been written largely by men and about men. The majority of ideas relate to the actions of men. The fact that most buildings were designed by able-bodied men accounts for the neglect of the principal needs of women and disabled people. Until recent years no public buildings had specific accommodation for baby-feeding and nappy-changing, and this necessary provision is by no means widespread even now. Few buildings today have easy access for parents with prams or heavy shopping, and many of them remain a barrier to disabled people. In the domestic sphere, the space allocated for traditional women's tasks such as cooking, washing and cleaning has been marginalized. For example, kitchens, bathrooms and washrooms often occupy a relatively small area compared to other rooms in the house. Only recently has it been generally acknowledged that these tasks are better performed with adequate space and light.

That which is valued as great art is almost exclusively male. Most women have either been denied the opportunity to fulfil their artistic creativity and thus to make a significant contribution to history or, when they have had the opportunity, their work has often been marginalized, trivialized or, in some cases, misappropriated. For example, the now acknowledged work of the seventeenth-century artist Artemisia Gentileschi was appropriated and claimed to have been produced by men for a long time. Until recently the work of the artist Gwen John, which is now highly acclaimed, was completely overshadowed by that of her brother Augustus. Composer Ethel Smythe, a contemporary of Elgar, had extreme difficulty in getting her works played (she conducted a choir of Suffragettes in Holloway Prison).

The same is true, to a lesser extent, in the world of literature. In order to compete intellectually in male-dominated Victorian England, Mary Ann Evans wrote her books under the pseudonym of George Eliot. And the male-sounding names Currer Bell, Acton Bell and Ellis Bell were necessary *nom de plumes* used by Charlotte, Anne and Emily Brontë in order to publish their poetry. Even today, women's impact in the world of literature is still restricted. Despite the work of the Women's Press and other publishing organizations, newspapers are still male-dominated and tend to review books mainly by male authors. In late 1989 *The Guardian* produced a 12-page literary supplement under the heading 'Christmas Books'. Eighteen people had contributed to it, and every one of them was a man. A similar feature was produced by *The Observer* at the same time, in which just six out of 24 books reviewed were written by women. Not only were the majority of books reviewed male-dominated, but the actual reviewers themselves were almost exclusively male.

This reflects what Nicci Gerard, deputy literary editor of *The Observer,* calls 'the influence of the metropolitan élite' who run newspapers. She could not account for why the male editors continued to ignore women as authors. She said, 'I think mostly they don't know they are doing it, in the same way that men don't see that all the pictures in the art gallery are by men. But women notice' *(Cosmopolitan,* May 1990, p.104).

LANGUAGE AND MALE DOMINATION

Language plays a major role in informing us about how society views women and men. There are many aspects of contemporary English language which reveal prejudicial attitudes – for example, the use of pronouns, word order and forms of address. Each helps to reinforce the dominant social values. Everyday language can be seen to support the status quo, i.e. the subjugation of women and the dominance of men.

One clear injustice with regard to language is the requirement for females to declare their marital status. Women are addressed as 'Miss' or 'Mrs' depending on whether or not they are married, but men, for whom Mr is the general courtesy title, need not reveal whether they are married. This situation has been mitigated to some extent in the past 20 years with the adoption of the non-specific female courtesy title 'Ms', although it is often wrongly used to describe only single women, thereby defeating the point of its intended usage. A further inequality concerns the fact that, after marrying, it is the woman who is conventionally expected to surrender her family name and adopt that of her husband.

Another example of the way in which contemporary English tends to demean the importance of women is in the continuous use of the pronoun 'he' in a general sense when 'he or she' would be the correct words to use. For example, one may read in a textbook, 'When the child goes into care, special attention is paid to *his* personal requirements in order that *he* is not too traumatized by the move away from home.' 'His or her' or 'he or she' could easily be substituted in the above sentence, thereby rendering the true meaning and giving females and males an equal footing. It is not only the apparent clumsiness of 'he or she' nor the grammatical incorrectness of 'they' when referring to the singular which encourages the use of this narrow form of expression. It is another instance of the general invisibility of women in society reflected in daily language usage. Even the Children Act 1989 referred exclusively to the child as male.

Another example is the use of the word 'man' in the generic sense to mean all human beings; words like mankind and manslaughter help to maintain the domination of men. The adopted, relatively recent use of neutral words such as 'chair', 'ploughperson's lunch' and 'post person', however ridiculous they initially sound, represent a breakthrough and help to promote social change. Usually words associated with men carry positive connotations, such as craftsmanship and sportsmanship. Fewer positive female-based words spring easily to mind, but examples include 'sisterhood' and 'motherhood'. The fact that there are many more derogatory slang- and swear-words associated with females than with males is evidence of basic misogyny, and while there is a word for men who hate women, in the dictionary there is no such equivalent word for women who hate men.

In a letter to a newspaper responding to a previous letter headed 'You can swear by it', Constance Moore wrote:

> What about the C-word? This is the only one that can still raise eyebrows and cause protest in my local pub, where the former (the 'F'-word) is heard 10 times a minute. The fact that the word, which is regarded by men as their ultimate swear-word and worst insult, is a simple description of female genitalia illustrates to me how very far feminism still has to go.
>
> *(Guardian,* 26 September 1996, p.15)

It is not only the meanings of words which betray male domination, but the way in which people interact and the way in which language is used. Consider the following extract from the beginning of Peter Smith's book *Language, the Sexes and Society* (Smith, 1985), which shows how, in subtle ways, the use of language in everyday encounters serves to perpetuate male dominance:

> Several years ago a well-known feminist author was interviewed on British television about her new book on language and the sexes, in which she argued forcefully that language is a man-made product, designed by and for the male half of the species to the neglect and exclusion of women. Her interviewers, besides the male programme host, were three male academics, two of them full professors of English. I had read her book myself, and was keenly interested in what she had to say as I was in the early stages of writing this book. I was to be surprised and disappointed, however, for the great majority of the words uttered in the 15-minute interview were spoken by men. In fact, although I did not take accurate measures I estimated at the time that the author spoke for less than her democratic share of three minutes, much less than one might have expected under the circumstances. This did not seem to be due to the authors' unwillingness or inability to contribute to the conversation – she had after all written the book. Moreover, I knew her to be a very intelligent and articulate person. I also noticed that she was interrupted in mid-sentence at least twice, although she was in her thirties and had completed a PhD, she was addressed by her first name by the host and other interviewers alike, and even at one point as 'my dear', unlike the others, who were always addressed by their formal academic titles.
>
> (Smith, 1985, p.1)

Similarly, schoolgirls who had experienced an experimental 2-year single-sex mathematics class remarked about the way in which they were inhibited or put down in the classroom by boys.

> I think it is better with all girls you are more confident – less frightened. If you get an answer wrong the boys laugh at you. I prefer single-sex maths groups because when you get a question right all the girls say 'that's good'. In a mixed group the boys say 'Oh! that's easy – anyone could have done that'.
>
> (Cohen, 1988, p.50)

THE WOMEN'S MOVEMENT

The impact of the modern Women's Movement which flourished during the 1960s and 1970s was considerable, leading to a more widespread public acknowledgment of the position of women in society. The movement is often referred to as 'Second Wave' feminism, to distinguish it from the political struggle of the suffragettes and suffragists during the end of the nineteenth century and the early part of this century. Today, the Women's Movement, although still influential, is largely fragmented, embracing as it does a wide range of feminist opinion.

During the 1960s and 1970s, groups such as 'Women's Aid', 'Women Against Violence Against Women' and the women's peace groups were founded. Other action-based groups concerning issues such as abortion, education, trade unions and the media were formed, and women campaigned both locally and nationally in order to heighten public awareness and improve basic services. Political magazines that were established at this time, such as *Spare Rib* and *Feminist Review*, continued until the mid-1990s to oppose male domination. As a result of the Women's Movement, traditionally marginalized issues which had always been important in women's lives, such as child care, reproduction and work outside the home were brought into the centre of political debate. The Equal Pay Act 1970 was passed in order to establish equality between women and men, and it became illegal to pay a woman less than a man for the same work.

Despite the intention behind this legislation, women still generally receive lower incomes than men. In 1995, women's average gross hourly earnings were 79 per cent of those of men. This figure relates partly to the fact that women are still predominantly employed in occupations which are less well paid.

The Sex Discrimination Act 1975 set up an independent statutory organization, The Equal Opportunities Commission (EOC), based in Manchester, and relating to England, Scotland and Wales (Northern Ireland has a separate commission). Its principal duties are as follows:

- to work towards the elimination of discrimination on grounds of sex in employment, education and consumer services, and on grounds of marriage in employment;
- to promote equality of opportunity between men and women generally;
- to keep under review the working of this Act and the Equal Pay Act 1970 (implemented in 1975) and, when they are so required by the Secretary of State, or otherwise think it necessary, to draw up and submit to the Secretary of State proposals for amending them.

The impact of the Sex Discrimination Act can be seen in the declarations of equal opportunities statements and formal practices of many public organizations which are beginning to have an effect. However, it has to be said that the Women's Movement generally and the legislation which was passed during its most active stages have not yet resulted in profound social change.

SEXISM

If sexism makes life difficult for successful and aspiring women, it makes the quality of life available to poor and powerless women almost intolerable.

(Campling, 1989, p.xi)

This statement may be extended to include black women and disabled women who, owing to their disadvantaged position in society, are more prone to the effects of both indirect and direct discrimination.

Sexism is still firmly entrenched within our society, ranging in degree from the overt to the subtle. A clear form of sexism would be a case where someone is denied admittance to or membership of a club or premises on the grounds of his or her sex – for example, the 212-year-old practice at Lords, the headquarters of the Marylebone Cricket Club and the English cricket establishment, to refuse admission to women (other than the Queen and cleaning and catering staff) to the pavilion during hours of play. In September 1998 the male membership finally voted to accept women as members. A more subtle instance of sexism includes the veiled putdown which occurs in everyday conversation, when women are referred to as 'dear', 'love' or 'pet' by men with whom they might not even be familiar. (It should be noted that in some areas such words are used in a non-gender-specific way in order to convey endearment.)

As well as being evident in ordinary interactions between individuals, sexism can be seen to be institutionalized in the practices and procedures of different organizations. Indeed, there are many similarities between racism and sexism in this respect, but whilst racism is directed against a numerical minority in the UK, sexism is principally directed against women, who currently represent 51 per cent of the population.

An example of institutional sexism is the current but now less frequently adopted practice of the House of Commons whereby it conducts its business through the night and the early hours of the morning. These all-night sittings have, for many years, deterred family-oriented women from considering a career as an MP.

The word sexism was coined by analogy with racism to denote discrimination based on gender. Originally sexism referred to prejudice exclusively against the female sex. It is now used in a broader sense to indicate the stereotyping of both females and males on the basis of their gender. Strictly speaking, both sexes are affected by sexism, but it is women who suffer most. 'This is because sexism does not merely encourage an artificial segregation of the sexes: it perpetuates the notion of male superiority' (Inner London Education Authority, 1985, p.4). That is to say, sexism is directed primarily against women because men hold power disproportionately within society.

EDUCATION

Girls and boys can be seen to be treated differently within the education system in this country. Traditionally, boys have been guided towards the science-based subjects whilst girls have been encouraged to study the arts and humanities.

The Sex Discrimination Act 1975 gave schools the drive to develop policies in order to combat gender-based inequality. Educational materials have been scrutinized for their sexist content and, where this has been identified, have been replaced by newly created, non-stereotyped materials. The National Curriculum 1989 provided for all girls and boys to be taught the same subjects. Deliberate efforts have been made to break down the traditional gender association with subject areas. Girls are being encouraged towards the sciences and boys are being encouraged to develop skills in domestic science, biology and office practice.

There has been a closing of the gap between the achievements of girls and boys, with girls doing better in maths and science, formerly considered to be 'boys' subjects'. In fact, girls generally do better than boys academically. 'Young women emerge from the education system out-numbering and out-performing young men at every stage, from GCSE to degree level' (Donnellan, 1996, p.30). However, there is still a gender division at both GCSE and GCE 'A' level (see Table 3.1).

The choice of subjects taken at school may determine the kind of occupation a young person enters,

and is likely to influence the area of study they undertake if they go on to university. Table 3.2 shows a more pronounced difference between the genders that emerges at higher education level, and demonstrates men's numerical dominance once the post-graduate stage has been reached. Less than one in five female graduates move on to postgraduate studies, whereas nearly one in three male students do so.

This fact reflects society's pressure for men to achieve outwardly and determine a career, whereas for a woman this is considered to be less important objective, given her centrally ascribed role as the family's principal caregiver. Many parents will encourage their sons into further and higher education and be less supportive of their daughters' ambitions. In turn, girls and young women may internalize this message and regard their careers as being less important.

Training is generally less available to women, who are more susceptible to the cut-backs in private and public budgets and the inability of colleges of further education to subsidize support for returners. They may be precluded from full-time college attendance by low income and lack of child-care resources.

It is noticeable that applications for social-care courses are almost exclusively female. The more general social-care courses attract the interest of some young men, but once selected, male students may feel under pressure to discontinue the course.

A young working-class man on a nursery nursing course was forced to leave after the second term. He had survived the banter from his friends and the awkwardness arising from belonging to a class of 24 female students. He was also coping financially on a small educational award. However, he succumbed to pressure from his father, who had not been keen on his son starting the course and who insisted that he should start earning money and find a 'proper job'. It is unlikely that such pressure would be placed on a young woman under the same circumstances.

The lack of male social-care and nursery-nurse students detracts from a balanced situation where young men and women can learn from one another. It also contributes to the maintenance of the dis-

Table 3.1 School examination results for 1994/95 (data expressed in thousands)

Subject	England GCSE Grades A*–C		Scotland SCE Standard Grades 1–3		Wales GCSE Grades A*–C	
	Females	Males	Females	Males	Females	Males
English	168.0	123.4	24.0	20.0	13.3	9.6
Mathematics	113.9	118.6	15.5	15.9	7.3	7.1
Single award science	6.9	4.1	1.8	2.4	0.3	0.2
Double award science	101.8	100.5	*	*	3.0	3.1
Biology	11.9	18.4	11.5	4.5	0.6	0.8
Chemistry	10.8	18.6	10.5	10.5	0.6	0.8
Physics	10.1	19.4	6.4	12.6	0.5	0.8
Design and technology[†]	73.8	48.4	1.2	4.7	10.0	6.7
Home economics	16.5	1.1	3.3	0.3	1.2	0.0
French	89.9	61.2	12.6	8.0	4.4	2.5
History	64.9	54.5	6.6	4.3	3.2	2.4
Computer studies	3.6	4.1	3.5	5.9	*	*

	GCE A-Level Grades A–E		SCE Higher Grades A–C		GCE A-Level Grades A–E	
English	38.7	16.8	13.3	9.4	2.2	0.8
Mathematics	14.0	24.3	6.6	6.9	0.6	0.9
Biology	17.9	11.3	5.3	2.5	0.8	0.5
Chemistry	11.0	14.6	3.9	4.4	0.6	0.7
Physics	4.6	17.4	2.7	5.3	0.2	0.7
French	12.9	5.5	3.0	1.0	1.1	0.3
History	15.5	12.5	3.3	2.0	1.1	0.7
Computer studies[‡]	1.5	6.2	0.6	1.8	0.1	0.6

* Not available.

[†] Craft and design in Scotland.

[‡] Technology in England.

Source: Department for Education and Employment, Scottish Examination Board and Welsh Joint Education Committee.

proportionate representation of women in all fields of social care.

WOMEN AND THE MEDIA

The media tends to reinforce the unequal position of women in society in two ways. It reflects exist-ing inequalities, so that it depicts women predom-inantly in their caretaking role and renders them invisible in more socially powerful positions. It further distorts the view of women, since it is largely controlled by men and there is an over-emphasis on what women look like. Images of women are often stereotyped in a limiting way which does not reflect the true diversity of women's lives:

Table 3.2 Students in higher education in 1994/1995

	Undergraduates		Postgraduates	
Subject group	Females	Males	Females	Males
Medicine, dentistry and allied studies	77 321	27 945	12 521	9228
Biological sciences	31 511	20 936	6744	6611
Physical sciences	19 811	35 863	4551	11 531
Mathematical sciences	5983	10 127	931	2597
Engineering and technology	15 970	96 646	3320	21 925
Social, economic and political studies	51 332	38 648	13 817	13 144
Business and administrative studies	75 685	77 033	19 039	34 130
Languages	49 259	21 093	6294	4737
All subjects	613 522	599 686	140 621	174 772

Source: The Higher Education Statistics Agency.

> despite some progress in the areas of TV drama and children's drama, women are still primarily portrayed in stereotyped roles as sex objects, mothers or victims. Girls' and women's magazines present a very limited picture of women's lives and choices. There is much concern about the commutative effect of increasing pornography and violence, and degrading images of women, on the lives of women and their position in society.
>
> (Equal Opportunities Commission, 1995b)

Newspapers, cartoons, films and television often depict women as having negative characteristics, having a narrow and specific range of interests, and being almost always white, heterosexual and able-bodied.

The media does not always aim to inform. Often it seeks to dramatize or to entertain in order to increase circulation or obtain more viewers or listeners. In doing so it creates distorted images – its sensationalized emphasis on 'perverts', 'sex maniacs' and 'monsters' helps to perpetuate the myth that there are no more than a very limited range of men capable of being involved in child or partner abuse. In addition, the lack of black women's prominence in the media, except for their misrepresentation as victims or social misfits, contributes to their general invisibility within society.

Since the early 1990s more women presenters have appeared on television, which to a certain extent reflects their improved access to positions within the media. However, it needs to be pointed out that women's images are still a significant factor, and that they are up against the dual barriers of sexism and ageism. In a letter to *The Guardian*, a reader wrote, 'There is still too much of what Anna Ford called body fascism, i.e. female presenters and reporters have to be attractive, have good, if not perfect figures, be young, i.e. up to fortyish. Male presenters can be any age, figure or hair colour.' Another reader added, 'I want to see fat women reading the news and presenting documentaries ... over half the women watching are size sixteen plus' (*Guardian*, 2 April 1990, p.22).

Exploitation of sex is more subtle nowadays. Referring to the deliberate use of camera angles, when shooting the reading of the TV news, Stuart Jefferies states:

> Men are often shot at a slight angle with one shoulder casually forward, the glance not quite three-quarters, or leaning on the desks, while women are mostly shot full-face, sitting primly and tensely. Men occupy more space than women: they

used to do it on the buses and now they also do so as they read the news.

(*Guardian*, 7 February 1997, p.2)

Women are still under-represented in the upper echelons of the press and broadcasting and in technological areas. In 1992, only 13.8 per cent of senior managers and 5.9 per cent of technical posts in broadcasting were held by women (Equal Opportunities Commission, 1995a).

In both the press and broadcast media, programming and editorial decisions are overwhelmingly taken by men and therefore reflect a male view of the world and what is important in it. A Fawcett Report on the 1997 election coverage found that, in one week of the campaign:

84 per cent of the people appearing on TV election news were men; 4 out of 5 election items were reported by men; and 93 per cent of professionals and experts called on for comments were men. Of the 135 politicians who appeared, 127 were men; not one Government spokesperson was a woman. There is clearly much for female voters to find off-putting.

(*Guardian*, 24 April 1997, p.17)

Black women are particularly under-represented in the media. Clare Gotham, journalist and broadcaster, when asked about major changes needed within the media said:

I'd like to see more black women and men holding the highly powerful media reins. I'd like there to be more black production companies run by women and more collaboration in programme making. That way there'd be less emphasis on skin-tone and safe tokenism, more on talent.

(*Guardian*, 5 April 1997, p.6)

WOMEN AND WORK

The principal reason women have for seeking paid work is the same as it is for men – that is, to earn money in order to provide for themselves and any family they may have. There are other non-financial benefits to be obtained from work outside the home, and these vary from occupation to occupation. In the more skilled areas of work, they may include a sense of satisfaction, intellectual fulfilment, career progression or a chance to develop personal and social skills. Not all jobs are stimulating – in fact, the majority are mundane and repetitive – but employment outside the home at least offers women a source of independence, and a chance to relate to other people and to feel that they are contributing to society. There have been several major studies on the debilitating effects of unemployment. The majority of these have focused on men. A study by Cochrane and Stopes-Roe (1981) showed that women in employment had fewer symptoms of depression than women who were not in paid work.

Many women and a small number of men choose not to work in order to remain at home so that they can look after their children. They find this work sufficiently stimulating and engaging. Other women may work outside the home part-time or on a job-share basis, and spend only a part of their week exclusively looking after children. Not all women want to spend all of their time looking after children and doing domestic duties. It can be an isolating and debilitating existence, particularly for single parents on low incomes. It has been established that many more women would work if better provision of child-care services existed for the under-fives.

- Women now represent just over 45 per cent of the country's work-force, and their proportion is growing.
- There are only 250 000 fewer women with jobs than men and 'women are now the primary source of income in as many as 30 per cent of households' (Donnellan, 1996).

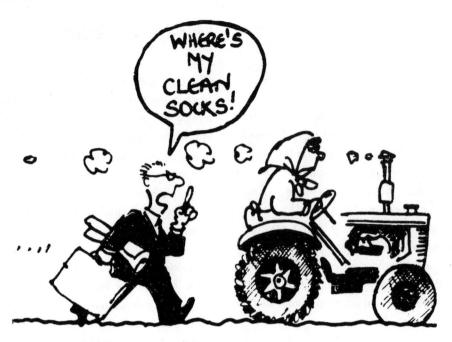

(Reproduced with permission from Spellbound Books, 23–25 Moss Street, Dublin 2.)

- There are cultural differences in the participation of women in paid work: '76 per cent of white women work outside the home, and 56 per cent of black women, of whom West Indian women are more likely to be economically active than Indian women, who, in turn, are more likely than Pakistani or Bangladeshi women to be economically active' (Labour Market Structure and Prospects for Women, University of Warwick, 1994, p.57).
- Women's increased participation in the workforce is replicated throughout Europe, 'where, for the last 20 years, women have accounted for the entire growth of the labour force and are likely to continue to do so in future years' (Labour Market Structure and Prospects for Women, University of Warwick, 1994, p.9).

Women have not always had such access to work outside the home. During the First and Second World Wars the myth that only men could do certain types of work began to be broken down. The wars required everyone to do his or her share of the work, regardless of gender. Vacancies created by the call of the armed forces meant that women were needed in a whole range of occupations, including munitions, public transport and work on the land. By the end of the war the expectation was that women would give up their jobs and return to their homes. Not all women did so, but the prevailing social attitude and governmental policies were opposed to the majority of them remaining economically active. Today over 50 per cent of all married women are now engaged in work outside the home, compared to 20 per cent in 1951 and 10 per cent in 1921 (Cohen, 1988).

Although women represent a large and increasing proportion of the work-force, working outside the home still involves discrimination against them. Women can be seen to be discriminated against in two ways, both vertically and horizontally.

Vertical discrimination refers to discrimination within the same occupation. For example, within the teaching profession women can be seen to be disproportionately represented in the lower-paid basic-grade teaching posts, and correspondingly under-represented in positions of seniority, such as headships.

From Table 3.3 it can be seen that secondary schools employ women and men in roughly equal numbers, yet men are three times more likely to be appointed to headships and twice as likely to reach deputy headships than women. Within the nursery and primary sector the contrast is more stark – headships are evenly shared between women and men, yet women fill over seven times as many basic-grade teaching posts as men.

Horizontal discrimination refers to discrimination across all occupations, and shows women to be over-represented in certain lower-status, largely service-related jobs, whilst they have restricted access to other more prestigious or better-paid occupations.

- Women are concentrated in relatively few occupations.
- Half of all women employees work in four occupational groups – clerical, secretarial, sales and personal service occupations.
- The majority (85 per cent) work in the service industries – health, where 81 per cent of workers are women, education (69 per cent women), hotels and restaurants (61 per cent women) and the retail trade (59 per cent women).
- Only 13 per cent of women work in manufacturing and construction industries, compared to 36 per cent of men. However, in clothing manufacture 73 per cent of workers are female.
- Overall, 70 per cent of women work in non-manual occupations.

- Certain occupations are predominantly female: receptionists (92 per cent), nurses (87 per cent), clerks and secretaries (75 per cent), welfare workers such as matrons of residential homes and community workers (74 per cent), cashiers (74 per cent), local government administration workers (73 per cent) and teachers (63 per cent).
- A substantial proportion of the female labour force is clustered in the clerical sector, which employs nearly one-third of women and only 7 per cent of men.
- Large concentrations of female workers are in the service sector groupings of catering, cleaning, hairdressing and other personal services, including social care and secretarial occupations.
- The main professional areas of employment for women are in the fields of health, welfare and education.
- In contrast, the range for men is more evenly spread, with the two greatest concentrations being in managerial posts (13 per cent) and metal and electrical manufacture and repair (17 per cent).

The 'glass ceiling'

In recent years the term *glass ceiling* has been coined to describe the invisible barriers which exist to prevent women from achieving their full potential and obtaining positions of seniority, not just at work but also in other positions of power and authority. In other words, women can see where they would like

Table 3.3 Full-time teachers in maintained schools in England and Wales in 1993

	Females			Males		
	Nursery and primary	Secondary	Total	Nursery and primary	Secondary	Total
Headteachers	10 661	1027	11 688	10 541	3689	14 230
Deputy headteachers	12 526	3111	15 637	5944	6152	12 096
Teachers	123 638	93 328	216 966	16 769	89 325	106 094
Total	146 825	97 466	244 291	33 254	99 166	132 420

Source: Equal Opportunities Commission 1996: *Facts and figures about women and men in Great Britain, 1996*. Manchester: Equal Opportunities Commission.

to go but not the hurdles that stand in their way. A 1990 report commissioned by the Hansard Society and entitled *Women at the Top* looked at 'identifying barriers to the appointment of women to senior occupational positions, and to other positions of power and influence and to make recommendations as to how these barriers could be overcome' (Hansard Society, 1990). Later, in 1996, in her Foreword to the follow-up study, *Women at the Top: Progress after 5 Years*, Lady Howe stated, 'Certainly there has been some progress, though no one would wish to claim it has been spectacular' (Hansard Society, 1996, p.2).

Women in government and public administration

Women have begun to make inroads into positions of power, most noticeably in 1997, when 114 women were returned to the House of Commons, doubling female membership, and five were given positions within the Cabinet. However, women still represented less than 25 per cent of the new intake of the House of Commons. Within the House of Lords, female representation is still minimal, having only risen from 6 per cent to 7 per cent between 1989 and 1995.

Within the Civil Service steps are being taken to overcome 'the historic under-representation of women', and a target has been set to achieve at least 15 per cent women across the senior open structure by the year 2000. In 1995 there were only three women Permanent Secretaries, representing 6 per cent staffing at this level.

Women and the law

The decisions taken by judges and magistrates have far-reaching consequences for all members of society, and the under-representation of women among their ranks limits the quality and vision of those decisions.

(Hansard Society, 1990, p.9)

The Hansard Society found that women were seriously under-represented among the judiciary. In 1990 women represented 1 per cent of High Court judges and 5 per cent of Recorders. By 1995, women represented 7 per cent and 15 per cent, respectively, in these positions. However, the report added 'that elsewhere within the judiciary there had been little improvement: there remain no women Law Lords, there is only one Lord Justice of Appeal, and the increase in the number of Stipendiary Magistrates brought little or no increase in the proportion that are women' (Hansard Society, 1996, p.10). Against this it should be stated that more women than men are entering the legal profession, and that women account for one-third of practising solicitors and one-fifth of independent barristers. However, 'women in 1995 remained more likely to be assistant solicitors than partners and more likely to practise outside leading barristers' chambers than within them' (Hansard Society, 1996, p.10).

Women and management

In 1990 the Hansard Commission reported that women's representation in management 'has slowly increased in the past two decades, but women at the very top are scarcely visible'. Five years later they found that 'the boardroom presence of women has increased in all areas, but they none the less remain a small minority'. In 1989, women senior managers accounted for less than 7 per cent of senior management, and in 1995 they accounted for just over 10 per cent.

The Hansard Society conducted a survey of women's views about the barriers that slow or halt women's progress into positions of influence (see Table 3.4).

Table 3.4 is divided into three groups of obstacles — those pertaining to organizational structures and practices, those deriving from women's familial roles, and those existing in men's and women's attitudes. Although 29 per cent of respondents felt that women's own attitudes held them

Table 3.4 Women's perceived barriers to progress

	%	n
Organizational barriers		
Inflexible working arrangements	15	18
Recruitment practices	19	23
Men recruit in their own image		
Men think women are risky		
Informal and subjective practices		
Use of old boys' network		
Male work cultures/work cultures that	10	12
do not encourage women		
Long-working-hours culture	10	12
Lack of role models/mentors/networking	13	15
Traditional roles		
Having to balance work and family roles	32	38
Taking career breaks	14	17
Real or perceived lack of mobility because	7	8
of family commitments		
Attitudinal barriers		
Prejudice of (older) male colleagues/managers	20	24
No lead from men at the top	3	3
Outdated attitudes	18	22
Women are not 'serious' about careers		
Women work only for 'pin' money		
Women cannot travel		
Undervaluation of women's management	10	12
styles		
Perceived lack of leadership skills		
Women are not 'tough'		
Women's own limitations due to:	29	34
Lack of determination to succeed		
Lack of confidence		
Family commitment		
Lack of willingness to take risks		
Lack of commitment		

Note that the table sums to more than 100% because respondents gave more than one answer.
Source: Hansard Society 1990: *Women at the top*. London: Hansard Society, p. 14.

back, this should be viewed within the context of male prejudice and outdated attitudes, as well as the practical difficulty many women experience in having to balance work and family roles. 'Despite efforts to dismantle practices that discriminate against women, there remain deeply rooted emotional and cultural discriminatory attitudes that influence women's advancement in organizations' (Hansard Society, 1996, p.15).

The position of black women is more starkly disadvantaged, as they are exposed to the combined effect of race and sex discrimination. It is harder for them to become managers. In 1994, *The Health Journal* claimed that 'If white women managers find a glass ceiling, the ceiling that presses down on black and ethnic minority women is a concrete one' (*The Health Journal*, November 1994, p.23). Again, referring to the Health Service, research at Warwick University showed that there were very few women in positions of management, and no black or ethnic minority women directors.

Women and academia

As mentioned earlier, women are sparsely represented within academic institutions. More women than men graduate, yet women represent less than 25 per cent of the lecturers teaching undergraduates in the old university sector, and no more than 5 per cent of professors. By 1995, 32 universities in the UK had become members of 'Opportunity 2000' – a group dedicated to achieving a more balanced work-force. These included Oxford and Cambridge, which signed up in 1993. As Table 3.5 shows, 'there is still some distance to go before women gain parity with men, but the journey at least appears to have been started' (Hansard Society, 1996, p.16).

Women and the police

The Police Service is understandably male-dominated, owing to the nature of much of its work and the fact that it deals mainly with other men as the chief perpetrators of crime. In 1995, women represented 16 per cent of the force, yet only 3 per

Table 3.5 Academic women: Oxbridge (data expressed as percentage values)

Oxford	1973–1974	1984–1985	1995
Lecturers	13	14	18
Professors	3	5	7

Cambridge	1973–1974	1986	1995
Lecturers	5	8	14
Professors	2	3	6

Source: Hansard Society 1990: *Women at the top*. London: Hansard Society, p. 17.

cent of the Chief Constables. Until quite recently there has been substantial evidence of sexism within the police force. Between 1994 and 1995 there were over 250 cases of alleged sexual or racial harassment, some of which were high profile and caught the attention of the media. Sgt Jane McGill stated 'To be a women in the police force until recent times has been very difficult. I have survived that experience for more than a quarter of a century because I chose to go along with it. I blame myself but I was not going to let it destroy me' (*Daily Telegraph*, 16 May 1996, p.3). Malcom Young thinks that sexism within the police force is hardly surprising because 'We have something like 160 years of an organization of essentially macho origin. Only in the last 20 years, since the Act, have we had anything like the idea that we have got to treat women differently. Only in the last decade have they had to face up to what it means' (*Guardian*, 9 October 1996, p.7). Progress towards equal opportunities has been led by the Metropolitan Police who have introduced such measures as abolishing the height requirement and removing the word woman or letter 'w' from reports indicating the gender of the officer.

Sadly, similar discrimination against women can be found within the Armed Forces, where women have encountered abuse in the dominant male 'canteen culture'.

According to Sgt Lynne Godall, who in 1995 won damages against the Ministry of Defence on grounds of sex discrimination, 'Women are either tarts or dykes to the squaddies, and to the senior officers they just do not have a place in a man's world' (*Independent*, 22 May 1996, p.2). Women are again under-represented at the top. In 1986 there were no women among the rank of Brigadier in the army, and none above the rank of Commodore in the RAF or the Navy. In 1996, the same was true, while now there are only two women at this rank, compared to six a decade ago (*Independent*, 22 May 1996, p.2).

INEQUALITIES IN PAY

Despite the passing of the Equal Pay Act in 1970 and the Sex Discrimination Act in 1975, the average gross hourly earnings for women continue to be significantly lower than those for men. Today women earn only 79 per cent of men's full-time hourly earnings. There are several reasons for this apart from the glass ceiling effect already examined. Women are clustered in 'women's jobs' which are undervalued and under-paid, they are less likely to be in unionized occupations, and they represent the bulk of part-time workers with low pay and less chance of working overtime.

The proportion of women among low-paid, full-time workers is similar throughout the European Union, as shown in Table 3.6.

Women from ethnic minorities are twice as likely (18 per cent) to be unemployed as their white counterparts (8 per cent), and more likely to be in low-paid occupations when they are in work. At a conference organized by Church Action on Poverty entitled the 'Forgotten 30 per cent', held at Westminster Central Hall in March 1997, Baroness Flather referred to ethnic minority women as the 'the most forgotten of the forgotten'. She went on to outline how many of them, particularly Indian, Pakistani and Bangladeshi women, were engaged full-time in low-paid, low-status occupations in restaurants, factories and as home workers.

Table 3.6 The extent of low pay and the concentration of women among the low paid in the European Community

Countries ranked by share of low-paid work-force	Percentage of workers in full-time employment receiving less than 66% of median wage		Percentage of women among low-paid full-time workers[*]
	All workers	Female workers	
Belgium	5	10	62
The Netherlands	11	28	53
Portugal	12	19	49
Germany	13	33	82
France	14	20	51
Italy	14.5	23	62
Ireland	18	29	51
Spain[†]	19	29	70
UK	20	41	63
Greece[‡]	na	26	55

[*] Workers receiving less than 66% of median wage.

[†] Less than 40% of the median wage. Also includes domestic workers who receive benefits in kind.

[‡] No estimate available for total share of labour force that is low paid, so Greece is not included in the ranking. As with Spain, the estimates include domestic workers, and also part-timers, but part-timers represent only a small proportion of the Greek labour force.

Source: Donnellan, C. (ed.) 1996: *Men, women and equality. Independence. Vol. 18.* Cambridge: Cambridge University Press.

In 1996:

- almost 10 per cent of women earned less than £3.00 per hour, compared to just over 5 per cent of men;
- 40 per cent of female employees and 20 per cent of men earned less than £4.50 per hour;
- 29 per cent of female employees and 14 per cent of men earned less than £4.00 per hour (Equal Opportunities Commission, January 1998).

The establishment of a national minimum wage in the UK is eagerly awaited by many who see it as a way of redressing the gender pay inequalities that exist today. 'The introduction of the national minimum wage will provide the government [with the opportunity] to tackle both the problems of low pay and the pay gap between women and men. We urge the government to seize that opportunity' (Kamlesh Bahl, OEC Chairwoman, *Equal Opportunities Commission News*, 26 January 1998).

PART-TIME WORK

Part-time work is, by tradition, poorly paid. 'In the UK 75 per cent of women part-time workers earn less than the Council of Europe's decency threshold hourly rate (Church Action on Poverty, 1996, p.2). Furthermore, part-time work often excludes benefits such as sick pay, annual leave and other arrangements that are customarily associated with full-time employment. The House of Lords Select Committee on the European Commission, which examined the problems of part-time work, commented:

Part-time employees, while contributing significantly to the development of the economy and to the flexibility of the productive system, are, as a group, still behind their full-time colleagues in regard to wage rates, access to training and promotion and the provision of other benefits. This is both economically self-defeating and socially unacceptable, not least when it reinforces types of discrimination, such as that between male and female employees.

(The House of Lords Select Committee on the European Commission, 1985, p.72)

Women, who represent 84 per cent of part-time workers, are forced into part-time work arrangements mainly because of their other responsibilities of caring for others and running a home.

CHILD CARE

Although there is a growing tendency for men to take more of a share in the care of children, the responsibility rests predominantly on the shoulders of women. It is still women who sacrifice career opportunities by withdrawing from the labour market for long periods to look after their children. It is women who reduce their paid working hours in order to be available for children outside school hours. It is women and not men who are most likely to take time off work on the occasions when their children are sick and both parents are working.

It is largely due to the lack of adequate child-care facilities that women are forced to sacrifice themselves in this way. With proper state-funded day-care facilities available, women would be more free to decide their own level of involvement in the labour market.

At present the UK has fewer publicly funded child-care services than any other EEC country except Portugal. In France, 95 per cent of children are in publicly funded child care, Italy has 80 per cent, Germany has 60 per cent and The Netherlands have 50 per cent. The majority of parents in this country are forced to make their own child-care arrangements. Consequently, most families rely on relatives or neighbours to provide informal care for their children.

The most common form of paid day-care provision is a child-minder. In 1994, 357 500 children were cared for in this way. A child-minder is self-employed, based at home and provides care, play and learning opportunities for children from babyhood to school age. The cost of using a registered child-minder is prohibitive to many families, and it is far more common for them to use non-registered ones – this relationship carries more risk to the child's welfare.

Local education authority nursery classes, nursery schools or primary schools provide a high proportion of the places available for children under the age of 5 years. However, children need to be 3 years old before they can start. Furthermore, the places are often part-time and unavailable during the school holidays. Nursery schools and classes are entirely paid for by the state and, of course, are normally very stimulating settings for young children. For this reason places are much sought after by parents. However, since there is no statutory requirement for local authorities to provide education for children under 5 years of age, except where the child has a stated specific need, the availability of vacancies depends on where the family lives and the political commitment of the local council.

Local council day-nurseries represent slightly less than 1 per cent of the total day-care provision, and are thus clearly unavailable to many families. Day-nurseries have been forced to place priorities on their intake and allocate according to the child's social need – children at risk are given priority, and socially disadvantaged children are accommodated whenever possible. This practice has served to alter the function of day-nurseries to some extent, and also to create a stigma for women who take their children there.

Today there are fewer day-nurseries than there were at the end of the Second World War, over 50 years ago. At the start of the war, in 1939, there were only 14 day-nurseries, but as the war progressed there was a dramatic improvement in child-care facilities, particularly in the number of day-nursery places. Within 3 years there were 1345 day-nurseries offering 60 000 places to young children. Shortly after the end of the war, in 1945, many of these newly created day-nurseries were closed down because it was no longer deemed necessary to assist women to remain in work outside the home. Women had to wait until the 1960s, when job opportunities became increasingly available again, before there was an expansion of day-care provision, but the immediate post-war level of nursery places was never matched. Today there are less than half as many public day-nursery places available as there were in 1945. These places have been reduced still further by the need for local authorities to generate income; some local authorities have offered up to half their day-care places to the fee-paying private sector. This has had the advantage of reducing some of the stigma at the cost of valued child-care places.

In recent years there has been an increase in the number of workplace nurseries, mainly in the public sector, in hospitals, town halls and colleges. 'On-site' crèches have obvious advantages to parents who work in these establishments, yet they are not numerically significant enough to provide many parents with alternative child care. Fewer than 10 per cent of firms provide any form of day-care. All other types of child-care provision involve parents in some expense, and this in itself can be prohibitive. Some families have to calculate whether it makes economic sense for the mother to take on a job because, in addition to having to consider the ordinary work-related expenses of travel, food and clothing, they need to calculate the cost of having their child or children looked after during the time she is at work.

Playgroups continue to be the main source of part-time day care. Au pairs and nannies offer support to children of high-income families only. Owing to the expense involved in child care, much of the existing provision discriminates against working-class women. In some areas these women have retaliated and developed their own community nurseries, or have pressurized councils into assisting them.

The UK compares unfavourably with most other European countries with regard to child-care pro-

vision, particularly for children over the age of 3 years.

> Most member states have achieved, or are moving towards, comprehensive coverage for children aged 3–6 years either in pre-primary schooling or kindergarten. Within the EU, there is a convergence around . . . three years of publicly funded provision prior to compulsory schooling at 6 (or 7 in the Scandinavian countries). The main exceptions to this picture are Ireland, The Netherlands and the UK, which combine early admission to primary school with limited or no pre-primary schooling.
>
> (European Commission Network on Childcare, 1996, p.130)

With the availability of proper day-care facilities, many more women who wish to work would be able to do so. There would appear to be a clear correlation between the participation of women in work outside the home and the availability of adequate child-care provision. For example, in Denmark, where the level of public child-care provision is high, over 75 per cent of mothers with young children are employed. In the UK, according to the 1994 British Social Attitudes Survey, '4 out of 5 non-working mothers said they would go out to work if they had the child care of their choice' (Department for Education and Employment, 1996), and 25 per cent of mothers who worked part-time said they would increase the hours they worked if they had better child-care arrangements.

The 1998 Budget introduced new measures to extend child-care provision to lower-income working families. This innovation was welcomed by The National Child-Minding Association. In a letter to the *Guardian*, Gill Haynes (Chief Executive of the National Child-Minding Association) said, 'For more than 20 years, the association has been campaigning for high-quality, affordable child-care for all. The Chancellor's child-care plans will make that a reality for thousands of families.' She went on, 'We are also delighted that the tax credit will only be available for registered child care. The message is that it is worth investing in training and development, toys, equipment and safety measures, because for the first time in history, a Chancellor is saying the job of looking after children is an important one' (*Guardian*, 19 March 1998, p.23).

DOMESTIC ROLES AND LEISURE TIME

The 1980s reputedly saw the emergence of the 'new man' – a male partner committed to equal responsibility in household duties and child care. Research has not always supported this observation, and some studies have shown that 'women have considerably less leisure time than men in all parts of the country, even in areas of high male unemployment' (*Sociology Update 1996*, p.26). It goes on, 'If new man ever existed he was very short-lived and disappeared when the children came along.'

These findings have been countered by the later works of Adrienne Burgess of the Institute of Policy Research, who argues that today a father's place is increasingly in the home. 'By 1995 women in Britain were spending 6.5 hours less per week on routine housework than their mothers had in 1961, due mainly to increased ownership of domestic appliances, while men doubled their time on housework over the same period. The time spent on child care also increased over time – fourfold.' She adds, 'So why does the British press regularly announce that the new man is a myth? Though tasks such as cooking and cleaning may not be shared equally, the reality is that in average families with young children both parents are "running from morning to night" ' (*Guardian*, 4 February 1997, p.2).

One reason put forward to explain the low contribution of working men towards their families is the long, often antisocial hours they are now required to work outside the home: '82 per cent of British fathers with children under 10 in two-parent families are full-time employed and are working an average of 47 hours, and this doesn't include time spent commuting'. Until the adoption of the European 47-hour rule, 'Britons worked the longest hours of all Europeans and 50 per cent of British workers said they came home exhausted' (*Guardian*, 4 February 1997, p.2).

The UK does not have many of the 'family-friendly' policies that operate in other countries of the European Union. For instance, 'the UK has a situation, shared only by Ireland, of no entitlement to parental leave and no access for employed parents to a limited supply of publicly funded services. Employed parents needing care for their children must make private arrangements' (European Commission Network on Childcare, 1996, p.130).

In contrast, 'in Denmark and Sweden, the policy is that parents should take a period of leave when children are under 12–25 months, after which their participation in the labour market should be supported through services and other means' (European Commission Network on Childcare, 1996, p.130).

Adrienne Burgess talks about a 'cultural over-valuing of motherhood and a devaluing of fatherhood within society' (Burgess, 1997a, p.208), and nowhere is this more clear than in the arrangements following family breakdown when mothers are consistently given sole or chief custody of children, and fathers are only permitted contact. This relationship may contribute in some way to the absenteeism among fathers, some of whom eventually cease all contact with their children, although this is quite rare.

WAKING UP WITHOUT YOU
This waking up without you is a pisser,
I know. But if I were there with you
your mother would expect me to kiss her,
write a cheque, say how much I miss her,
all keeping my hands strictly out of view.

Tonight when the monsters are prowling,
I'll come back and help chase them away,
and though your mama may be scowling
I'll bath you and give you a towelling
dry, and a story, then bed, and I may

even play Dennis the Cowboy. Then fuss
around saying goodnight to your mother,
then come back here to my flat on the bus.
You're the best thing that's happened to
either of us;
we just can't get on with each other.

(Nigel Planer, *Unlike the Buddha*, Jackson's Arm, Sunk
Island Publishing, 1997. Reproduced with permission.)

Over the past 10 years fathers' support groups
such as 'Families Need Fathers' have campaigned
politically in order to improve the rights of fathers
to continue to bring up their children. They have
argued that 'contact is a demeaning, alienating and
artificial concept' (Baker and Townsend, 1996)
implying that one parent is more capable than the
other of loving the child or children of a relationship. Arthur Baker and Peter Townsend have sum-
marized the arguments for 'shared residence'
arrangements whereby children may spend between
30 and 70 per cent of the time living with each of
their divorced parents. They point out that in
places where this has been tried, research has
shown that sole or joint custody made no difference
to the children's adjustment subsequent to divorce
(Baker and Townsend, 1996, p.224). As Adrienne
Burgess points out, parents need to work together
after divorce because 'the single most important
indicator of maladjustment in children is their parents' active hostility to one another' (Burgess,
1997a, p.178).

WOMEN AS CARERS

In addition to the fact that women are primarily
responsible for the care of young children in our
society, they are also the people most likely to be
involved in caring for a dependent friend or relative.
In fact, there are more women caring for dependent
adults than there are women looking after children
under the age of 16 years. Hunter Davies described

his part in looking after his mother who was suffering from Alzheimer's disease: 'I admit I did little
except pay the endless helpers and moan when they
did not turn up, or cut corners when it was my turn.
My sister and my wife carried and cared most.
Women do. No that's not sexist. That's looking
coldly around the planet.'

Caring for a dependent relative can be a full-time
activity – some may need attention 24 hours a day.
Support services do exist and are provided by the
local authority Social Services Departments but the
availability of these heavily demanded services
varies from region to region. Limited financial assistance is also available through the Department of
Social Security (DSS) in the form of attendance and
mobility allowances. For many carers, however, this
support is meagre by comparison with the personal
sacrifices they have to make.

On a personal level, because of their commitment to the person being cared for, some carers may
forgo the opportunity to develop other loving relationships. It is common for a woman to devote a
great many of her younger years to tending the
needs of a dependent adult and, because of the
demands involved, ultimately to subjugate her own
needs. Caring for others can be an isolating activity
because it usually takes place within the relative's
own home, and physical caring tasks and the associated routines are often very time-consuming. In
addition, a carer's need to be private may also be
threatened:

My husband has never been the same since he was
in hospital with atrophy of the brain. He follows me
everywhere all day, knocking on the bathroom door
when I go to the toilet. There is no hiding place. I feel
I am losing my mind. This happened only a year after
my mother died aged 98 here at home, confined to
bed for many years. I need to get a break, but so-
called nursing homes are too expensive, and I have
no money. There is nowhere else for him to go, even
for a few days.

(*Guardian*, 10 December 1994, p.10)

Whilst some carers undoubtedly derive satisfaction from the position they are in, a prolonged, isolating, caring relationship can psychologically undermine a woman's confidence in other social situations because of her withdrawal from society in general. Various studies have highlighted the debilitating effect of unemployment, including the psychological harm experienced by those who become isolated in their own home. These studies have almost exclusively focused on the plight of men who are out of work. Less attention has been paid to the many women who are similarly isolated from mainstream society.

It is a mistake to believe that all carers find themselves in the caring role as a result of their own choosing. They may volunteer to provide care, but this is often done in order to avoid the unsatisfactory alternatives. Society places the burden of care quite firmly on women's shoulders. The principle is so deeply instiled that women may perform the task primarily because they need to avoid the guilt they would otherwise be made to feel.

The task of caring for relatives is not exclusively undertaken by women; men, too, are carers. Studies have shown that men are more likely to be involved when they are looking after wives who have become dependent. This arrangement does not normally require a dramatic shift in the living situation. In the case of parents who are being cared for by their children, it is usually the daughter who responds to the demand for care. This situation is also true for the in-law relationship, where a wife or partner is more likely to provide care for her father- or mother-in-law than any of her husband or partner's brothers. Furthermore, men are less likely to be involved in a caring relationship where the dependent person is suffering from any form of incontinence.

WOMEN AND VIOLENCE

Most women have painful emotional and/or physical experiences of coercion. It is merely one of the ways in which women's subordination is enforced, privately in the home, or publicly on the streets, in workplaces and in state departments.

(*Spare Rib*, February 1990)

Within our society women constantly face the threat of, or actually experience, physical violence from men. This may range from verbal harassment to physical abuse, leading ultimately to rape or murder. It may take place in any setting – at work, in public places or, more commonly, within the home. Much of it goes on undetected since, for a number of reasons, it does not get reported to the police. The precise extent of violence that women have to contend with is unknown. However, it is clear that many women can expect to be sexually or physically abused either as children or as adults in their lifetime.

Sexual harassment is a common experience for women. UNISON encouraged its members to seek advice from union officials if they experienced what they considered to be harassment during their working hours. The Union's guidelines state: 'The European Union defines sexual harassment as "unwanted conduct based on sex affecting the dignity of women and men at work" ' (UNISON, 1997, p.4). It can include:

- physical contact, ranging from unnecessary touching through to sexual assault or rape;
- demands for sexual favours;
- sexual propositions;
- unwanted comments on dress or appearance;
- leering and suggestive gestures;
- the display of pornographic pictures or pin-ups.

Whatever form it takes, sexual harassment can make women feel offended, embarrassed, degraded or humiliated, and in a work setting it can deleteriously affect a woman's work performance and may actively damage her career or promotion prospects.

Outside the workplace, women are exposed to physical and sexual abuse in everyday public settings, even within populated surroundings. In August 1989, Leah Geller wrote to the *Guardian* about how she had been sexually molested on a crowded tube train in London, telling how 'in appealing for support from fellow passengers – not a single pair of eyes would acknowledge the incident'. She described her assailant: 'He was about 6 foot 2, and was wearing an expensive, blue pin-striped suit. He was about 40, his dark hair greying. His face was distinct with sharp facial features.' She added, 'What I saw, or see in retrospect, was an image of arrogance and power' (*Guardian*, 2 August 1989).

Learning The Hard Way (Campling, 1989) contains the contributions of 57 mainly working-class women and their struggle to survive and achieve in a male-dominated world. The following extract underlines the everyday nature of abuse to which women are subjected in public places by men:

> I was sitting in the pub with my women friends. Mistake number one: never take up men's space – especially in large numbers (there were three of us). And never approach the pub on your own.
>
> At first the banter was innocuous and wildly original: 'Hello darlin'. What's a nice girl like you doing out on her own?' (Apparently my friends were invisible.) 'Let's have a bit of service here. Isn't anyone going to serve the little lady?' (Is this the chivalry I've heard so much about?)
>
> 'Wot's the matter?' 'Lost your voice? Thought you ladies didn't know how to keep your mouths shut' he laughs. 'Nice pair of knockers', another one joins in. 'Bet she could show us a thing or two.' A hand reaches for my breast, another clutches at my thigh.
>
> 'Fuck off you arseholes' I shout with some degree of terror and go back to my seat at the table. Jenny gets

> the drinks by going next door into the lounge and standing by an old man with a stick, who looks harmless enough. He beams on her breasts and allows his arm to brush against hers. Could be an accident. (Am I becoming paranoid?)
>
> Meanwhile back in the bar, Sir Lancelot (the 'chivalrous' one) and Neanderthal Eddie (his Oppo) amble over to our table. By this time we are the centre of attention, with every male eye fixed on the fun.
>
> 'Wot's the problem girls? We're only trying to be friendly. Wot you talking about? Maybe we might have a few thoughts on the matter.'
>
> 'Look – why don't you just piss off,' says Pam (who is braver than me) 'and leave us alone'.
>
> 'Leave you alone? I wouldn't touch you with a bargepole, you ugly bitch.'
>
> (Campling, 1989, p.6)

According to the writers of the book, such instances are one of the consequences of the proliferation of the image portrayed in advertising, the media and in pornography, that women are sex-objects and that they are permanently sexually available, so that men, 'however insignificant and undesirable', feel entitled to pass sexual comment and make judgements on women.

It is very difficult for women to go out unaccompanied to pubs or to the cinema or the theatre without attracting unwarranted attention or harassment. Walking through the city centre or waiting to use public transport can be unsafe. Because of their fear of violence, many women remain at home, particularly after dark. Consequently their social lives are curtailed, especially the lives of those women who do not have partners.

> There is a widespread misconception of domestic violence as a personal and relationship problem rather than a social and institutional one rooted in gender inequality. There is insufficient recognition of sexual,

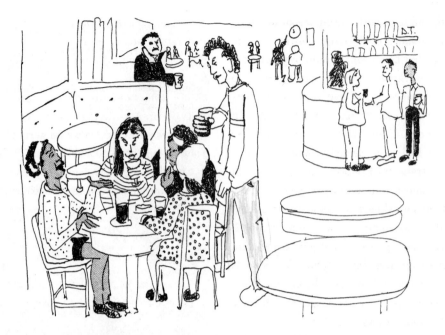

Men commonly feel entitled to invade women's public space.

emotional and psychological abuse; and failure to acknowledge a complex pattern of violence against women and abuse of children.

(A National Agenda for Action. Policy Paper 6, 1995 *Violence Against Women*, p.1)

In addition to the violence against women that takes place in public, there is the abuse of women that is carried out within the home. It is common for women who experience violence from their partners, initially at least, not to do anything about it. They neither report it to the authorities nor attempt to leave their partners.

Women may not want to report abuse to the police or to the Social Services because they are mistrustful of these organizations and fear the consequences of reporting domestic violence against themselves or their children. Many are concerned for their partner, whom they do not want to get 'into trouble', either because of fear of reprisal or for reasons of compassion. 'Sometimes the police would come, when the neighbours called them, if they heard me scream. But I'd just tell them it was all right and that we'd sorted it out. He'd have killed me if

they had arrested him' (*Observer*, 20 October 1996, p.5). Some abused women still love their violent partners and hope to enable them to change. Others are emotionally dependent on their violent partner because they have become systematically isolated and now regard their man as the only person in their world.

Other reasons why women are loath to report incidents of partner abuse are that they feel they may be ignored, blamed or treated unsympathetically. They may sense the collusion of others who do not wish to become involved in their domestic circumstances: 'No one saw me. I was fine, I was grand. I fell down the stairs. I walked into a door. I hit myself with the heel of a shoe. I looked older than my age; what age was I anyway? It was my little secret and they all helped me keep it' (Doyle, 1996, p.188).

Recently it has become evident that there is a reduced tolerance of domestic violence both by women and by society as a whole. This is indicated by an increase in the number of reported incidents and the commitment of police forces to become involved as necessary. Many police forces have their own female-staffed domestic violence units. In October 1997, Lord Irvine, the Lord Chancellor, announced the introduction of two measures aimed at tackling domestic violence. Courts will be able to make two types of order against a person accused of violence:

- an Occupation Order, enabling the court to banish the offender from the home;
- a Non-Molestation Order, forbidding the offender from harming the victim.

As we have said, despite the danger to themselves, some women are reluctant to leave their violent partners. They may feel guilty and somehow responsible for what is happening to them. Other women will have strong religious or cultural reasons for not wanting to leave their partners; they may fear disapproval within their own communities, or they may be morally opposed to breaking marriage vows. Whatever personal reason lies behind a woman's reluctance to leave a violent home, a major obstacle faced by most abused women is the absence of a realistic alternative. The houses of friends or relatives can only be a temporary solution, and women's refuges are grossly underfunded and numerically inadequate.

In 1975 the Parliamentary Select Committee on Violence in Marriage estimated that one refuge place was needed for every 10 000 members of the population. By the 1990s it was clear that the Committee had underestimated the need:

> There are currently under 1700 family places in refuges in England: only one-fifth of the recommended supply except in London, where around 4/10 of the recommended places are available, far short of the 1975 standard. 6550 new family places (650-700 refuges) are required to make good this shortfall.
>
> (Frayne and Muir, 1994, p.19)

Local authority temporary accommodation is also sparse and often substandard, particularly in major cities. The long wait for permanent council housing faced by abused women persuades many of them to return home even though their lives may be threat-ened. The majority of calls to the Women's Aid Federation are referrals for accommodation. The problem of finding a new home is more difficult for black and Asian women, who may face racism. Mama (1989) points out that it took between 18 months and 3 years for the black and Asian women in her London-based study to obtain permanent rehousing. She says that black women's access to public housing is severely circumscribed because many of these women are ignorant of the provision available, some are unable to speak English properly, and they are put off by the bureaucratic process and the fact that structural racism mitigates against them.

WOMEN AND PORNOGRAPHY

> Pornography is a celebration of rape and injury to women; it's a kind of union for rapists, a way of legitimizing rape and formalizing male supremacy in our society.
>
> (*Guardian*, 30 September 1979, p.4)

It is not possible to establish an absolute causal link between pornography and the incidence of male violence against women, although many people feel that a close correlation exists and that violence does not occur in isolation from the rest of society. The suggestion that 'hard porn' in particular leads automatically to violence and/or rape has never been scientifically proven and would be very difficult to establish conclusively. However, it is strongly felt that since pornography reduces women to sexual objects, it degrades and dehumanizes them and allows men to perceive them as being always sexually available. Against this it is argued that pornography acts as a release for men and dissipates potential aggression. Certainly soft pornography is viewed by many as being harmless. Mr Robert Adley, MP, said in a House of Commons debate, 'If a man gets hot and steamy, these pictures act as a release not a stimulation to rape' (*Observer*, 16 March 1986).

Another MP, Mr Peter Temple, argued, 'Everyone should be free to look at page 3, we are not in the business of petty censorship. These pictures are amusing' (*Observer*, 16 March 1986). Both men were speaking in the debate following the first reading of Clare Short's Indecent Displays Bill 1986, which unsuccessfully sought to ban sexually provocative pictures of women.

Just as there is no overall agreement about the effect of pornography on its users and the rest of society, exactly what constitutes pornography is not universally agreed upon either.

The Campaign Against Pornography and Censorship (CAPC) defines pornography as:

> the graphic, sexually explicit subordination of women through pictures and words, that also includes one or more of the following: women portrayed as sexual objects, things or commodities, enjoying pain or humiliation or rape, being tied up, cut up, mutilated, bruised or physically hurt, in postures of sexual submission or servility or display, reduced to body parts, penetrated by objects or animals, or presented in scenarios of denigration, injury, torture, shown as inferior, bleeding, bruised or hurt in a context which is sexual.
>
> (*Guardian*, 15 February 1990, p.38)

This rather comprehensive definition would include all representations of women, ranging from 'hard porn' through to 'soft porn', including what have become known as 'page-3 pictures' of partially clad women which are to be found daily in certain tabloid newspapers.

Pornography needs to be distinguished from erotica, although for many people there will always be a thin dividing line between the two. *Erotica* has been defined by the CAPC as 'sexually explicit materials premised on equality'. For example, non-violent, non-degrading explicit sex scenes in films may be considered erotic rather than pornographic when they are the product of the relationship of the people involved. However, the attention of the camera, whether it zooms in, lingers or withdraws in order to allow the viewer to make the choice, can itself determine whether something is presented as pornographic or erotic. Erotica, whether it is depicted in books, pictures or films, is generally considered to be healthy and/or stimulating since it is not based on a distortion. Pornography, as the CAPC points out, is less about sex and more about power. 'It reflects and reinforces inequality and injustice, manipulating sexist and racist stereotypes and perpetuating the power men have over women.'

The CAPC is concerned with challenging the acceptability of pornographic images. 'Images which silence women and children by denying them a personality, images which perpetuate the myth that "women are asking for it" when they are harassed, abused and raped; images which portray enjoyment of violence, images which are often an actual record of the rape of, or violence against, women and children. Images which enable men to perceive women and young girls as sexually available'. These images are all around us. Hard pornography is readily available in local shops, and soft pornography permeates the whole of the media and advertising industry to such an extent that the degradation and dehumanization of women is institutionalized. The images and representations reflect women's unequal status in society.

Pornography also exploits men because it peddles the idea that men can control and possess the women portrayed in the magazines and films. According to Ian Warwick of the Sheffield Men's Awareness Project, 'Brought up in a world where men are supposed to be strong and independent, sex brings fear of vulnerability. Pornography reasserts our security and identity. Perhaps this is why pornography more often leads to masturbation than to intercourse. While masturbating a man can control his own sexual pleasure, unaffected by the sexual desire of his partner' (Ian Warwick, 1996, personal communication). A similar sentiment was expressed by Peter Baker in a letter to the *Guardian*, 'Teaching me that women were essentially objects for my own lustful purposes and that good sex was quick, impersonal and purely penetrative, pornography helped prevent me from easily forming permanent relationships with real women' (*Guardian*, 8 May 1990, p.21). Ian Warwick adds 'that within pornography, nowhere do men express tenderness, love and caring, nowhere do men experience closeness, warmth or the feeling of being loved' (Ian Warwick, 1996, personal communication).

WOMEN AND SOCIAL CARE

As we have already established, it is women who undertake to perform the majority of paid care. Women, too, perform the majority of unpaid care. The NHS and Community Care Act 1990 was based on the assumption that women will continue to perform their traditional roles.

Around 90 per cent of nurses are women, as are nearly all home helps and infant teachers. Within social work itself, most workers are female (80 per cent of staff in care homes for older people, 75 per cent of those who work in children's homes, and the majority of field workers and medical social workers are women). However, senior and managerial roles are more commonly performed by men, so whilst the grass-roots care is carried out mainly by women, policies and decision-making are generally shaped by men.

Joyce Brand, who retired early from social work after 25 years working for a local authority, feels that the impact of the 'contract culture' has shifted the focus away from care, 'now that we are being encouraged to ask whether an elderly person has antiques that could be sold by her family to provide for her care' (*Independent*, 9 April 1997, p.19). The new business-style culture appeals more to men than to women, who still represent 'the vast majority of field social workers'. They have no difficulty in working to BASW's definition of social work; that is, 'the enforcement of human well-being and the relief and prevention of hardship and suffering through working with individuals, families and groups.'

However, most senior managers are male, and to them such a philosophy is not nearly so attractive. 'How much more enjoyable it is to think of performance indicators, internal markets and financial management.' To substantiate her impressions, Brand says, 'The statistics are stark: seven out of eight staff in social service organizations are women; most people using the service are women; but seven out of eight managers in these organizations are men (*Independent*, 9 April 1997, p.19).

One consequence of this imbalance is that social services policies are often based on society's dominant male values, which may operate against the interests of women. Women's propensity to act as carers has often been exploited by Social Services Departments (and Social Work Departments in Scotland) which have failed to support women in caring situations, regarding their role as 'natural', whereas they have been more inclined to support a man in similar circumstances. Consider, too, the general inadequacy of the allowances normally paid to foster carers, the assumption being that fostering is no more than an extension of domestic labour. A foster mother's motivation would be considered suspect if she sought reward for her work over and above the cost of the child's upkeep. Lesbian mothers and black women have additional and understandable reasons for fearing intervention from white, male-dominated social-work organizations.

Another long-term consequence of caring roles being carried out almost exclusively by women is the reinforcing effect that this will have upon the next generation. Eugen Hckejos cites the example of 4-year-old Tommy living in Islington: 'Next month he will start nursery. In Islington, 97 per cent of nursing staff are female. When he moves to primary school he will be welcomed by the teaching staff which if it is any thing like the national average will be 80 per cent female. Should his mother have problems requiring help from the Social Services he will again see only women in the caring role as, similar to other authorities, Islington's pool of social workers is 82 per cent female.'

There is little chance for Tommy to encounter a caring male during his contact with Social Services, as many male staff are allocated to deal with drug- or alcohol-dependent clients, or those with HIV/AIDS, and they are often preoccupied with tasks considered to be too dangerous for Islington's female workers. He asks, 'Will Tommy learn to care if he has no access to role models?' (*Guardian*, 20 March 1996, p.2).

Not only do women represent the majority of social carers, they also constitute the bulk of social work clientele. The situation is almost completely reversed within the probation service, which is largely staffed by men who work predominantly with male offenders. The probation service works mainly at the 'soft end' of the penal system, and deals mainly with 'perpetrators' rather than 'victims', and therefore involves an element of social control.

The situation is different in Scotland, where there is no probation service as such and the work is carried out by Social Work Departments. Consequently, more women than men are involved in work with offenders, because there are more women social workers.

There are several reasons why women represent the majority of social work clients, some of which have already been discussed. Owing to the responsibility society has bestowed on women to be concerned primarily with the care and well-being of others, many women present themselves at Social Service Departments (and Social Work Departments in Scotland) because of, or on behalf of, other family members. They may seek help with their children, for a dependent relative or for the whole family. Women, too, as we have seen, are more likely to experience mental illness in its various forms and to be victims of domestic violence, and they may need help because of this.

Women's lower earning potential or their inability to obtain paid work because of domestic commitments means that they are more likely to experience material deprivation and the effects of poverty. Consequently they may require social work support. Indeed, due to the fact that more women are on fixed incomes, either as pensioners (among whom women form the great majority), disabled people or, because they are on income support, as single parents, or that they are on low incomes

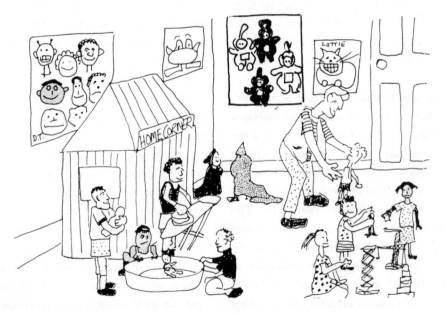

Staff gender and the activities in which children are permitted to take part can serve either to reinforce or to break down stereotypes.

because of the lowly regarded nature of the work that they do, they are more likely than men to need support from welfare agencies.

Jalna Hanmer and Daphne Statham in their book, *Women and Social Work: Towards a Woman-Centered Practice* (Hanmer and Statham, 1988), suggest that social work directs itself towards recognizing the fact that it is essentially a female-dominated profession and that women, both as workers and as clients, can draw strength from this. They feel that within social work it is important that more women reach positions of authority in order that they can have an influence on policy. Furthermore, they feel that policies could be made which emphasize the similarities women have with one another, and that the division between worker and client should be minimized. Instead of being seen as 'elderly', 'disabled' or 'mentally ill', female clients would be seen as women first. Women clients would thus be empowered by the corresponding lack of stigma, and by their closer association with their helper.

CONCLUSION

This chapter has focused on the unequal position of women in society. We have seen that women are undeniably structurally disadvantaged and that they have less access to privilege, power and life-chances than men. Whilst women's position within society has improved over the past 30 years or so, due mainly to the increased awareness brought about by the resurrection of the feminist movement in the late 1960s, progress has only been gradual, and women remain fundamentally oppressed. As carers it is important that we recognize this fact in order that we are better able to support our female clients and colleagues.

We have examined the socialization process and highlighted the instances and effects of sexism at both the individual and institutional level. We have seen that much of the contribution which women make to society goes unrewarded (it is undervalued and is often taken for granted) and that, moreover,

this negative attitude towards women is deeply ingrained within our culture. It is the same worldwide. It has been calculated that if women's labour was properly valued it would be worth around the order of US$11 trillion, nearly half the global output (*Financial Times*, 28 August 1995, p.18). However, in more recent years a more respectful representation of women has developed, as well as a greater acknowledgement of the contribution that they make to society and the difficulties which our society creates for them. In an interview with Murray Davies in the *Daily Mirror*, Glenda Jackson talked about why she was giving up her acting career in order to become a Labour candidate in the next election. She had recently been selected to represent the Hampstead and Highgate constituency. In answer to the question, 'Why choose an actress?' she answered, 'I'll tell you why. Because to be an actress, I have first to be a woman. I have been a daughter, sister, mother, wife, a shopper, a cleaner, a gardener, a home economics expert, a driver, a dressmaker, a cook, a nanny and a professional career woman. It would be very difficult to find a man who had done all that' (*Daily Mirror*, 29 March 1990, p.18).

In 1996 the Equal Opportunities Commission (EOC) celebrated 20 years of progress in challenging inequalities between women and men. It reported on the developments since the introduction of the Equal Pay Act and the Sex Discrimination Act at the end of 1975 and listed the symbolic landmarks, some of which are reproduced in Table 3.7, that occurred during this period. The work of the EOC, the Northern IREl and EOC and the Women's Commission continues today in the pursuit of equality between women and men.

In 1996 the EOC produced a list of significant achievements by individual women throughout history, calling the list *First Among Equals*. Part of this list is reproduced in Table 3.7. Since then there have been more milestones reached. For instance, Marjorie Scardino became the first woman Chief Executive Officer of a company (Pearsons) on the *Financial Times* listing of the top 100 traded securities in the UK.

Table 3.7 First Among Equals

First among equals – through the glass ceiling

Women at the top

1972	First woman judge to sit at Old Bailey: Rose Heilbron QC
1973	First woman on London Stock Exchange: Susan Shaw
1979	First woman Prime Minister: Margaret Thatcher
1979	First woman President of British Medical Association: Josephine Barnes
1983	First woman Lord Mayor of London: Dame Mary Donaldson
1984	First woman General Secretary of a big trade union: Brenda Dean, SOGAT
1984	First woman Law Commissioner: Brenda Hoggett
1992	First woman Speaker of the House of Commons: Betty Boothroyd
1992	First woman Director of the Crown Prosecution Service: Barbara Mills
1993	First woman Civil Service Commissioner: Ann Bowtell
1993	First woman head of MI5: Stella Rimmington
1995	First woman member of Bank of England's Court of Directors: Frances Heaton
1995	First woman Chief Constable: Pauline Clare, Lancashire Constabulary
1995	First woman executive director under 30 of a top company: Lisa Gordon, Chrysalis

First among equals – breaking new ground

Women into 'men's jobs'

1975	First woman jet airline captain: Yvonne Pope
1977	First woman firefighter: Mary Langdon
1979	First full-time woman coastguard: Sue Nelson
1981	First woman station-master: Pennie Bellas
1981	First black woman TV newscaster: Moira Stewart, BBC
1983	First black woman train-driver, Anne Winter

First among equals – the games people play

1977	First woman to ride in the Grand National: Charlotte Brewer on Barony Fort
1977	First woman football referee of all-male match: Jenny Bazeley
1992	After a 5-year battle, Susan Thompson becomes Britain's first ever woman professional pool player, with the EOC's help
1993	The first woman boxing Master of Ceremonies, Lisa Budd, settles her sex discrimination claim, with EOC support
1994	First woman linesperson in a Football League match: Wendy Toms
1995	EOC helps Beverly Davis establish that she can stand for election to the National Executive Committee of the Rugby Football Union
1995	Sophie Cox granted permission from the Rugby League to play for Rochdale Town Under 11 Schools Team and played for her team at Wembley on 28 October

1. Who are the 'dinner ladies'?

Observe the differences in gender roles in your place of work or college. Make a list of all the occupational positions within your establishment, either full-time or part-time, and divide them into those performed by females and those performed by males. Consider the status related to each of the posts. Include administrative, domestic, kitchen and caretaking staff and all social care/teaching and management staff. What conclusions do you draw? (You could extend this study from your own place of work to include the whole agency.)

2. Community resources

Investigate within your own community the number and range of community resources and provisions available exclusively for women (or ethnic minority women). Comment on your findings and suggest why it is important that women should have separate provision to men. Consider other areas where community provision could be made more available to women.

3. Pornography versus erotica

Each member of the group should select a few items from the media (pictures, 'news' stories, cartoons, video extracts) or from literature (stories or poems) or from art (paintings, drawings or postcards). With the help of some of the information given in this chapter, try to categorize these items along a continuum between acceptable and unacceptable image, either as 'pornography' or as 'erotica'. Discuss your reasons with other members of the group.

4. Team meetings

One problem with team meetings is that some people, often men, tend to dominate the discussion, either by constantly interrupting their (female) colleagues or by talking over them. Plan how you would raise this as an agenda issue for your next meeting, and try to produce constructive suggestions as to how the team members can create an environment in which everyone can be heard and will feel safe to express themselves in their own style.

5. Who does what at home?

The 1980s and early 1990s reputedly saw the emergence of the 'new man' – a partner willing to do an equal share of domestic and child-care tasks. How true do you think this is of most families? Who normally does the work in your home? Is it still structured along sexist lines? Make a table of the various domestic duties and estimate the time spent by males or females on those jobs within your household over a short period.

1. What can be done in order to attract more men into social care/nursing? Why do you think it is important that more men become involved in this field either as paid workers or as volunteers? What possible long-term consequences would there be should more men become involved in social care?

2. What can be done in order to enable women to feel safe outside the home on their own after dark?

3. Men are 'sexist' by their very nature and it is impossible for them to change?

4. The feminist movement in the UK has not fully represented and reflected the history and interests of working-class white women or black women in this country.

5. Social-care and social-work students on work placements and also student nurses should be able to ensure that they are supervised by someone of the gender of their own choosing.

6. How far does a lack of confidence and poor self-image contribute to the absence of women from the more senior managerial positions within social care or social work?

FURTHER READING

Academic sources

Burgess, A. 1997: *Fatherhood reclaimed: the making of the modern father.* London: Vermilion. An up-to-date book that outlines the unique value that fathers have for their children. It challenges stereotypes and examines ways in which men can be more positively involved with the care of their children.

Hanmer, J. and Statham, D. 1988: *Women and social work – towards a woman-centred practice.* Birmingham: British Association of Social Workers. A book which clearly outlines the relevance of gender to social care, emphasizing what women social carers have in common with women clients, as well as what distinguishes them from each other.

Langan, M. and Day, L. (eds) 1992: *Women, oppression and social work.* London: Routledge. This book looks at the effects of oppression on women as workers and clients. It examines the different manifestations of oppression, including racism, sexism, ageism, heterosexism and material deprivation.

Keith, L. (ed.) 1994: *Mustn't grumble – writings by disabled women.* London: The Women's Press. A collection of writings and poems on disability and illness written by a number of disabled women with a wide range of experiences.

Mama, A., 1989: *The hidden struggle – statutory and voluntary sector responses to violence against women in the home.* London: London Race and Housing Research. A London-based detailed account of black women's experience of violence, homelessness and the response of the voluntary and statutory 'caring services'.

Oakley, A. 1972: *Sex, gender and society.* London: Gower/Temple Smith. A classic study that attempts to establish the 'real differences between men and women', and whether these are culturally or biologically determined.

Other literary sources

Doyle, R. 1996: *The Woman who walked into doors.* London: Jonathan Cape.

Emecheta, B. 1987: *Second-class citizen.* London: Fontana.

Grant, L. 1998: *Remind me who I am, again.* London: Granta Publications.

Hall, R. 1982: *The well of loneliness.* London: Virago.

Hornby, N. 1995: *High fidelity.* London: Victor Gollancz.

Walker, A. 1990: *The colour purple.* London: The Women's Press.

Films and plays

Campion, J. 1990: *An Angel at my Table.* New Zealand.

Friel, B. 1990: *Dancing at Lughansa.* London: Faber.

Leigh, M. 1995: *Secrets and Lies.* UK.

Scorsese, M. 1974: *Alice Doesn't Live Here Anymore.* USA.

4

Racism, black people and discrimination

Who am I?

Who are we?

Our goal should be a society in which we appreciate and value our differences; one where everyone can learn, work and live free from racial prejudice, discrimination, harassment and violence. That is the vision we must strive towards for Britain, as part of global cultural diversity.

I am what I am.

We are what we are.

(Sir Herman Ouseley, Chairman of the CRE. Foreword to *Roots of the Future*. Commission for Racial Equality, 1996, p.vii)

INTRODUCTION

Racism is an immensely complex subject and one which, perhaps more than any other, is likely to evoke strong feelings whenever it is raised. People may feel strongly because they have experienced and continue to experience the effects of racism in their everyday lives, or they may feel angry simply because of the social injustice of racism. Some individuals may feel threatened and act defensively whenever the matter is mentioned, for fear of their own actions being criticized or condemned. Others will remain confused and uncertain about an issue which they feel to be inflated in importance since it has barely touched their lives.

Before we go on to look at racism and the various definitions associated with it, we need to acknowledge as a starting point that the UK is a racist society and has been so for centuries, and that racism is evident both at the individual level and in society as a whole.

This chapter aims to examine the complex issue of racism in as simple a way as possible in order that we can try to understand the phenomenon and consider its influence within society today. We can also try to understand our own position as individuals and see how racism affects us and those for whom we care.

DISCUSSION OF SOME OF THE TERMS USED

Throughout history attempts have been made to classify human beings into groups – as certain racial types distinguishable by their physical characteristics, cultural patterns and modes of behaviour. It would seem that the aim of such classification has been to demonstrate that one *race* or group of people is in some way superior to others, and to justify or facilitate the creation of a structural hierarchy.

Superficial differences between people do exist, but these are nothing more than indicators of how the human race has adapted to its various climatic surroundings during the evolutionary process. For example, dark pigmentation offers the skin more protection against the sun and is consequently a characteristic of those people whose ancestors lived in hot countries. Observable physical characteristics have no other significance, and there is no evidence that one race of people is in any way superior to another.

In fact, the very concept of 'race' is imprecise because there can hardly be such a thing as a pure race, given the increasing mobility of people throughout history. For a pure race of people to exist today, it would need to have led a very insular and self-contained existence – in a vacuum, isolated from an ever-expanding and increasingly interdependent world. All 'races', are therefore made up of a mixture of different people, and the notion of a pure race is not valid. However, the term 'race' remains a powerful social concept which is widely understood and used.

Racialism and racism

These two words are generally considered to be interchangeable, and in everyday usage they convey broadly the same meaning. However, one of the key organizations that represents the interests of ethnic minority people in the UK, the Institute for Race Relations, distinguishes between them. *Racialism* refers to individual prejudiced beliefs and behaviour. Any individual who prejudges another person on the grounds of his or her skin colour or cultural differences and acts accordingly is considered to be a *racialist. Racism* refers to the situation where racialist views are interwoven into the structure of society so that society's major social, economic and political institutions systematically perpetuate the philosophy of racial superiority. *Racialism* then refers to individuals and *racism* refers to the way in which society is structured and operates. However, despite this distinction, the words 'racialist' and 'racist' are commonly used interchangeably to describe individuals in everyday speech.

Not everyone's definition of racism will accord with that of the Institute for Race Relations. In fact there is a wide diversity of interpretation. A common and strongly held view is that *racism equals prejudice plus power.* In other words, racism is a combination of individual racial prejudice and society's support. In the UK today the political, legal and economic institutions are predominantly staffed by white men and some white women, so that social policies reflect the ideas of the white majority, and the 'black perspective' is largely absent. The practices and procedures of so many of our organizations are consciously or unconsciously racist in that they operate unfavourably towards and therefore discriminate against people from ethnic minorities. As we shall see, this accusation applies to all of the caring services, as well as to business and industrial institutions. At the same time it needs to be pointed out that genuine attempts are now being made to counteract racism within these various organizations.

According to the above definition it would be impossible for a black person to be racist in a white-dominated society (although it is possible for one ethnic group to act in a racist way towards another ethnic minority group). Correspondingly, a white person could not be racist in a black-dominated society. This is because the structure and institutions of a society reflect the dominant ideology of the majority people. However, the problem with the definition 'racism equals prejudice plus power' is that it implies that *all* white people in a white-dominated society are automatically racist, despite any attempts they may make towards combating their own racism. It is true to say that all white people who are brought up in the UK are almost bound to be racist to a certain extent because of their conditioning. They have been subjected to a socialization process which values white skin colour more highly than black. This is not to say that white people have chosen to be racist. In fact the process is much more subtle, occurring subconsciously during their formative years and being reinforced throughout their lives. In order to combat this process, white people need to make a conscious effort to eradicate racism within themselves and to oppose it within society. Daphne Statham, Director of the National Institute for Social Work, represents a stance commonly held among white people. 'My position is', she said, 'that however liberal I like to see myself, having been brought up white and benefiting from that status, I must be racist. It is my response to try to overcome it in my job and in my relationships with other people. I make mistakes and I have to learn from them' *(Social Work Today*, November 1987). (In 1998 these sentiments still represent Daphne Statham's stance with regard to the effect of being brought up as a white woman in racist society, and the need to combat this.)

Furthermore, as an ideology racism has been used in many different societies to support the oppression of various minorities at different stages throughout history. At its most extreme, the practice of discrimination and persecution has led to genocide, a clear example during this century being the wholesale murder of millions of Jews and other minorities, including black people, disabled people, gays and gypsies, by the Nazi regime during the Second World War. The more recent mass murders carried out in Bosnia, Rwanda and other parts of the world under the gruesome title of 'ethnic cleansing'

are modern reminders of the ultimate horror of racism.

Until its formal abolition in 1994, racism was most starkly apparent in the apartheid structure of South Africa, where black people were denied many basic human rights and were forced to live in separate restricted townships where they suffered extremes of deprivation, while the minority white people had almost exclusive access to privilege and power. In the UK, racism is clearly not so extreme nor always so blatant, yet it is still prevalent.

Blackness and whiteness

The words 'black' and 'white' are not really accurate when they are used literally to describe skin colour, for few people could properly be described as either black or white given the extensive gradations of skin colour – most people fall somewhere in between. However, for the purpose of classification, *black* normally refers to those people whose family origin is African or West Indian (African-Caribbean) and *white* refers to people of European (or North American) descent, while *Asian* includes people who originate from the subcontinent of India. Within the UK, apart from the Chinese and Irish, minorities are not generally regarded as being sufficiently numerous to be categorized by themselves, and so for convenience they are included in one of the above categories.

This form of classification is obviously very crude and unsatisfactory, not least because it obscures the enormous cultural diversity between people of the same country, let alone that between people of different countries. For example, the term 'Asian' can be seen to be a blanket term, which broadly covers identifiable groups of people but includes a range of countries (such as Bangladesh, Hong Kong and Sri Lanka), a range of religions (such as Sikhism, Buddhism, Christianity and Islam), a range of languages (such as Urdu, Gujarati and Sinhalese) and an infinite variety of other customs and styles. Similarly, as Dudley Rhodes, a Barbadian, was quoted as saying:

> There are a number of black people here who come from a variety of islands, and to lump us together as one group who have got the same causes and the same difficulties is insulting, is denying my culture, is denying my heritage.
>
> (*Social Work Today*, November 1987)

To some extent the term '*ethnic minority*' was introduced in recognition of the great variety of different cultures. Ethnic minorities are thus all those groups of people whose land of origin is not the host country. It must be remembered that 'minority' is only a relative concept – a Pakistani becomes a member of a minority only when he or she settles outside of Pakistan; globally speaking, however, white people are a minority.

In 1997, an Organization named 'English Rights Scotland' was formed to support English people living in Scotland who had experienced 'racial abuse'. Increased levels of anti-English discrimination and hostility had been reported to all of Scotland's Racial Equality councils. One person who had experienced constant verbal abuse in his workplace said, 'the difficulty is getting people to realize this kind of behaviour is not acceptable – whether it is a black person or an English [*sic*] person, it is still racial abuse' (*Guardian*, 30 August 1997, p.4).

In the UK, when we talk of racism we are almost exclusively speaking about discrimination based on skin colour, since this is the most visible difference between people. This is not to say that racism is not directed at other minority groups including, for example, Irish, Jewish, Polish and Greek people, and others. However, it is agreed that their experience of racism, although similar, is less severe than that of black people because of their closer physical similarity to white people. Their language and cultural differences are not immediately apparent from external observation. For example, a white Irish person with a regional accent may not face discrimination until after he or she has spoken.

Since the 1960s the word 'black' has been used to convey a more positive identity of people of African-Caribbean origin. 'Black Consciousness' and 'Black is Beautiful' are two examples of positive statements of blackness made during this period. Similarly, the word 'Asian' now serves to distinguish further between black people, and provides a more distinct identity for people from the Indian subcontinent.

As well as the examples listed above, there is yet another use of the term 'black'. It is used in a wider political sense as an umbrella term to describe all of those whose life-chances are reduced in an equivalent way. For example, white-skinned Irish or Polish people could be considered 'black' on the occasions when they are discriminated against in the job market or a housing situation. In this generic sense 'black' is synonymous with the term 'ethnic minority'.

According to Banda Ahmad, Director of the Race Equality Unit – Personal Social Services, at the National Institiute for Social Work: 'For those who define themselves as black:

- it is a declaration of struggle for equality and justice;
- it is an acknowledgment of similar experience of racism and racial discrimination in Britain;
- it is a challenge to white perceptions of blackness being inferior and getting rid of negative connotations;
- it is redefining the white definition of black, which has historical links with slavery and colonialization;
- above all, it is a positive statement'.

(*Social Work Today*, 11 May 1989)

Tokenism

Organizations may be accused of being tokenistic when they appoint a member of a panel or employ a worker who is black merely in order to give the impression of balance, where the change is superficial and does not represent full implementation of equal opportunities policy.

ORIGINS OF RACISM

The roots of racism are to be found in the past. Influences in the development of racism can be traced in the English language itself, and from this the justification of supporting the practice of the African slave trade and the policy of imperialism.

The English language

Throughout English literature and within the English language there has been a long-held association between the word 'black' and something which is intrinsically bad – the devil, black magic, blackmail and black-ball. This is illustrated in the following anecdote. A black military bandsman was strolling down the Strand during the seventeenth century when he was accosted with the question, 'Well, blackie, what news the devil?' He knocked the questioner down, remarking, 'He send you that – how you like it?' (quoted in Fryer, 1984, p.88).

Whiteness, on the other hand, has stood for 'goodness', 'virtue' and 'cleanliness'. Clear examples of the association of 'white' with 'purity' are to be found throughout the literature. Consider, for example, Shakespeare's use of such associations in *Othello*. The Duke summarizes the character of the dark-skinned, noble Othello thus:

> ... is far more fair than black.

Again, later in the play, Othello agonizes over Desdemona's supposed unfaithfulness:

> I'll have some proof.
> Her name, that was as fresh
> As Dian's visage, is now begrimed and black
> As mine own face.
>
> (*Othello*, Act 3, Scene 3)

In his emphasis of the beauty of Desdemona he says:

> It is the cause.
> Yet I'll not shed her blood,

Nor scar that whiter skin of hers than snow,
And smooth as monumental alabaster.

> (*Othello*, Act 5, Scene 2)

Images that associate the colour black, darkness and the night, the devil and evil abound throughout Shakespeare and other works, written both before and after his time. They have their origins in early medieval beliefs and the symbolic use of darkness and light in the Bible.

Given this link with medieval superstition, it is possible that people began to ascribe these negative connotations to dark-skinned people when they were first encountered in large numbers. Similarly, the idealized, flattering associations with whiteness could just as easily have been internalized by white people and contributed to the feelings of superiority necessary for racism to take root. It is likely therefore that racism found its earliest expression in our existing language. It was to begin to flourish with society's involvement in a lucrative slave trade and subsequent colonialization.

Slavery

The system of slavery met the needs of an expanding British economy for a period of 150 years, spanning the seventeenth to the nineteenth centuries. The buying and selling of black women and men was a profitable business, and it formed part of a sophisticated triangular trade arrangement between Britain, Africa and the Americas (Fig. 4.1).

On the first leg of the journey Britain shipped manufactured materials such as tools and textiles to Africa. These goods were sold in exchange for young Africans, who were then transported to the West Indies and the Americas in order to work on the new sugar and cotton plantations. The traders only took the healthiest of the African people – the youngest and strongest – in the interest of maximum profits. The harrowing, overcrowded travelling conditions which the slaves had to endure were so severe that many of them failed to complete the journey. Those who did survive were sold to plantation owners and

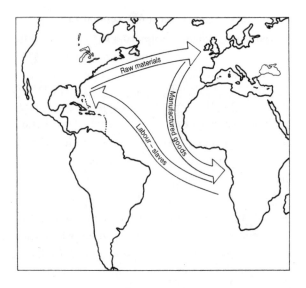

Fig. 4.1 The slave triangle.

forced to work long hours and undertake arduous tasks. Devoid of their basic human rights, the slaves were often kept in chains and subjected to the whims of their masters.

The product of their labour, mainly sugar and cotton, was then shipped back to Britain to meet a growing demand. Some slaves were brought back to Britain and sold into servitude to wealthy families, where owning a black slave denoted elevated social status.

The whole system, based on the treatment of human beings as commodities – as things to be bought and sold – generated huge profits for all those concerned in the trading. These profits made a considerable contribution to later industrial development in Britain, particularly in the expansion of the ports of Bristol, Liverpool and London. Any guilt stemming from those who acknowledged or were involved in this inhumane and degrading practice was offset by the material gains it produced.

> I own I am shocked at the purchase of slaves,
> And fear those who buy and sell them are knaves;
> What I hear of their hardships, their tortures, and groans
> Is almost enough to drive pity from stones.

> I pity them greatly, but I must be numb,
> For how could we do without sugar and rum.
> (W. Cowper, *Pity for Poor Africans, 1788,* cited in Fryer, 1984: *Staying Power*, London: Pluto Press, p.39. Reproduced with permission.)

For the system to have been tolerated and to have lasted so long, it needed some form of moral justification. This was supplied by racism – the belief that Africans were inferior to white people. They were regarded as barbaric, even subhuman, capable of only dull, menial work, and needing to be enslaved and manacled because they could not be trusted with their own freedom.

Slavery was officially made illegal in this country in 1833, by which time the lives of millions of Africans had been destroyed. African slavery eventually came to an end, but not simply as a result of righteous indignation. By this time there had been many slave insurrections, the system was becoming less profitable and there were easier gains to be made elsewhere. The owners of capital turned their attention to the exploitation of other countries in the world through colonialism.

Colonialism

Alongside other European countries, Britain became involved in colonial expansion – the conquest and exploitation of other countries. Britain was in a position to expand and develop a vast empire because of her powerful armed forces. Military superiority implied cultural superiority, and Britain and other European countries were able to repress cultures far older than their own. Colonial expansion took place in three main ways.

First, the British and other Europeans invaded, settled in and imposed their authority on a host country, pushing aside the native people. One consequence of this action that is apparent today is the disaffection felt by the Maoris in New Zealand and the Aborigines in Australia, who are now minorities in their own countries and whose cultural heritage, ancestry and relationship to the land have been all but lost in the wake of the establishment of a white, European-based culture. Theories of white superiority justified the wholesale slaughter of many indigenous peoples.

In 1988 the late Aboriginal political activist, Burnum Burnum, travelled from Australia in order to plant an Aboriginal flag on the White Cliffs of Dover and symbolically claim England for the Aboriginal people, with the declaration, 'We wish no harm to England's native people. We are here to bring you good manners, refinement and an opportunity to make a Koompartoo – a fresh start.' This personal gesture was made at the same time that people in Australia were celebrating the country's Bi-Centenary of British Settlement. 'To non-Aboriginal people, 1788 marked the start of "settlement". But to Burnum Burnum's people, it was an invasion that sent a civilization that had prospered for 40,000 years into rapid and devastating decline' (*Independent*, 20 August 1997, p.11).

In other instances, in countries such as South Africa and Zimbabwe (formerly Rhodesia), the original inhabitants remained the numerical majority, but the British and other Europeans settled, having eventually defeated the native peoples and taken their land. The indigenous people were then used as cheap labour, and the ruling whites used force to maintain their position of privilege.

The third and most common form of colonialization occurred in countries such as India and the West Indies, where the British did not settle in large numbers, but instead ruled the countries from afar. Britain became known as the mother country, and at the height of the Empire ruled over 25 per cent of the world, an area so vast that it was claimed that the sun never set on the British Empire.

Colonized countries were rich in raw materials and cheap labour, which were exploited by Britain. Opponents of colonization now point to the economic dependence with which many former colonies are left because their economies have changed from self-sufficient agricultural communities to economies that are dependent on the international fluctuations of their main cash crop.

Supporters of the process of colonialization point to the great benefits bestowed on the developing countries, including road and rail networks, and the establishment of legal and political institutions and commercial systems. However, such benefits as did accrue were not always a result of altruism. They were often incidental, a consequence stemming from activities generated by the pursuit of profit.

Moral 'backing' for colonization was, in effect, initially supplied by the church. Black people were considered to be 'heathens' and 'savages' in need of enlightenment and civilization. Later came scientific or pseudoscientific explanations aimed at justifying white supremacy. Some scientists measured skulls in order to try to demonstrate differences in the brain capacity of black and white people. Others focused on the proportions and shape of the skull and nose in order to establish intellectual superiority between 'races'. They were unsuccessful. A more recent study conducted by psychologist Arthur Jensen attempted to prove that white people had higher IQs than black people. His results were discredited because, among other things, they took no account of environmental factors.

More recently, in 1996, Christopher Brand's book *The 'G-Factor': General Intelligence and Its Implications*, which attempted to outline a racial theory of intelligence, was withdrawn by the publishers, John Wiley, who wanted to be 'disassociated with a book that makes assertions that we find repellent'. The author's own University Principal, Sir Stewart Sutherland, denounced the work as 'false and obnoxious'(*Guardian*, 1 May 1997, p.2).

In a discussion on racism it may seem a little surprising to devote so much attention to issues of the past. The significance of this lies in the effect that past attitudes, with their roots in centuries of slavery and colonization, still have on our present lives. The racism of the past permeates our culture today. It is in everything we come across – the books we read, the lessons we receive at school, the messages we obtain through the newspapers, magazines, television and films, and the policies and practices of different organizations.

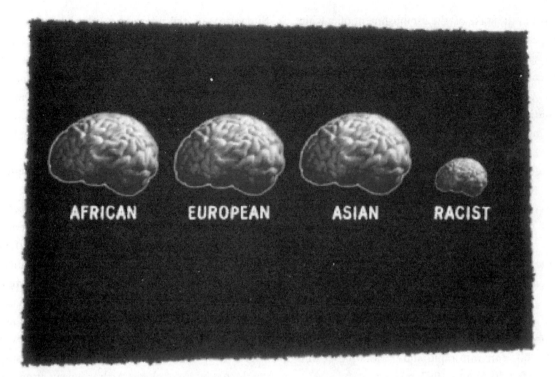

Fig. 4.2 Size matters. (Reproduced from Commission for Racial Equality, with permission.)

> If you want to understand British racism – and without understanding it no change is possible – it is impossible even to begin to grasp the nature of the beast unless you accept its historical roots. Unless you see that 400 years of conquest and looting, centuries of being told that you are superior to the 'fuzzy-wuzzies' and the 'wogs', all leave their stain on you all: that such a stain seeps into every part of your culture, your language and your daily life: and nothing has been done to wash it out.
>
> (Salman Rushdie, *The New Empire Within Britain*, *New Society*, 9 December 1982)

BLACK PEOPLE IN BRITAIN

There is a long history of black people living in Britain. Early records make reference to black soldiers in the Roman army of occupation, but black people have always been a minority in this country.

Post-war settlers

It was not until comparatively recent times that black people began coming to this country in relatively large numbers. The arrival of the 'Empire Windrush' on 22 June 1948 brought 492 Jamaicans, described in one newspaper as 'five hundred pairs of willing hands'. This marked the beginning of a period of increased black immigration to this country, made possible for several reasons, including the passing of the 1948 Nationality Act which granted British citizenship to all members of existing and former British colonies. Some say that the Act was introduced in gratitude to the colonies who helped during the Second World War. Others argue that black people were invited primarily to meet the needs of a growing economy. After the devastation of war, the economy picked up through the 1940s and continued to grow throughout the 1950s.

In response to the need to find workers, particularly for the essential services, the Conservative Government of the time decided to recruit from abroad. The recently established National Health Service and London Transport, for example, canvassed directly in Jamaica and other Caribbean islands. The advertisements themselves eulogized the nature of the work and the prospect of life in Britain. It was hardly surprising then that many West Indian people took up the challenge and welcomed the opportunity of full-time work and the chance to escape the poverty and high unemployment in their own countries. Over the years people from other countries, particularly the Indian subcontinent and East Africa, also came to Britain to seek work and to flee the poverty or political uncertainty of their own lands. At this time all immigrants, as Commonwealth citizens and British passport-holders, were entitled to come to Britain to live and work. Furthermore, they were encouraged to do so by the government.

In the minds of many of the immigrants, the trip to Britain was a short-term venture to enable them to save money and support their families back home, and so improve their basic standard of living. Whatever had attracted them to Britain and whatever they had been led to believe, it is doubtful they expected to encounter racism on the scale that greeted them.

> I love me mudder and me mudder love me
> We come so far from over de sea,
> We heard dat de streets were paved with gold
> Sometime it hot and sometime it cold.
>
> (B. Zepheniah, *I Love Me Mudder*. From *The Dread Affair – Collected Poems*, Arena, 1985, p.36.)

Early difficulties

Immigrant black people faced a number of difficulties when they came to this country at the end of the Second World War. Housing was expensive and rented accommodation was often denied them on the basis of their skin colour or race. Notices saying 'No blacks' or 'No Irish' were commonplace. A few years earlier, in 1943, the Captain of the West Indies cricket team, Sir Learie Constantine, was refused accommodation at the Imperial Hotel in London on the grounds that his colour might offend the other guests. However, when he successfully sued the hotel, he set a precedent and made some inroads into the operation of the 'colour bar' which had been a major issue for some time. The 'colour bar' is a term that refers to the prejudicial exclusion of entry to various private facilities on the basis of colour. It was used by the proprietors of hotels, golf clubs, night clubs and guest houses.

Black people were similarly openly discriminated against in the job market, despite the fact that many of them were skilled workers. They found work mainly in the more menial and lower-paid occupations. As a consequence of these factors there was a strong tendency for black people to settle in the poorer industrial towns and inner-city areas. In a sense they continued to remain cheap 'immigrant' labour.

Once they were established in these deprived and physically decaying areas, the new immigrants were then associated with these surroundings and blamed for the squalor that was truly a result of society's neglect. This association fuelled the racist argument that black people created the decay and decline of certain districts. Furthermore, a worsening of the economic conditions, a rise in unemployment, and an unresolved and deepening housing crisis exacerbated relationships between black and white people.

Black people were obvious and visible targets for the anxiety felt by white people about job and housing shortages, and they were an easy and convenient scapegoat for the social dissatisfaction of the times. This insecurity was fanned by politicians and the press, most famously in the 'rivers of blood' speech made in 1968 by the late Conservative MP Enoch Powell. In his speech he alluded to impending racial violence and the 'swamping' of British culture by 'foreigners'. This theme has periodically been restated, notably by Margaret Thatcher, who referred to 'swamping' in 1979, and more recently by Norman Tebbit MP who, in 1990, questioned the loyalty of black British people with the infamous cricket test speech. He argued that people of Caribbean, West Indian, Indian, Pakistani and Sri Lankan origin would rather support the cricket teams of these countries than England, and thereby insinuated a lack of 'Britishness'.

In 1997 Lord Tebbit revived this argument at a fringe meeting of the Conservative Party Conference, claiming that multi-culturalism was a 'divisive force' and that, referring to black people born in this country, 'one cannot be loyal to two nations'. His views were denounced by the party leadership.

The government responded to the difficulties faced by black people in Britain by attempting to give them some form of protection through the passing of race relations legislation. At the same time, government intervention caused further hardship to the black community through a series of immigration laws which restricted the entry of black people into Britain in a way that could hardly have been envisaged in 1948, and thereby reinforced the idea that black people were a problem.

RACE RELATIONS

The rights of all minorities were formally recognized by the passing of the Race Relations Acts of 1965 and 1968, which were later replaced by the 1976 Act. This legislation sought to make all forms of racial discrimination illegal. The 1976 Act distinguished between 'direct' and 'indirect' discrimination.

Direct discrimination consists of treating a person less favourably on racial grounds – for example, by rejecting all job applicants who do not have British nationality, or by refusing to consider any black job applicants. Treatment based on racial or national stereotypes can constitute direct discrimination (*Racial Equality and the Asylum and Immigration Act 1996*, Commission for Racial Equality, 1997g, p.5).

Indirect discrimination involves the imposition of a condition or requirement which applies equally to everyone, but which is more difficult for people from particular racial groups to satisfy, and which, when balanced against the discrimination that results, cannot be justified – for example, by requiring an inappropriately high standard of English (Commission for Racial Equality, 1997g, p.6).

It was one thing to outlaw overt racist practice, but it was another to eliminate it completely. Some people felt that the Race Relations Act 1976 increased rather than decreased racial tension because somehow black people were seen by some whites as being favoured. Another criticism was that the Act dealt only with overt racism, and had no power over its more subtle forms.

IMMIGRATION LAWS

The Government itself has been charged with racism over its immigration policies. A series of Acts passed between 1962 and 1996 have redefined the status of former British Commonwealth citizens and systematically restricted the rights of black people to enter Britain. The 1981 Nationality Act dispensed with a 900-year right of *ius soli* (the right of soil) – the automatic right of a child born on British ground to be a British citizen. The 1988 Immigration Act restricted non-citizen residents' rights to bring in dependents.

Immigration laws have created undue hardship for many black families because members have been subject to excessive delays while their applications for entry to Britain were being processed. In extreme cases, some Asian women suffered the indignity of having to undergo vaginal examinations in order to establish the validity of their claims to enter Britain – a practice that was stopped in 1979. At a press conference following the report of the Joint Council for the Welfare of Immigrants, Jeremy Corbyn, Labour MP for Islington North, said, 'It's disgusting the way non-white arrivals to the UK are treated. These people are put through long delays and a series of long interviews, often after coming on long flights' *(Guardian, 18 July 1990).*

According to the Commission for Racial Equality, people of some nationalities are more likely than others to be refused entry into Britain. Some ratios of refusals to acceptances were as follows:

- Jamaicans – 1:65;
- Africans – 1:167;
- Europeans – 1:600 (except Poles, for whom the refusal rate was 1:66);
- South Asians – 1:675;
- US citizens – 1:3,437.

(Commission for Racial Equality 1997c, p.3)

Until recently, Britain was a net exporter of people. Almost every year from the mid-nineteenth century more people left the country than arrived in it. Since 1983 the trend has been reversed, and now more people come to Britain than leave it (Table 4.1).

The net increase in residents coming to the UK can be explained by an increase in migration from the European Community and 'other foreign' areas *(Social Trends* classification). Primary immigration from the Caribbean and India and Pakistan ceased long ago. Today most black immigration is of a secondary nature – that is, immediate relatives joining a family that has already settled in this country. New entrants to Britain are predominantly white.

Table 4.1 Migration in and out of the UK in 1994

	Inflow	Outflow
British	118	108
Non-British	135	82
European Union	29	22
Old Commonwealth	20	12
New Commonwealth	32	16
Other foreign	55	32

THE EVERYDAY EFFECTS OF RACISM

I say I'm a black person who lives in Britain. Although I hold a British passport I still don't say I'm a British citizen. I will only say that when I believe I'm treated justly and get fair treatment from this society.

(John Fernandez, college lecturer and a Goan who has lived in Britain for over 20 years, *Asian Times,* 3 March 1989)

No one is born a racist. Racism is learned. However, its influence is felt at a very early age. Young children are aware of the differences in colour between themselves and other children, and they soon recognize which colour is more highly valued by society. There have been examples of young black children scrubbing themselves 'in order to become white'. This point was made by the Commission for Racial Equality, who state in *From Cradle to School* (Commission for Racial Equality, 1989) 'We know from research evidence that by the time they enter primary school, white children may well be on the road to believing they are superior to black people. Black children may believe that society is not going to show them the same respect and esteem that white people receive'. The Commission for Racial Equality adds: 'Such attitudes are not innate, but learned. What is learned before the age of five in race relations is therefore of critical importance to the stability of the next generation and to society as a whole.'

For this reason it is vital that playgroups, nurseries, childminders and schools oppose the dominant culture and message of society and provide young children with surroundings which instil equal tolerance and respect for all cultures. This was emphasized in the 1989 Children Act Guidance 'Children should have the right to be cared for as part of a community which values the religious, racial, cultural and linguistic identity of the child' (Chambers *et al.,* 1996, p.3).

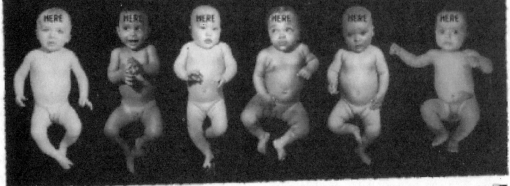

Fig 4.3 There are lots of places in Britain where racism doesn't exist. (Reproduced from Commission for Racial Equality, with permission.)

There are many ethnic minority children in various child-care settings who do not see either themselves or their culture reflected in their surroundings. All children need positive cultural images and role models, and to have their history acknowledged and their identity respected. Particular requirements concerning dietary needs, skin and hair care, religious and other cultural needs have to be met, and all festivals have to be acknowledged and celebrated. Much of this is already firmly integrated into the day-to-day structure of nursery and school provision.

In some cases where all of the staff and children are white, objections have been raised to the development of anti-racist practices on the grounds of it being inappropriate. Such objections miss the point of anti-racism. Children are growing up in an increasingly diverse, multicultural society. As individuals, all children need to cherish and respect their own cultural heritage and be open to embrace the rich diversity of other cultures devoid of any artificial notion of inferiority or superiority. As the Commission for Racial Equality points out, 'it is important to acknowledge that racism damages all concerned; black children may internalize racist messages while white children too are limited by a narrow, ethnocentric environment which denies them the opportunity to develop positive attitudes towards other people and ways of life. Being proud of one's culture is not the same as believing it to be superior.'

The task facing those working with the under-fives is to recognize and eliminate discrimination, and to maximize each child's motivation 'by encouraging his or her sense of being included, personally, racially and culturally, in all aspects of the learning experience'. This is important in order to avoid 'another generation of white children developing a belief that they are superior to or somehow more British than their black peers because of a very narrow, old-fashioned notion of what being black means'.

INSTITUTIONAL RACISM

There are disturbing facts and figures extracted from all areas of British life which indicate substantial evidence of widespread *individual* and *institutional* racism. Individual racism, or *personal racism,* is more easily identified and dealt with, but institutional racism, i.e. the practices and procedures of organizations, including businesses, voluntary organizations, and central and local government departments, is less easily located. Institutional racism is sometimes referred to *camouflaged racism*, meaning that it is not open and visible, but is concealed in practices and procedures.

Sir Herman Ousley, Chairman of the Commission for Racial Equality, commenting on the twentieth anniversary of the Race Relations Act, stated: 'Perhaps one of the reasons why insufficient action is taken to remove discrimination is the lack of understanding and awareness of institutional discrimination, barriers caused by the way things have always worked in organizations'. (From *A mind to work*, Christian Socialist Election 1997, p.4).

Discrimination in employment may be indicated by a failure to create conditions where black people can develop, unrepresentative interviewing panels, failure to advertise job vacancies to all members of the community, and failure to be flexible in terms of leave needs for religious festivals, or to allow more consecutive days (within leave entitlement) to enable visits to families who live outside the UK. These policies are examples of institutional racism and, together with the occurrence of personal racism, in which black people are deliberately excluded by individuals, they begin to account for the under-representation of black and Asian people in many areas of activity throughout the UK today.

BLACK PEOPLE AND POSITIONS OF POWER

It is possible to confirm that we live in a racist society simply by looking around us. That is not to say that we will witness clear instances of racial abuse, but rather we need only consider the lack of prominence of black people in society. In other words, racism is characterized by the absence of black people from positions of power and authority in our

society. In some ways this reflects their general social class position as well. It is well known that working-class people are not often in positions of power and authority.

As can be seen from Table 4.2, black people number over 3 million and represent 5.5 per cent of the population of the UK. They form 6 per cent of the total work-force. By the law of averages, one would expect this percentage to be reflected in all occupations, but this is not the case.

At the general election in 1987 a record number of four black MPs were returned to the House of Commons out of a total of 654. The only previous election of a black MP, Shapurji Saklatrala, was over 60 years ago. In 1996, the then Prime Minister, John Major, admitted: 'The present mix of the House of Commons does not remotely reflect the mix of the country as a whole, either in terms of Asian candidates, West Indian candidates, or indeed the male and female balance of the population' (*Guardian*, 29 May 1996, p.3).

At the 1997 general election the number of MPs increased to nine (out of 659), but this figure is still a distinct under-representation of the black community. Significantly, there were no black cabinet appointments in the new Labour Government.

A similar picture of black under-representation emerges when we look at the number of black councillors, top civil servants, bank managers, bishops and managing directors, who are almost exclusively white and male.

Within the Civil Service black people represent 0.34 per cent of the senior positions (grades 1–5) and Asians represent 1.13 per cent. At senior management level (grades 6–7) the proportions are 0.52 per cent and 1.59 per cent, respectively. However, lower down in the administrative grades black and Asian people are better represented, together forming 7.67 per cent of all administrative assistant posts.

This under-representation of black and Asian people, particularly at managerial level, is replicated in most other industries and government departments.

Table 4.2 Resident population by ethnic group for the UK in 1991

Ethnic group	Number[*]	Percentage of total population	Percentage of total ethnic minority population
All ethnic groups	54 889	100.0	
White	51 874	94.5	
Ethnic minority groups	3015	5.5	100.0
Black groups	891	1.6	29.5
Black Caribbean	500	0.9	16.6
Black African	212	0.4	7.0
Black other	178	0.3	5.9
Indian	840	1.5	27.9
Pakistani	477	0.9	15.8
Bangladeshi	163	0.3	5.4
Chinese	157	0.3	5.2
Other groups			
Asian	198	0.4	6.6
Non-Asian	290	0.5	9.6

Source: Office of Population Censuses and Surveys 1991 Census, published November 1993, the first to include a question on ethnic groups.

[*] Thousands.

> We cannot be a beacon to the world unless the talents of all the people shine through. Not one black High Court Judge or permanent secretary; not one black army officer above Colonel. Not one Asian either. Not a record of pride for the British establishment. And not a record of pride for Parliament that there are so few black and Asian MPs.
>
> (Prime Minister Tony Blair,
> Labour Party Conference,
> 1 October 1997)

BLACK PEOPLE AND THE CRIMINAL JUSTICE SYSTEM

The Law

As mentioned above, black and Asian people are grossly under-represented within the judiciary.

Table 4.3 illustrates this at all levels, and most notably at the highest level, where all judges are white.

'On 31 July 1996 ethnic minorities accounted for 5.8 per cent of solicitors on the roll of the Law Society and 6 per cent of all barristers (representing an improvement over the 1989 figures of 1.3 per cent and 5.3 per cent, respectively)'(*Guardian*, 2 October 1997, p.17). 'Seventy per cent of all judges have been to public school and two-thirds to either Oxford or Cambridge Universities. There has been a rise in the number of black and Asian students entering the legal profession. However, in order to become a High Court Judge at least 15 years experience is required, so change in the courts looks as if it will continue to be slow' (*Guardian*, 2 October 1997, p.17).

In 1995, a relatively high proportion (8.2 per cent) of new appointments of magistrates were either black or Asian, but there were no black justice clerks, and only 17 out of 370 deputy justice clerks and 21 out of 1470 ushers were from ethnic minorities.

The lack of black and Asian judges and court officials has ramifications throughout those who

Table 4.3 Holders of judicial office of ethnic minority origin as at 1 May 1998

Post	Of ethnic minority origin (*n*)	Total	%
High Court Judges	0	97	—
Circuit Judges (including Official Referees)	5	553	0.9
Recorders	13	854	1.5
Assistant Recorders	11	375	2.9
Assistant Recorders in Training	2	106	1.9
District Judges	4	335	1.2
Family Division District Judges	—	18	—
Deputy District Judges	12	740	1.6
Stipendiary Magistrates	2	89	2.2
Acting Stipendiary Magistrates	4	84	4.8
Chairman of Industrial Tribunals (full-time)	3	77	3.9
Chairman of Industrial Tribunals (part-time)	5	195	2.6
Full-time Chairman of Social Security Appeals tribunals	2	57	3.5
Part-time Chairman of Social Security Appeals tribunals	11	497	2.2

Source: Lord Chancellor's Department.

The database may be incomplete as data for the ethnic origin of candidates for Judicial Office have only been collected since October 1991.

work in the courts, including solicitors, probation officers and social workers. This predominance of white, male, middle-class and middle-aged officials can only damage the confidence of the people who appear before judges and magistrates, many of whom are younger and disproportionately from ethnic minority and working-class families.

Offenders

- In 1994/1995, 8 per cent of people starting probation orders and 9 per cent of those starting combination orders were of ethnic minority origin; 42 per cent of black, 43 per cent of Asian and 28 per cent of white offenders were sentenced without the judges having seen a pre-sentence report from the probation service (Commission for Racial Equality, 1997i, p.3).
- In 1995, black people represented 17 per cent of the prison population, an increase of 3 per cent since 1989.
- It can be shown that black and Asian offenders are more likely to proceed through the criminal

justice system and are more likely to be incarcerated than their white counterparts. This is particularly the case for young black men. It has been pointed out that 'there are more young black men in prison than in higher education (Ali Brown, *Independent*, 31 May 1997, p.18).

Staff in prisons

- Only 5 out of 1013 prison officers at governor grade were black or Asian.
- 2.4 per cent of officers at basic grade were black or Asian.

Probation officers

The proportion of ethnic minority probation officers rose from 2.6 per cent in 1989 to 7.6 per cent in 1995. There was also an increase in the number of senior probation officers during this period, from 0.2 per cent to 3.4 per cent, yet in 1995 there were no black or Asian people among 54 chief probation officers.

Black people and the police

The police are alarmingly under-represented by black and Asian people at all levels:

- in 1989 there were 1306 ethnic minority officers in a force of 122 265 (1.06 per cent);
- in 1995 there were 2223 ethnic minority officers in a force of 127 222 (1.75 per cent);
- 158 ethnic minority officers were sergeants;
- 36 were inspectors;
- eight were chief inspectors;
- one was a superintendent.

The white male domination of the police force perpetuates itself because many black and Asian people are reluctant to join an organization which they mistrust and see as inherently racist. The following figures were obtained from *Policing and Race in England and Wales* (Commission for Racial Equality, 1997e).

- 22 per cent of people stopped and searched by the police in 1994/1995 were from ethnic minority groups. In London, 37 per cent of people stopped and searched were from ethnic minorities. (People from ethnic minorities represent 5.5 per cent of the population of Britain and 20 per cent of the population of London.)
- 42 per cent of African-Caribbeans who owned a car had been stopped by the police, compared to 18 per cent of white people who owned a car.
- 64 per cent of African-Caribbeans arrested in the Metropolitan police area were referred for prosecution in 1899/1990, compared to 42 per cent of Asians and 36 per cent of white people.
- 17 per cent of black interviewees in 1994 believed that the police did a very good job, compared to 24 per cent of whites.
- 65 per cent of black pedestrians stopped by the police in 1994 were dissatisfied with the police, compared to 48 per cent of Asians and 30 per cent of the overall population.

Furthermore, the male-dominated 'canteen culture' is both sexist and racist and directed, respectively, at women and black colleagues. According to the Police Complaints Authority 'there was an apparent inability to manage some "gross disharmony" between officers' (*Guardian*, 4 July 1997, p.2). In addition to any racial harassment within the Police Force, there 'were 440 complaints of racial discrimination made against the police, an increase over the previous two years, resulting in the dismissal of four officers'(*Guardian*, 4 July 1997, p.2). Black people were also over-represented among those who died unexplained and inexplicable deaths in police custody (*Guardian*, 4 July 1997, p.2).

BLACK PEOPLE AND THE ARMED FORCES

The under-representation of black and Asian people is similarly illustrated by examination of the make-up of the armed forces:

- in 1994, ethnic minorities represented 1.1 per cent of the Royal Navy;
- in 1994, ethnic minorities represented 1.5 per cent of the Army;
- in 1994, ethnic minorities represented 1.4 per cent of the Royal Air Force;
- 13 out of 100 black applicants were accepted by the Army;
- 5740 out of 21 361 white applicants were accepted by the Army;
- in all services black people are over-represented at or below the level of corporal.

Racial abuse has been endemic within the armed forces:

> The armed forces is a tribal organization and that makes it difficult to accept new ideas and people. That is a good thing for bonding and creating a fighting spirit but it is no good when it comes to civil behaviour.
>
> (Breaking the thin black line, *Guardian*, 5 March 1997, p.3).

Several black soldiers have received compensation for being the victims of racial abuse within the army. One mixed-race soldier, Scott Enion, was the subject of racial abuse from his own officer, while on active service during the Gulf War. He said, 'It was quite ironic really because here I was fighting for Queen and Country and I was getting abuse from my own sergeant'. The Army has recently examined its recruitment and other procedures in an attempt to attract and keep more ethnic minority members. Scott Enion feels that black people will continue to stay away until the Army makes racial abuse a specific offence. He added:

> At times I used to listen to the abuse and feel ashamed. But it wasn't the black side of me that I was ashamed of, it was the white side of me.
>
> (*Guardian*, 5 March 1997, p.3)

BLACK PEOPLE AND EMPLOYMENT

> Ingalan is a bitch deres no escapin it
> Ingalan is abich y'u haffi know howfi suwive in it
> Well me dhu day wok an mi dbu nite wok
> mi dhu clean wok ant mi dhu dusty wok
> dem seh dat black man is very lazy
> but if y'u si how mi wok y'u wouldu sey mi crazy.
>
> (Lynton Kwesi Johnson, *Ingalan is a bitch* in *Tings and Times: Selected Poems* (Bloodaxe Books, 1991))

The overall employment picture further attests to the existence of racial barriers, whether we examine the professions and occupations where ethnic minorities are least visible, the industries where blacks and Asians are more often employed, or unemployment rates.

As the poster designed for the Commission for Racial Equality (Fig. 4.4) crudely indicates, black and ethnic minority people are often over-represented in the more menial lower-paid occupations. This fact is apparent to anyone visiting many inner-city hospitals, fast-food outlets, theatres, cinemas and art galleries, particularly in London, where black and Asian people are disproportionately employed as

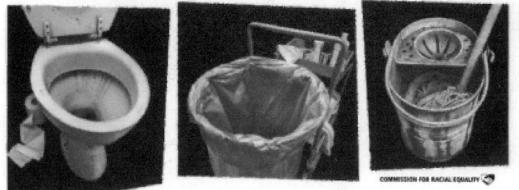

Fig. 4.4 Who says ethnic minorities can't get jobs? There are openings everywhere. (Reproduced from Commission for Racial Equality, with permission.)

service, domestic or security staff. Furthermore, black and Asian workers are more likely than white people to do shiftwork and to work in temporary, seasonal or casual employment.

Table 4.4 shows the occupations in which ethnic minority workers are engaged. It can be seen, for instance, that 34 per cent of Pakistani Bangladeshi men were employed in the distribution, hotels and restaurant industries, compared to 17 per cent of white men. Ethnic minority workers are often found in industries where employment conditions are poor and unsupported by trade unions. Correspondingly, on average, they are less well paid. In 1994, full-time white employees earned on average more than men from all minority groups (*Social Focus on Ethnic Minorities*, p.42).

Black people find it more difficult to obtain employment than white people and, once in work, are less likely to progress as quickly, if at all. The following facts have been extracted from the CRE Employment and Unemployment Factsheet (Commission for Racial Equality, 1997j).

- White applicants are more than four times as successful as black applicants when answering job advertisements.
- Ethnic minority groups experience more than twice the level of white unemployment (18 per cent vs. 8 per cent in 1995/1996).
- It was three times as difficult to get an interview for a job if you were Asian, and five times as hard if you were black.
- Black and Asian employees are having to wait longer than whites for promotion.
- Industrial tribunal cases continue to show discrimination in appointments to professional and managerial grades, just as they do for access to unskilled and casual vacancies.

Furthermore, in a TUC survey conducted in 1997, the following information was revealed.

- 14 per cent of callers to a hot line said that they were more likely to be disciplined than their white colleagues.
- 12 per cent said they were regularly overlooked

Table 4.4 Employment by gender and industry in spring 1995

Great Britain						Percentages
Employees	Manufacturing	Distribution hotels and restaurants	Transport and communication	Banking finance and insurance	Public administration education and health	All industries* (=100%) (thousands)
Males (16–64 years)						
Black	22	18	12	10	25	130
Indian	32	22	13	14	13	178
Pakistani/Bangladeshi	31	34	—	—	—	75
Other ethnic minorities	17	29	9	13	23	108
White	31	17	9	14	15	10 702
Females (16–59 years)						
Black	—	15	—	12	57	146
Indian	29	28	—	13	23	140
Pakistani/Bangladeshi	—	—	—	—	45	30
Other ethnic minorities	—	27	—	11	38	101
White	13	23	3	15	38	9517

* Includes construction and other industries.

Source: Social Focus on Ethnic Minorities, p.42.

for promotion, while better jobs were given to white workers with fewer qualifications and/or less service.

- 12 per cent said that overtime was allocated on the basis of race, with white workers getting more overtime opportunities than black staff.
- large numbers phoned to say that they were the subject of direct abuse, and that when they complained to their bosses they were often told it was their fault and that they needed to make more of an effort to fit in (*Independent*, 10 July 1997, p.4).

BLACK PEOPLE AND THE MEDIA AND ENTERTAINMENT INDUSTRY

The old men running the industry just have not got a clue. They've got to come to terms with the fact that that Britain's no longer a totally white place where people ride horses, wear long frocks and drink tea.

(Marianne Jean-Baptiste, *Guardian*, 13 May 1997, p.2)

Marianne Jean-Baptiste was the first black British person to be nominated for a film Oscar (*Secrets and Lies*), but was excluded from the group of 20 top young actors invited to the Cannes Film Festival fiftieth anniversary celebrations.

The invisibility of black people in the media was most marked in the 1997 TV advert for Vauxhall Astra cars when, of the 2000 babies featured, only one was black and he or she was on the back row. According to Dr Beula Ainley, 'Newspapers also fail to provide a balanced coverage of ethnic minorities with blacks rarely being shown outside their designated roles of sportsman, entertainer or criminal'.

Of the 5000 journalists working on national newspapers, fewer than 20 are black or Asian, and there are only 15 black or Asian journalists on the provincial newspapers, which employ over 8000 journalists. Broadcasting offers better opportunities to non-white people, there being 300 black and Asian people employed in 1997 (*Observer*, 7 July 1997, p.3). This under-representation means that a black perspective is often absent from national comment. Of course, black and Asian people have established their own newspapers – for example, *The Voice* and *The Asian Times* – in an attempt to publicize black and Asian issues, but they are not read widely outside the black and Asian communities.

October 1997 saw the tenth anniversary of black history month, and was marked with a number of events celebrating black people's contribution to the arts and other fields. Taking part was actor Paul Barber, who said, 'I know all about the Saxons and the Normans but nothing about black history because I wasn't taught any at school' ... 'One of my ambitions is to eventually play a black man from British history' (*Evening Standard*, 13 October 1997, p.16).

Supermodel Naomi Campbell said of the advertising industry, 'You've got to understand, this business is about selling, and blonde and blue-eyed girls is what it sells'. A study of TV advertising carried out by the Glasgow media group in 1997 showed that superficially black people were proportionately represented in leading roles in TV adverts, starring in 5.3 per cent of them. However, on closer inspection it was revealed that 'White actors get more lines than their black, Asian or Chinese colleagues. Whites are much more likely to be cast as middle-class professionals, non-whites as sportspersons or to appear in exotic dress or as musicians' (*Observer*, 24 August 1997, p.5). The study also found that 'the most frequently shown white main lead shows a man with responsibility having fun. The most frequently shown non-white advertisement has a poor man doing nothing' (*Observer*, 24 August 1997, p.5).

The media, particularly television, plays an important part in portraying that which, it pleases it to think, our society values. It reflects and creates images. With regard to ethnic minority people, many of these images have been and remain negative. Some impressions of black people are grossly stereotyped cartoons, or they are portrayed as subjects of 'jokes', or they are disproportionately associated with 'trouble'. This type of presentation is not always balanced with positive associations, and black people are not commonly depicted in responsible, authoritative roles. There are very few programmes provided for minority communities, except during off-peak hours, and even these are often directed at an English-speaking audience.

> We live in a multilingual society. But this fact could never be derived from watching television or listening to the radio. There are over 12 languages other than English, spoken in England by a very large number of people. These languages are: Chinese, Arabic, Punjabi, Urdu, Bengali, Gujarati, Hindi, Polish, Italian, Turkish, Greek and Spanish.
>
> (Twitchin, 1988, p.45)

However, the situation is slowly improving, as television companies become more aware of their responsibilities towards all groups in society. Even so, until they operate true equal-opportunity policies they will continue to marginalize black people to a nation that watches an average of 27 hours television per week.

BLACK PEOPLE AND EDUCATION

It has been known for some time that the teacher's expectation of a learner is crucial to that person's progress. This was acknowledged in the education inspectors (Ofsted) report in September 1996. It criticized teachers for misinterpreting black boys' energetic and enthusiastic behaviour as aggressive or threatening, and stated, 'Teachers expected them to achieve little at school. Asian pupils, meanwhile, were seen as quiet and compliant. Not surprisingly, both groups of pupils tended to live up to their stereotypes' (*Independent*, 6 September 1997, p.3). Teacher expectation is not the only factor affecting ethnic minority children's achievement – other factors include social class and poverty.

It can be seen from Fig. 4.5 that only 21 per cent of black children in the study obtained five or more

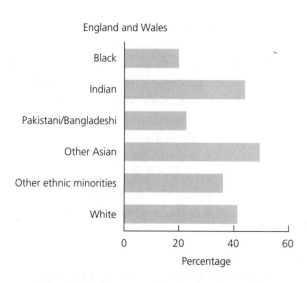

England and Wales

Fig. 4.5 Pupils aged 16 years achieving five or more GCSEs at grades A to C at the end of compulsory education, spring 1994. (*Social Focus on Ethnic Minorities*, 1996, p.34. Reproduced from Commission for Racial Equality, with permission.)

GCSEs at grades A to C. In contrast, the Indian group achieved similar results to the white group, with 45 per cent of pupils achieving at this level, while 51 per cent of other Asian groups gained five or more GCSEs at grades A to C.

The degree of school failure of black pupils can be measured not just by examination rates, but also by exclusion rates. It is now estimated that black boys are six times as likely to be excluded from schools as their white counterparts. Black girls, too, are suffering disproportionate levels of exclusion (*Guardian*, 11 October 1996, p.3).

Young people from ethnic minorities are more likely to stay on after compulsory education has ended. This may in part reflect the difficulty that some black and Asian young people face in finding employment. In the 1994 Youth Cohort Study by the Department for Education and Employment, 65 per cent of Indians and 61 per cent of the Pakistani/Bangladeshi group were still in full-time education, compared to 38 per cent of the white group.

Indians have the highest proportion of young people (6 in 10) with a qualification of at least NVQ level 3 or equivalent. Four in 10 are qualified at the

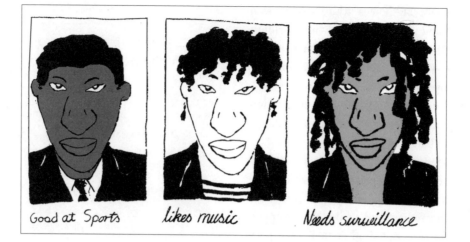

UK School report by Tam Joseph. The faces are painted red, white and blue from left to right. (Reproduced with permission from Sheffield Galleries & Museums Trust.)

same level from both the black and the white group, but only three in 10 of the Pakistani/Bangladeshi group are qualified at level 3. (The Foundation Learning Target level for the year 2000 is that 60 per cent of people under 21 years of age should be qualified at NVQ level 3.)

In 1995/1996 at higher education level, 12 per cent of white women had a higher qualification, compared to 13 per cent of ethnic minority women. However, this figure masks the disparity between the level of education of the different ethnic groups. For instance, over 30 per cent of black African women had a higher education qualification, compared to 6 per cent of their Caribbean counterparts, and nearly 25 per cent of Chinese women had a higher education qualification, compared to only 3 per cent of Bangledeshi women (*Guardian*, 4 February 1997, p.8). 'Black Caribbean men (6 per cent) and Bangladeshi men (7 per cent) were more than half as likely as any other group of men to obtain higher education qualifications' (Commission for Racial Equality, 1997a).

Educational achievement has obvious implications for personal growth, a sense of worth and self-respect, to say nothing of its practical influence on obtaining a worthwhile career of a person's choice. It is all the more important that all children are encouraged to fulfil their potential, and that racial barriers are removed. 'If ethnic diversity is ignored, if differences in educational achievement and experience are not examined, then considerable injustices will be sanctioned and enormous potential wasted' (Donald MacCleod, *Guardian,* 10 September 1996, p.4).

INDIVIDUAL RACISM

Individual racism takes many forms, ranging from looks to verbal abuse, assault, and in some cases even murder. Racism is an ongoing threat to all ethnic minority members in the UK, and it occurs in every-day situations. According to Brian Jacobs, 'For minority groups racism is something which is part of everyday life and it is they, therefore, who are best placed to understand the full implications and effects of it.' (Jacobs, 1988, p.6).

Everyday occurrence

Some black social care students from a London further education college discussed routine experiences of racism.

- Samantha spoke of how a white female shop assistant, whose hand she had inadvertently touched whilst paying for her purchase, unself-consciously withdrew her hand and wiped it against her overall.
- Eloise cited a similar example of being rudely forced away after offering assistance to an elderly white woman who had stumbled.
- Another student, Ramone, feels angry that each time she goes into a department store or large shop she is immediately singled out and asked 'Can we help you madam?', while other shoppers are free to browse and shop at their own pace. (This was a common occurrence for many black women in the group.)
- Others mentioned the experience of being the subject of a lengthy security check, even for cheques made out for very small amounts.
- The group also talked of instances where white women were seen to clutch their handbags closely to themselves in the presence of a black person.
- Hannah, who came to Britain in 1956, felt that racial prejudice had diminished. She remembers the signs 'No Blacks, No Irish' and the difficulties she had in obtaining basic living accommodation when she first came to this country. She talked, too, of her initial puzzlement at the behaviour of young white boys who would approach her and ask her the time. When she looked at her watch and told them, they would then go away disappointed. She later discovered that young English boys expected her 'as a black woman' to look at the sun in order to find out the time.

For other black people racism is still very much a reality. It means being at a job interview and knowing you will not be chosen, or having a vacant seat next to you on a crowded train. For one young man, Andrew, 'it is something I can feel the moment I enter a room'.

The effects of everyday racism can be debilitating, as care home manager Jocelyn Mignott says:

> I get tired of people calling me coloured because they feel it sounds better than black. I get tired of being the only nice black person people have ever met. I get tired of being mistaken for someone else. Take a good look at black people – we don't all look the same. I get tired when relatives of my residents look through me and search for a white officer. I get tired of people who think that to be white is 'normal'. I get tired of people who pay lip-service to the abhorrence of racism yet fail to confront it in their everyday lives.
>
> (*Social Work Today*, 28 March 1988, p.28)

Black people and racially motivated harassment and violence (Fig. 4.6)

> Racial incidents are under-reported. In 1995/96 the police recorded 12 222 racial incidents in England and Wales, an increase of 3 per cent over the previous year; of these, 4 per cent involved serious physical violence.
>
> (Commission for Racial Equality, 1997e, p.2)

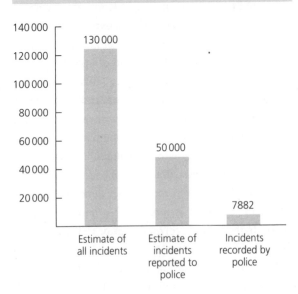

Fig. 4.6 Racial incidents in England and Wales, 1991. (*Home Office Research Findings*, No.39. Reproduced from Commission for Racial Equality, with permission.)

According to the New York - based human rights watch, 'Britain has the highest rate of racially motivated crime in Europe, with nearly one in five crimes suffered by ethnic minorities being linked to the colour of their skin' (*Community Care*, 19–25 June 1997, p.17).

There has been growing acknowledgement of the seriousness and widespread existence of racial abuse. In September 1997, the Home Secretary, Jack Straw, announced that in future judges will be able to pass heavier sentences for any crime which has a racial element. This followed a threefold increase in the number of racial incidents reported to the police between 1988 (when separate statistics were first kept) and 1996. It also followed a number of murders of young black men carried out in separate incidents where the unprovoked attacks were seen to be entirely racial. The brutal deaths of Stephen Lawrence, Michael Menson, Ali Ibrahim Abu Zaid and others serve to remind us all of the horrific extremes to which racism can lead.

Racially motivated offences are more likely than other offences to be carried out by more than one offender – 38 per cent of Indians, 37 per cent of Pakistanis and 14 per cent of African-Caribbeans said that they were victims of four or more assailants. Such offences were more likely to be carried out by white people (98 per cent of racially motivated crimes against Pakistanis), and they were more likely to be perpetrated by men (responsible for 80 per cent of racially motivated offences) (Commission for Racial Equality, 1997f).

There are signs that the authorities are taking action to combat racial violence and harassment. More sensitive handling of abuse allegations is being shown by the police authorities, and Housing Departments are taking action against perpetrators who live on council estates. 'A London Housing Unit survey in June 1997 found that half of London's 33 councils had taken successful legal action against tenants' (*Community Care*, 19 June 1797, p.19). The successful 'Let's kick racism out of football' campaign was launched in 1994, at the professional level, where it was recognized that

although 25 per cent of players in the premiership were black, only 1.6 per cent of the supporters were. Now the message has spread to the amateur level, where local authorities such as Hounslow have threatened to ban from using council pitches any football club that breaks their anti-racism charter. Club secretary and footballer Peter Laxton said, 'Fighting and abuse was a regular occurrence in the league practically every week a few years ago, but it has got better now' (*Guardian*, 12 June 1997, p.4).

CHANGING RELATIONSHIPS BETWEEN BLACK AND WHITE PEOPLE

During the 1960s there was an expectation that black immigrants would assimilate themselves into the established British way of life in the way that immigrants to Britain had done throughout history, i.e. black people were expected to fit into the existing social structures.

By the 1970s, this emphasis on assimilation was recognized as a denial of the value of the contribution that black people made to society. Within educational settings in particular, the importance of people's cultural backgrounds was being recognized and incorporated under the umbrella of multicultural education. Children learned to appreciate differences in food, dress, music, customs and religious festivals. The effect of multicultural education generally increased people's awareness of the rich cultural diversity of modern Britain. However, it did not appear to lead towards a decrease in racism. Put simply, informing people about 'saris, samosas and steel bands' was not confronting the institutional racism of society.

The late 1980s and early 1990s saw a change of emphasis, and the development of anti-racism as an approach aimed at addressing the institutions and organizations within society which, by their very practices and procedures, deliberately or unwittingly perpetuate racism. Many organizations have now made anti-racist statements. In addition to making any racist act a punishable offence, by examining issues such as staff recruitment and selection and by scrutinizing working procedures, organizations are able to rid themselves of those practices which hitherto worked towards excluding black people. For example, colleges with an anti-racist policy will monitor the ethnic origins of students and compare these with the population of the catchment area, consider the ethnic background of the staff at all levels within the hierarchy, and see how this reflects the local population. Educational materials are continually being examined for their possible racist influence and also with the purpose of ensuring that there are positive black images to which black students can relate. Anti-racism is, after all, about social justice. It seeks to eradicate institutional barriers to equality of opportunity that operate against all British citizens whatever their skin colour.

EQUAL OPPORTUNITIES

Owing to the under-representation of ethnic minority people in local authority and voluntary services, many public bodies have sought to redress this balance by implementing equal opportunities policies. Such policies recognize that belonging to an ethnic minority is in itself a positive attribute, particularly when the nature of the work concerns working with ethnic minority communities. Membership, knowledge and understanding of another culture, as well as proficiency in one of Britain's several living languages other than English, is of great value to any organization that wishes to work closely within the community. With regard to staff recruitment, less emphasis may be placed purely on academic qualifications, but relevant life-experience is sought after and acknowledged. Professional standards remain the same but in a situation where, for example, several candidates for a single job are equally qualified academically and only one of them is a member of an ethnic minority, that person is likely to be offered the post in recognition of his or her additional value to the organization.

Positive action can be regarded as a development of equal opportunities which concentrates on equality of outcome. The principle allows an organization to discriminate in favour of a recognized

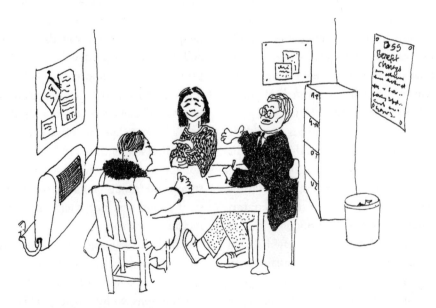

Having knowledge of another language and of another culture is a positive attribute for any health or social work organization.

disadvantaged group. For example, prior to the general election of 1997, the Labour Party established a number of women-only lists at certain constituencies in order to increase the number of women candidates and ultimately to increase female representation in Parliament. This strategy was successful in that there are now a record number of women MPs, although there is some way to go before equal gender balance is achieved. Significantly, there were no black-only lists and the number of black MPs is still disproportionate. In general, positive action aims to reduce past discrimination and to enable previously disadvantaged employees to compete for jobs on an equal footing.

BLACK PEOPLE AND ACHIEVEMENT

You may write me down in history
With your bitter twisted lies
You may tread me in the very dirt
But still like dust
I rise
. . .
From a past rooted in pain
I rise
A black ocean leaping and wide
Welling and swelling and
Bearing in the tide
Leaving behind nights of
Terror and fear
I rise
. . .
Into a day-break miraculously clear
I rise
Bringing gifts that my ancestors gave
I am the hope and the dream of the slave
And so – wow
There I go.

(Maya Angelou, 1986, *Still I Rise.*
In *Complete Collected Poems.* London: Virago, p.41)

This contribution (made by immigrants to Britain and their descendants) is incredibly wide and varied – from the economy, politics and the public service to the law, medicine, the arts and even our cooking. It is a contribution which today forms part of our national identity, and it adds immeasurably to the richness and creativity of modern Britain.

(HRH Prince of Wales, in foreword to *Roots of the Future. Ethnic Diversity in the Making of Modern Britain*, Commission for Racial Equality, 1996)

It is only relatively recently that the long and continued contribution of black people to society has truly begun to be acknowledged. The 'Roots to the Future' exhibition and accompanying book, developed by the Commission for Racial Equality in 1996, explored the part played by immigrants and their descendants in every aspect of the British way of life. It did not merely outline the role of the now better-known black people such as Olaudah Equiano, Samuel Taylor Coleridge, Mary Seacole or Ignatius Sancho, but it also described the hidden contribution of the forgotten black women and men – the soldiers, secret agents, engineers, doctors, chefs, architects, social reformers, scientists and poets. Similarly, it outlined the role of Jews, Huguenots, Poles, Irish and countless other white immigrants who helped to make Britain what it is today.

More recently, the CRE publication *No Limits* (Commission for Racial Equality, 1997d) described the many achievements of ethnic minority women throughout history. It stated:

Individually, ethnic minority women have been pioneers in their own right, pushing back boundaries and breaking racial and gender barriers. Collectively they have provided invaluable, and often unrecognized labour, working in services and industries such as textiles, retail, health and education. Often, too, they have been at the forefront of the pursuit of equality and social justice.

(Commission for Racial Equality, 1997d, p.8)

It then highlighted the specific contributions made by Second World War secret agent Noor Inayat Khan, suffragette Sophia Duleep Singh, political newspaper editor Claudia Jones and Grunwick strike leader Jayaben Desai.

Today, black people continue to make a valuable contribution to society at all levels. There are growing numbers of high-profile achievers in industry, entertainment, sport and fashion. According to Louis Gates Jnr, 'the emergence of a black British culture can now be seen. Black people have turned marginality into an art-form – life-form really – and they have done so at the level of youth culture, of music and of dress. They have styled their way into British culture' (*Guardian*, 19 July 1997, p.1).

Of course, countless numbers of black people also continue to contribute to society both in the outside world of work, in the professions and other occupations, and at home, supporting their families and other individuals in the community.

However, whatever the sphere of activity in which they are engaged, black people's achievements take place in the face of racial barriers which need to be removed. This was recognized by Robert Ayling, Chairperson of British Airways, who recently warned, 'We have thrived, improved and become more wealthy by taking the best of the immigrant community and utilizing their skills. If we can't break down racial barriers between people, we won't work successfully as an organization' (*Independent*, 31 May 1997, p.18).

BLACK PEOPLE AND SOCIAL CARE

In a society where racism is not a side-issue, social work and the social work profession cannot, by definition, be unaffected by racist ideology. It should come as no surprise therefore to find racism operating in the institutions, structures and practices of social work as well as in the personal values of social workers.

(Cook, 1994, p.3)

It is now widely recognized that both Social Services and National Health Service provision have in general failed to meet the needs of the black community. In 1978, the report of a joint working-party made up of the Association of Directors of Social Services (ADSS) and the Commission for Racial Equality stated that the response by Social Services Departments to ethnic minority communities was 'patchy, piecemeal and lacking in strategy'. More recently, in 1989, studies conducted by the Commission for Racial Equality, based mainly on areas with a high ethnic minority population, showed that not all local authorities had fully committed themselves to equal opportunities in service provision – policy implementation was still in its early years. In other words, there had been little advance during the 11 years between the two reports.

More recently, a report entitled *The Social Services Workforce in Transition, 1997* has shown that, while white staff have tended to view their department's equal opportunity policy more positively than black staff, 'Few black staff believe equal opportunities are a reality in Social Services, whatever the rhetorical mutterings' (*Community Care*, 24 July 1997, p.18).

The fact that services have not effectively reached black people is evidence of institutional racism. By and large the policy of Social Services Departments and the NHS has been shaped by white, middle-class males who represent the majority of senior and higher management positions. Within Social Services, ethnic minority people are grossly under-represented at the decision-making level. In 1990 there were only two black male directors of Social Services, and no black women directors. In July 1996 there were still only two black directors (both male) of Social Services Departments out of almost 200 such departments throughout the country, and four assistant directors. There has yet to be a black female director of Social Services.

Black people are under-represented throughout the fieldwork sector and at the managerial level within residential and day-care work. Members of ethnic minorities, particularly women, are more commonly employed in the more basic social care roles of care assistant/officer, home-carer and home-help. This situation is paralleled within the National Health Service, where much of the basic care and domestic work is carried out by black women, and once again black people are less directly involved in decision-making.

Institutional racism within the NHS is evident in the way in which black people are treated in the same way as white people. Because of this there is very little knowledge about diseases specific to black people, and a reluctance to encourage research in this field. This is most clearly illustrated in the case of genetically transmitted diseases such as sickle-cell disease, which until recently has always been regarded as a rare tropical disease of little significance in the UK. There are in fact many sufferers of this disease among people in the UK. It is estimated that 1 in 10 people of African or Caribbean descent has sickle-cell trait (Sickle Cell Society, 1997).

The NHS was criticized in a recent report by the Commission for Racial Equality on the appointment of doctors, which found that people with non-British-sounding names often failed even to obtain interviews, in contrast to similarly qualified people with British-sounding names. The report concludes, 'Although almost every respondent had an equal opportunity policy covering the recruitment and selection process, in almost every case there was a gap between policy and actual practice' (*Community Care*, 24 July 1996, p.19).

Many black carers are themselves subject to individual racism in the form of racial abuse which is sometimes directed against them by patients or clients. This may coincide with society's racism if the management of an establishment has failed to acknowledge the existence of racism, and therefore failed to developed strategies for its elimination. In such circumstances a black worker may be tempted to ignore abuse rather than voice his or her objections and risk being labelled a trouble-maker. When an establishment implicitly condones racial abuse, an employee with the reputation of being a trouble-

maker can find that this adversely affects their job and promotion prospects.

Black staff also experience racism from their own colleagues and managers. 'This was reported by 27 per cent of all black staff, rising to 54 per cent among social work staff and 43 per cent among managers. Furthermore, of those who reported racism, most felt the help available from the employer was less than they needed' (*Community Care*, 9–15 October 1997, pp.20–21).

Josephine Kwhali, former Assistant Director of Lambeth Social Services, and now Director of Focus, a social-care training consultancy, refers to the 'decades of failure of the social work profession to meet the needs of black people' (*Social Work Today*, 17 October 1989). She adds that much serious damage has been done to black families, particularly Afro-Caribbean families, 'in the name of social work intervention'. The disproportionately high numbers of black children who are received into care and the large numbers of black youths who are sent to detention centres are evidence of the harsh consequences which social control agency policies have had on black families. These policies have been founded on prejudicial assumptions about the ability of black families to cope. Cultural differences have often not been acknowledged or explored, and differences in child-care practices have been stigmatized as being automatically inferior or inadequate.

Many black people have been mistakenly labelled as mentally ill by white psychiatrists who have not fully understood the cultural context of their clients' behaviour. This point has been well made by Roland Littlewood and Maurice Lipsedge (1982), whose study on ethnic minorities and psychiatry stemmed from a concern that people from 'Eastern Europe, the Caribbean and South Asia were often admitted to the hospital by their family doctors or by the police under a "section" of the Mental Health Act – that is, as involuntary patients. On arriving in hospital they frequently received the diagnosis of schizophrenia and were seldom offered psychotherapy, usually being treated with pharmaceutical drugs' (Littlewood and Lipsedge, 1982, p.45). The authors go on to say 'we then looked at how the schizophrenia diagnosis was being made and realized that it often conveyed a doctor's lack of understanding rather than the presence of "key symptoms" by which this condition is conventionally recognized by British psychiatrists. Patients appear to be unintelligible because of their cultural background' (Littlewood and Lipsedge, 1982, p.46).

In 1989 Alison Whyte reiterated this point. She asked, 'How can a white, middle-class, male psychiatrist know how a young Afro-Caribbean man expresses grief or how an Asian woman deals with depression?' However, she goes on to state that the answer is not simply one of educating psychiatrists about culture. The problem lies within the racism which permeates our society and what Errol Francis, Director of the Afro-Caribbean Mental Health Association, calls 'the long route to the hospital'. 'The point at which a person is diagnosed,' he says, 'is the last port of call on this route.' If a person is socially disadvantaged and emotionally upset, then every contact with the police, the housing department, the Department of Social Security, social services and other agencies can compound their distress and eventually lead to mental illness (Alison Whyte, in *Community Care*, 20 September 1989 p.23).

Residential social services provision has also been shown to have ignored the particular needs of black people, although there are signs that this situation is being seriously addressed by the more enlightened authorities. In 1988, The Wagner Report commented, 'we have, however, formed the strong impression that ethnic minority communities are almost without exception particularly ill-served by the residential sector and that special provision for them in all its forms is in every way inadequate and in many places virtually non-existent' (National Institute of Social Work, 1988a, p.11). Since then, both the Children Act 1989 and the National Health Service and Community Care Act 1990 have alluded to the need to provide services which reflect a person's cultural need and identity. However, there is no widespread evidence that black people's needs are yet being fully met.

Some ethnic minority communities have learned to expect little support from welfare agencies, due to previous negative experiences. Indeed, among some communities there is a deep-seated mistrust. There is also widespread ignorance of the range and type of services available. Language can be a barrier to some people, and they are not always reached by the information and publicity which are directed essentially at the white, English-speaking public. Among some cultures there is a great reluctance to ask for help, even if the services available are known. This reticence may stem from pride, fear of losing self-respect, or suspicion of white-dominated organizations, or a combination of these and other reasons. However, according to Jocelyn Mignott, officer in charge of a local authority old people's home, the greatest barrier to services reaching all those in need is the assumption held by the caring organizations:

> There is a racist-orientated myth that should be written on the tombstone of every black, elderly person who dies, cold, alone and poor, unaware of the services which could have advanced their later years – they look after their own.
>
> (*Social Work Today*, 24 March 1988, p.28)

The assumption that ethnic minority communities are composed entirely of caring, close-knit, extended families which do not need or require support has meant that many Social Services Departments have failed to make ethnically sensitive provision for the communities which they serve. For example, despite the growing proportion of black elders in this country, very few of them attend local authority day-centres or care homes. They are often put off, partly by the absence of other black service users and partly by the predominance of traditional British activities and fare. Instead, many black elders have turned to the voluntary organizations, the church or local community groups that offer to meet their specific needs.

Some black communities argue for all black services to be delivered by or for black people who, after all, know best about the needs of the service users within their own community. Robin Queshi, Director of Glasgow-based Positive Action in Housing, is campaigning to create housing associations run by people from the communities which they serve, so that Scottish housing policy can incorporate more of a multicultural approach. He says, 'To achieve real integration, you have to have separation at the beginning. We want the government both to support funding for black-led housing associations and to encourage empowerment of our communities. Right now white people are deciding what is best for blacks and they are making a mess of it' (*Big Issue*, 10–16 April 1997, p.35).

Similarly, with reference to social services, Josephine Kwhali points out that black people know what is best for them, and should be given more of a role in developing services that will meet the needs of black service users. It has been recognized that many black community services are, owing to their relative size and minimal resources, not always able to compete with established white independent organizations when tendering for community care commissions.

Josephine Kwhali and others have called for the development of a black-focused sector, not as an alternative, but in order to extend the range for black people who have 'had a bellyful of inappropriate services' (The UK Purchasing Guide, October 1996, *Community Care,* p.5). She points out that in some authorities, such as Hammersmith and Fulham, this has already taken place. These authorities have community care resource centres for Afro-Caribbean and Asian communities, mental health provision and luncheon club facilities. These are well resourced, and are run and managed by black organizations.

Mohan Luthura has said that the widespread development of a black sector would have to be included as part of the economic development process 'if plurality of provision is going to be a reality'. (Luthura, 1997, p.270).

The failure of many Social Services Departments to recruit adequate numbers of foster carers who are representative of the community they serve has meant that many black and ethnic minority children have remained in residential care for longer than was necessary. Within institutional settings the needs of black children have often been neglected – for example, the need to receive proper

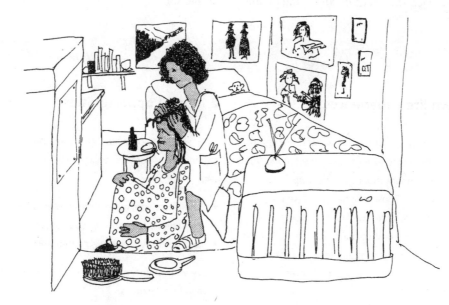

Black children in residential care must have their personal needs met and their cultural identity reaffirmed.

attention with regard to hair and skin care, to meet dietary and cultural requirements and, above all, the need to have their ethnic identity affirmed and respected. Similarly, within foster placements many black children have suffered the disorientation of being brought up by white carers who, however loving they may have been, have not been sympathetic to the children's cultural needs.

In recent years there has been a growing awareness of the damage done by insensitive social work practice, and as a result of this many authorities and voluntary organizations are beginning to establish anti-racist policies and practices. Within some organizations these practices have become integral to the services delivered, while in others they have yet to be implemented. The heightened profile of the black perspective has developed at a time of immense social work change bought about by the Children Act 1989, the National Health Service and Community Care Act 1990, and the developments in training, including the revised Diploma in Social Work, Project 2000, and the vocational qualifications of SVQ and NVQ.

It is to be hoped that anti-racism forms an integral part of these developments, for while the caring services fail to reach the needs of all of the people who make up society, they continue to discriminate against them.

CONCLUSION

We have seen that racism exists throughout society and that it adversely affects the lives of black people daily in many varied ways. At its most extreme it takes the form of physical violence. At other levels it can just be 'felt' by the victims, in the manner in which they are treated and in the way they are looked at or addressed in everyday situations.

It is reasonable to conclude that everybody is to some extent racist, given the influence of being brought up and conditioned by society. It is further suggested that in the UK white racism is the problem. However, it is too simple to suggest that racism is therefore solely a white person's problem. Dialogue between black and white people needs to continue and to be encouraged in order to allow change to occur. As carers, whatever our skin colour, we need to examine our own feelings and attitudes and consider what part we play in the maintenance of racism.

EXERCISES

1. Your own life experiences

Get into small groups of about four or five and discuss the similarities of your broad life experiences – the schools you have attended, the neighbourhood you grew up in and the friends you had, etc. Consider what you have in common. In particular, consider the first time you came across somebody of a different colour to yourself. How did you feel? Were you conscious of the difference in skin colour? Share these observations of the early events in your life with others.

2. Equal opportunities

Does your employer have an equal opportunities policy? If so, find out where the policy is located and with regard to race:

- familiarize yourself with its contents;
- consider its relevance to your organization;
- find out how it is implemented and monitored.

Share your understanding of the policy and its implications with your colleagues.

3. Care environment

> Hospitals are frightening and confusing places for old people from any background; much more so if the staff cannot understand what you are saying and cannot make themselves understood; if you can't eat the food and your body is exposed and handled in a way in which you find shaming and distressing.
>
> (A. Norman 1985: *Triple Jeopardy: Growing Old in a Second Homeland*)

Consider the sentiments expressed in the above statement and apply them to your own work setting. In your care team consider practical ways in which your establishment (or placement) can avoid inflicting such humiliation and distress.

4. Ethnic mix of an organization

Study your own organization. Find out the ethnic make-up of the community in which it is situated. Compare this with the proportion of ethnic minority people employed by your organization or college and the 'racial' mix of the service users or students. Note the level of employment with regard to status and responsibility.

5. Find out about another culture

With regard to any ethnic group, find out all you can about the following:

- dietary needs and preferences;
- special hygiene habits;
- religious practices and festivals;
- practised social activities;
- range of life-styles;
- traditional family structure;
- gender-ascribed roles.

QUESTIONS FOR ESSAYS OR DISCUSSION

1. African slavery and British colonialism are irrelevant to an understanding of racism in Britain today.
2. In Britain only white people can be racist, and black people can only be racialist.
3. How can the caring services more effectively meet the needs of ethnic minority groups?
4. What can individuals, regardless of their own skin colour, do about combating racism?
5. Jokes about minorities are inevitable and harmless. They serve to lighten any potential discord between cultures.
6. Just as it is impossible for men to rid themselves completely of sexism, so it is impossible for white people to eradicate their own racism.

FURTHER READING

Academic sources

Commission for Racial Equality 1996: *Roots of the future: ethnic diversity in the making of modern Britain.*
London: Commission for Racial Equality. A detailed look at the varied contribution made to the development of Britain by immigrants and the presence of ethnic diversity throughout history.

Dalrymple, J. and Burke, B. 1995: *Anti-oppressive practice, social care and the law.* Buckingham: Open University Press. An accessible book that illustrates how the law may be used to support and empower service users.

Dominelli, L. 1988: *Anti-racist social work.* London: Macmillan. A clear account of the value of and need for anti-racist social work.

Fryer, P. 1984: *Black people in Britain.* London: Pluto Press. A comprehensive account of the long history of black people living in Britain, the difficulties they have had to overcome and the significant contribution they have made to society.

Jacobs, B.D. 1988: *Racism in Britain.* London: Christopher Helm. A look at how minority groups have organized themselves to defend their interests in a society that is so often hostile towards the notion of equality of opportunity.

Luthra, M. 1997: *Britain's black population. Social change, public policy and agenda.* Aldershot: Arena. An up-to-date picture of black people's lives in Britain and an analysis of social change.

Other literary sources

Miller, A. 1989: *Focus.* Harmondsworth: Penguin.

Morrison, T. 1989: *Beloved.* London: Picador.

Ngcobo, L. 1988: *Let it be told – black women writers in Britain.* London: Virago.

Roy, A. 1997: *The God of small things.* London: Flamingo.

Sapphire. 1996: *Push.* London: Secker & Warburg.

Wilkomirski, B. 1996: *Fragments – Memories of a childhood 1939–48.* London: Picador.

Films and plays

Jewison, N. 1967: *Heat of the Night.* USA.

Schmultz, O. 1988: *Mapantzala.* South Africa.

Spielberg, S. 1995: *Schindler's List.* USA.

Van Peebles, M. 1970: *Watermelon Man.* USA.

5

Other oppressed groups

INTRODUCTION

Society is divided along a number of other lines in addition to the three major ways already dealt with in detail. It is possible to be a member of a minority on grounds of age, health, disability, life-style or sexual orientation, as well as on other criteria, while also being disadvantaged by social class, gender and race. Thus people may experience *multiple oppression* because they are disadvantaged by being a member of more than one minority. For example, a black, working-class boy experiences discrimination in what is known as 'double jeopardy' – first, from his colour, and secondly, from his class position. Similarly, the term 'triple jeopardy' can be used to describe the marginalized position of black elderly women, who are thereby discriminated against on the three grounds of race, age and gender. The term 'triple jeopardy' was coined by Alison Norman to describe the situation of black elders in the UK today. She states 'they are not merely in double jeopardy by reason of age and discrimination, as has often been stated, but in *triple* jeopardy, at risk because they are old, because of the physical condition and hostility under which they have to live, *and* because services are not accessible to them' (Norman, 1985, p.1). To extend the point further, a gay, elderly, working-class, disabled black woman would experience discrimination on six counts. The opposite is also true of course – a young, heterosexual, middle-class, able-bodied white man has the most to gain from society.

In order to look more closely at some of the other ways in which society is divided, we have selected 13 minority groups. In the first edition of this book we chose to discuss eight minority groups, but we have now added five other groups, namely *carers, asylum-seekers, homeless people, unemployed people* and *offenders.*

Carers, however they are defined, can be seen to be marginalized, and this is evident in their comparatively low status and the lack of support available to them. In particular, carers (formally known as 'informal carers') who are looking after a friend or relative, can be said to be oppressed. Refugees have a history of oppression, often in the country from which they have fled and in this country, too. In recent years social policies and more stringent entry requirements have made life very difficult for asylum-seekers. Offenders and prisoners and their families form another oppressed group. They attract little sympathy and support because they are viewed, in a similar way to other minority group members, as having contributed to their marginalized status, and are therefore regarded as deserving of exclusion.

It is known that over 300 000 people in England and Wales are registered as homeless with local authorities. This figure does not include the majority of single homeless people, many of whom sleep rough in our towns and cities. Homeless people represent a sizeable minority. Unemployed people, too, represent a sizeable group which in recent years has become almost an institution, so much so that it is taken for granted that unemployed people should exist in such large numbers. Their circumstances have been exacerbated by rapid changes in technology and business strategies, such as downsizing.

All of the groups discussed in this chapter are oppressed and socially excluded. We acknowledge that some may have chosen their life-style and may also have been aware that a partially 'marginal' existence might be the result of this decision, the obvious example being that of travellers. However, the majority are victims of political, economic and social processes which result in their being treated as 'outsiders' by society. Although free choice is a factor, once travellers have chosen their life-style the same excluding processes operate.

Such processes include prejudice, discrimination and stigma directed at the groups discussed by members of the wider society and by its institutions (including the National Health Service, Education Service, and Social Services and Housing Departments). A common consequence of these processes is that once society has *victimized* the members of these groups, it then often goes on to *blame* them for their marginalized position. Consider the following examples.

First, unemployment has increased since the 1970s, partly as a result of the decline in large manufacturing industry and more recently due to other changes in technology and a lack of governmental commitment to fuller employment. Many unemployed men and women who are nearing retirement age have found it impossible to obtain alternative employment. Similarly, traditional job opportunities are often no longer available to school-leavers. However, both young and old alike have been stigmatized and have frequently had to bear negative labels through no fault of their own.

Secondly, older people are also blamed for being victims of the ageing process. Because they are no longer economically active they are undervalued. Their past contribution to society is forgotten and their current contribution is ignored. The fact that they require services is often resented by others, and elders themselves can internalize society's image of them as 'burdens'.

Thirdly, many people who experience mental health problems do so as a result of the stress that they experience in their personal lives. However, having a mental health problem is often regarded as a sign of weakness or social failure, and people who experience such problems are blamed because they do not always appear to cope as well as others.

As mentioned earlier, marginalized groups fundamentally lack power. We have seen, for example, how stigma can only be attached to the less powerful by the more powerful. William Ryan has said, 'The primary cause of social problems is powerlessness. The cure for powerlessness is power' (Ryan, 1976, p.250).

Power relationships fluctuate according to changes in the relationship between particular groups of people and wider society. Today there is evidence of more public understanding and empathy towards minority groups. Furthermore, all of the groups we have selected have sought more power for themselves and have adopted a more assertive profile. This has manifested itself in a number of ways. Many self-help groups have been formed to promote their own particular interests, a great deal of publicity and informative material has been produced and there has been an increase in the use of the media, and action has been taken to push for policy and practice changes, in order to influence the personal social services and other welfare agencies.

Examples of such changes can be seen in the application of concepts such as 'role valorization' and 'integration' for people with learning disabilities, and 'community care' policies for a wider range of service-users. This offers a more respectful and independence-promoting alternative to automatic institutional care, although it should be pointed out that residential provision is still appropriate for some people.

There has also been an emphasis on greater user involvement and choice for all client groups. These progressive policy and practice developments have been officially endorsed by recent legislation and a series of charters and codes of practice produced by a wide range of care organizations.

It is not the aim of this chapter to provide a detailed causation of the various impairments experienced by some of the groups discussed, nor does it attempt to discuss in any depth the ageing process, or to provide a detailed history of travellers throughout the world. Such material can be found elsewhere, and there are some indications in the 'Further reading' section at the end of the chapter. Instead, we have concentrated on the social effects of oppression and marginalization on those particular groups which we have selected.

5.1 CARERS

The word *carer* strictly applies to a person providing care for someone at home. However, the description may be extended to include all people who provide 'hands-on' care for service-users in the community in a variety of settings, such as nursing and residential care homes and resource centres. A wider interpretation of the meaning of the word 'carer' may be applied to all those who work within the caring and health professions and who have direct contact with patients and clients. This broader definition will include nurses, social workers, probation officers, those engaged in therapy services, and others. All carers, in particular those people who are caring for a dependent relative or friend, may be said to be in some way oppressed.

This is evident in the lack of adequate resources and support available to carers at whatever level they operate. The absence of adequate support for carers of adults is mirrored by the lack of affordable child-care provision available, and the absence of any significant family or community policies that would make child care more manageable. The lack of resources and proper support reflects the *undervaluing of care* within society.

THE UNDERVALUING OF SOCIAL CARE, HEALTH CARE AND SOCIAL WORK

Social care, health care and social work are all undervalued in our society for a number of reasons, including the following:

- within a male-dominated structure of society care is not a priority;
- care is labour-intensive, and its true cost could not easily be met within a capitalist framework;
- care is not an economically productive activity;
- care is not generally regarded as being skilled;
- care is regarded as a moral duty or vocational occupation.

Social care, health care and social work may be said to be carried out by the following different practitioners and providers:

- *'informal' carers and volunteers* – who receive no remuneration for the support which they provide. People who are caring for a friend or relative at home constitute the largest number of individuals who may be described as carers. Few of them have had any training, and many receive little support as they perform their often very demanding role;
- *health and social carers and support workers* – such as health support workers, care 'assistants', home care-workers, home-helps and community support workers, all of whom may well have a 'professional' and responsible attitude to their work, but are unlikely to have completed any formal professional training. They are more likely to be engaged in, or have undertaken, NVQ Health and Social Care work-based assessment either at level 2 or 3, or both;
- *professionals* – such as nurses, social workers, occupational, speech and other therapists, community

workers, probation officers and others in the caring professions, the majority of whom have undergone professional training and are qualified.

Each of these groups of carers may be seen to be oppressed.

Carers looking after a friend or relative

> I want to start by saying that I do not think I was born to be a carer – I am not very good at it and do not have a very mature or resilient attitude to caring. I take no pride in looking after my husband, in keeping him happy and clean and groomed the way he would have liked, and I am too tired nowadays from always trying to keep one step ahead of him to make as much effort as I once did to talk and reminisce with him.
>
> (Council of Relatives to Assist in the Care of Dementia, 1994, p.1)

The above quotation highlights the point which so many 'informal' carers share – few of them have set out to provide exclusive care for a loved one, and in most cases they have simply responded to the circumstances of a relative or friend becoming seriously ill or disabled and needing support (Rowlands, 1998). Very often the carer is a partner providing care for a long-time or life-long mate, or a daughter or son providing support for a parent or in-law. In all cases, carers begin the task without necessarily having had any experience, let alone training. For some people, caring is a positive experience that brings them closer to the person they are caring for, while for others it is a simply a painful ordeal performed out of love and duty.

With different levels of ability and preparation, 'informal' carers often have to shoulder the main responsibility of providing care. Depending upon where they live and the networks to which they belong, carers may receive varying amounts of support, but for many of them, however gladly the task may be performed, it is often an isolating activity which can demand a huge personal sacrifice.

Numbers of carers

According to the General Household Survey of 1995, there are now 5.7 million carers (Rowlands, 1998). This represents a fall in the number of people who identified themselves as carers. Following the General Household Survey of 1990 there were estimated to be 6.8 million carers. However, since then there has been much more publicity about the role of carers, and the concept of a carer has become clearer. Formerly, some people considered themselves to be carers if they spent up to an hour a week supporting a friend or relative. Nowadays, the word 'carer' is understood to refer to a more substantial commitment, and the current figure of 5.7 million is composed of the 'heavy end of caring'. This means that approximately one in eight adults looks after a friend or relative who cannot cope without help because of sickness, age or disability. Furthermore:

- carers represent a larger labour force than the NHS and Social Services combined;
- some 1.5 million people provide care for more than 20 hours per week;
- almost 60 per cent of carers are women;
- between one-fifth and one-third of carers have provided care for more than 10 years;
- a relatively small proportion of carers (up to 51 000) are under 18 years of age, most of them caring for a parent (Carers' National Association, 1997, p.1).

Young carers

A young carer is defined as:

> a child or young person (under age 18) who is carrying out significant caring tasks and assuming a level of responsibility for another (adult) person, which would usually be taken by an adult.
>
> (Department of Health, 1997a, p.1)

Growing numbers of young people are providing care for a family member. They may be involved in the following tasks, as identified by a recent study:

- personal care;
- physical care;
- paperwork;
- practical care;
- keeping them company;
- taking them out;
- giving them medicines;
- keeping an eye on them;
- looking after siblings;
- role reversal' (i.e. bringing themselves up);
- 'emotional labour' (Social Services Inspectorate, 1997, p.3).

Young carers may support adults with physical disabilities, mental health problems or problems with substance abuse. The nature of their work will vary. Often the practical element of the care that they give may be the most straightforward to supply. It may be more difficult to provide emotional and psychological support.

It has been recognized that, although each young carer is different and able to cope with different levels of care, many of them are particularly vulnerable. They may gain some maturity, satisfaction and sense of worth from their responsible role, but this may be achieved at a cost to their own growth and development.

Some recurrent problems associated with young carers are outlined below:

- isolation from peer group and extended family, due to the amount of time that they devote to caring;
- impaired educational development – 20 per cent of young carers are missing school and 28 per cent show signs of educational difficulties;
- lack of time for usual childhood activities, again due to the amount of time spent caring for an adult;
- conflict between the caring role and the child's own needs, leading to feelings of guilt and resentment. The average age of young carers is just 12 years;
- feeling that there is nobody there for them, and that professionals are working with the adult;

only 5 per cent of young carers had been assessed under the Carers (Recognition and Services) Act 1995 according to a survey carried out by the Carers' National Association in 1998;

- lack of recognition, praise and respect for their contribution – 57 per cent of young carers are girls, and their contribution may simply be 'expected' of them;
- feeling stigmatized – this could be due to any of the disadvantages that often accompany disability, such as poverty;
- feeling that no one else understands their experience – caring can be quite isolating;
- lost opportunities and limited horizons – the time and commitment that are devoted to caring restrict the young carer (Social Services Inspectorate, 1997, p.5).

Despite the difficulties outlined above, it is wrong to view a young person's caring for an adult as being an exclusively negative experience that robs them of their childhood. Children often derive satisfaction from their caring role and from their responsibility and influence within the family. They may feel loved and needed, and gain insight and maturity, self-esteem and independence. However, it is vital that they receive support and that their social life and educational development are not adversely affected.

Legislation exists to provide support for young carers, namely the Children Act 1989, the National Health Service and Community Care Act 1990 and the Carers Act 1995. However, as has been indicated, there are not always sufficient resources available to implement the Acts in full.

Owing to heightened awareness of the plight of young carers, more is now being done to support them through the establishment, nation-wide, of different projects which are variously aimed at raising awareness, identifying support mechanisms and encouraging joint working between voluntary and statutory care agencies. Such projects provide practical advice and support, drop-in facilities, 'time-out' sessions, peer-support groups and individual counselling.

Adult carers

They are not, of course, in the employment statistics, despite many working longer hours than most employees, and they apparently contribute nothing to our national wealth, as they are not included in the conventional definition of gross national product. Yet they are worth at least 30 billion each year, according to modest estimates of their value.

(Malcolm Wicks, *Guardian*, 3 April 1996, p.7)

Emotional difficulties

Carers have to try to deal with the emotional demands of tending a loved one and perhaps of having to stand by as they gradually deteriorate. Depending on the severity of the illness of the person being cared for, the carer may have to assume new and unwanted roles. For instance, they may increasingly have to take decisions on behalf of their loved one. These may range from the many simple, everyday decisions that we are accustomed to making for ourselves, such as when to eat, when to rest and when to go to the toilet, to more complex decisions such as the amount of personal care to organize or, ultimately, where the person being cared for should live.

The act of caring itself often distances the carer from their own network and can make them feel isolated in their activity. In addition, the physical and mental strain of permanently caring for another person, the distress of sometimes observing personality changes and physical deterioration, and the need to appear strong for the person they care for, can generate untold stress for any carer. The following is an extract from the account of a doctor's wife, who is still caring for her husband who was diagnosed 5 years previously as a 'younger' sufferer from Alzheimer's disease.

At times I have plumbed the depths of despair – indeed I never knew it was possible to feel so ill and physically sick from stress and on the occasions take

antidepressants sometimes for months at a time. It is a cycle of worry, grief, exhaustion, self-pity, respite – the consultant who prescribed the drugs says there is nothing to be done for me or my husband. I know there is nothing physically wrong with me; it is the consequences of the situation and the fact there is so little support for either of us that makes me feel the way I do.

Five years ago I was gripped by fear; now it has turned to numbness. I worry that I have lost the ability to feel. I have become insensitive to others' suffering and am intolerant of the children's what I see as trivial problems, and cannot offer them the support a mother should. When a very dear friend, herself widowed in her thirties, died last summer after a seven-year battle against cancer, I found I couldn't even cry at her funeral. It seems I am so numb I can only cry for us. Or to be precise, for me. Selfish as this may sound, all the pity and deep sorrow I felt for him when we first faced this daunting challenge has evaporated a little more with each passing year; I am numbed by what is happening to him but full of self-pity for me and I know that is wrong.

(Council of Relatives to Assist in the Care of Dementia, 1994, p.4)

Lack of support

The absence of sufficient support is the lament of all carers. Local authority social services may carry out an assessment of the person being cared for, and varying levels of support may ensue. Voluntary organizations such as Cross-roads and the Leonard Cheshire Foundation provide services, as do the social services themselves. Alternatively, services may be bought in from the private sector.

However, not all carers are aware of all the services that are available to them, and those who are may receive support only up to a certain minimum level. Indeed, not all carers recognize themselves as 'carers' who are entitled to help and support – they see themselves as merely performing the duties and obligations of a loving relationship.

Lack of support is often a greater problem for members of ethnic minorities, especially if they speak very little English.

> I used to be all alone with Somailya while my husband was at work. . . . Having no one else to turn to I knew it was my responsibility to find out about help available from services. It hasn't been easy and I have struggled for years. Not knowing the language has meant that I could not go directly to services to ask for help but had to always arrange to make contact with someone who could speak English. My husband was at work at night and too tired in the day. My son was at college. So it was not easy finding someone to translate for me.
>
> (*Improving services for Asian people with learning difficulties,* Mental Health Foundation, 1996, p.20)

Figures show that black and ethnic carers make less use of the facilities available, and this may also be because those services are inappropriate for them.

Naseem Khan writes that 'for black and Asian carers, the situation has specific features that many feel have still to be fully recognized. On the one hand, there is the isolation, the loss of old familiar support mechanisms and a comprehensible cultural matrix. On the other, there is – ironically – a stereotype of black and ethnic communities that can impede provision. These groups, it is said, are better than white communities at looking after their own elders. So a sensitive service, it can be argued, should not try to duplicate what is believed to have been set up informally' (*Guardian*, 10 September 1997, p.9).

She adds that black carers can be reluctant to send their charges to day centres because 'the food is not right' or there is 'no space for saying regular Muslim prayers'. Similarly, all health visitors and home-helps need to be aware of certain appropriate ways of behaving such as 'taking shoes off in an Asian person's home or not shaking hands with men if one is a woman'. Finally, she says, 'It's not just

about halal food and skin care, it's about a delivery service that is totally equable'.

When care is provided by organizations, carers need to know that good-quality, reliable support is being offered. They expect their loved one to receive the same standard of care and attention that they themselves provide. Only when the substitute care is of a high quality can the carer properly enjoy any period of respite.

Carers have the right to expect appropriate support, but this is not always the case. Stanley Sheinwald, in a letter to *The Carer*, revealed his own experience:

> I look after my wife Gillian, who suffers from an advanced state of multiple sclerosis causing her to become easily confused. Recent Social Services changes mean evening calls are now undertaken by outside agencies, which has caused utter chaos.
>
> Every night we have a different care worker, so there is no continuity. I have to show each worker where everything is and how to handle my wife, which does not help me at all.
>
> These care workers are not trained in dealing with mentally and physically disabled patients. I find this most distressing. Some of the agencies use students waiting to go to university who are not trained and do not understand nursing. Surely social services has a duty to make sure that carers have trained careworkers and to ensure continuity is maintained. In the past I have always had a call between 7.30 and 8.00 p.m. Lately they have arrived as late as 10.00 p.m. – after my wife has gone to bed.
>
> (*The Carer*, January 1998, p.8)

Financial difficulties

Most carers may experience financial difficulty in order to carry out their task. This is inevitable where care is full-time and the carer has had to give up his or her paid occupation in order to look after a sick or disabled person. Any welfare benefits that are available relate solely to the needs of the person being cared for, and do not compensate the carer for his or her loss of earning.

In *Caring for Dementia* (Council of Relatives to Assist in the Care of Dementia, 1994), the point is made in more detail:

> working as a carer is unpaid and brings no status or contract of employment. Many people give up their paid job or reduce their hours to care for someone. They miss out on job opportunities and face the prospect of financial hardship because they have no chance to build up savings or a pension. What is more, carers often cash in insurance policies or eat into their savings to help meet the extra costs of caring.
>
> (Council of Relatives to Assist in the Care of Dementia, 1994)

The financial hardship will normally intensify the longer the caring relationship exists, and will therefore adversely affect carers who are engaged full-time in long-term caring relationships. As the Carers' National Association emphasize, the financial cost of caring for someone may be far-reaching: 'The economic consequences are horrendous, because you lose an income now and build up poverty for yourself in the future' (*Independent on Sunday*, 15 March 1998, p.4).

THE CARERS' (RECOGNITION AND SERVICES) ACT 1995

To a certain extent the Carers' (Recognition and Services) Act 1995 formally acknowledged the plight of carers, and it entitled them to a separate assessment in order to establish their need for support. However, the Act was implemented in 1996 without any extra funding, so it has yet to make a profound impact. At least the Act has symbolized the raised profile of those who care for an adult at home, and is a tribute to the many years of campaigning

carried out by carers' organizations such as the Council of Relatives to Assist in the Care of Dementia (CRAC Dementia) and the Carers' National Association (CNA).

Many authorities are busy trying to raise the profile of carers. For instance, the Social Services and Health Commissioning Agency for Westminster had, as one of its priorities for 1996, the establishment of a carers forum in order to reach a wider number of carers, and to improve the information and support available to them. In the Community Care plan it published some of the issues raised through consultation with carers.

Where a local group of the Carers' National Association exists, carers may meet for support. Alternatively they may form their own group. The value of a support group for carers lies in the opportunity to express themselves and to share their

- Carers want to be represented in joint planning
- Carers want to be involved in planning, service delivery and monitoring
- Carers from black and minority ethnic communities may have particular difficulties in accessing services (and in recognizing themselves as carers)
- Advocacy schemes and support groups are needed for carers
- More research information is needed about carers' needs
- There is a need to improve GP recognition of carers
- Carers have difficulties in getting assessments
- Carers want more choice and control over respite and relief care
- Carers say that they need more services based in the home
- Carers want accredited assessors to assess the carers' needs
- Carers feel that they are under pressure to keep people at home for longer than they want

Fig. 5.1 Issues raised by carers to Westminster Social Services, Health and Housing in 1996. (Reproduced from *Community Care Plan for Westminster 1996*, p.27.)

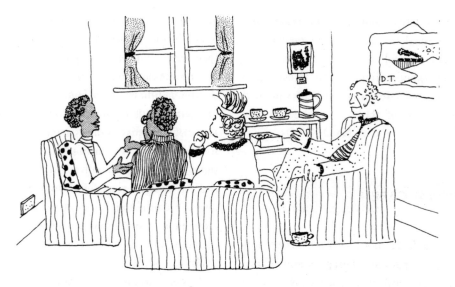

Carers can derive mutual benefit and support from regular meetings.

problems and learn from each other. For some the group can be a great source of confidence and support. In particular, Nick Fielding outlined the special value of an all-black carers' group, one of several black, Asian or Chinese carers' groups which have been set up throughout the country:

> The group gives the opportunity for its members to discuss their problems and to share them – realizing that someone else has to deal with similar issues can often be uplifting. It also allows the members to socialize, share recipes and discuss issues relating to the black community or home background which they may feel constrained to mention in an predominantly white group.
>
> (*Community Care*, 11 January 1990, p.15)

HEALTH AND SOCIAL CARE WORKERS

The work undertaken by paid care staff, including home-helps, care workers, support workers and health support workers, complements and overlaps the contribution of both those who care for a friend or relative at home and professionally trained workers. Yet it attracts some of the lowest rates of pay and is performed in some of the poorest working conditions in the country. It is almost exclusively carried out by working-class women, a disproportionately high number of whom are from ethnic minorities, and much of the work is part-time or on a short contract. Increasingly it is being performed by agency care staff who may experience even poorer conditions of service, including lower overall pay, lack of sick or holiday leave and job insecurity. Indeed, the increased use of temporary agency care staff is often disruptive for the service-user, who may be forced to accustom him- or herself to accepting care from yet another stranger for an indeterminate period. Reliance on agency staff may also reduce the effectiveness of team work and ultimately adversely affect client care.

The care task is commonly assumed to be unskilled, yet if it is carried out properly it demands a high level of commitment, skill and awareness. The practical task of providing personal care may at some times be routine, strenuous, repetitive and even unpleasant. However, in order to ensure that a service-user's dignity, culture and identity are respected, and that the person being cared for participates as much as possible in their own care, carers need to use good communication skills, show compassion, sensitivity and understanding, and demonstrate physical and emotional resilience. It is a skilled and complex role that many adults, mostly men, would be neither willing nor able to perform.

To a certain extent care work has been validated and the skilled nature of the work has been recognized with the introduction of NVQs/SVQs.

PROFESSIONAL CARE

At the professional level, social workers, nurses, probation officers, occupational therapists and others, along with teachers, now experience a low level of public regard. They are relatively poorly paid compared to other professionals, such as solicitors, accountants and architects. In terms of pay and working conditions they have fallen a long way behind their fellow public servants, e.g. their counterparts in the police force, and their salary structure does not match that afforded to many workers.

Nurses have traditionally been poorly paid and have always worked long and unsociable hours. This is reflected in the high staff turnover rate and high vacancy rate in many health settings. In January 1998, a UK record low level of recruitment take-up was announced, with the recognition that 'young women and men were now taking their skills elsewhere'.

A high proportion of social workers, particularly those who are graduates, have been engaged in several years of full-time or part-time study, before and after their 2 years of professional training, yet they are unlikely to be paid as well as many of their university contemporaries. The fact that professional social work training is expected to be completed within 2 years of full-time study, compared to 3 years throughout most of Europe and other parts of the world, shows a disregard for its complexity and value. Some social work functions, notably diagnostic, intake and care management, may now be carried out by people who have not necessarily received any formal social work training. The recent decision to withdraw the requirement

for probation officers to complete the Diploma in Social Work can be seen as an undervaluing of the care component of their work.

The media should bear some responsibility for the low public profile of nursing and social work. It has quite rightly been ready to highlight instances of abuse of care that have occurred within nursing and social work settings, but it has castigated (with hindsight) social workers both for action they have taken and for actions that they might or 'should' have taken. Health and social work includes risk and judgement. Consequences cannot always be predicted, so inevitably it is possible to make the wrong decision, which may have a tragic outcome.

It is easy to pillory individuals with no regard for the context in which decisions are made. Instances of successful, purposeful intervention that result in enabled independence, of which there are many, are not considered to be newsworthy events, and therefore do not appear in print.

THE PRIVILEGE OF CARE

Why, if such work is so undervalued within society, do so many people involve themselves in the care of others, either through their paid work, as nurses, social workers, support workers and home carers, or voluntarily, by caring for a friend or relative? It may be claimed that any job satisfaction gained from successful intervention in the life of another, that results in a person achieving an enhanced degree of independence or an improved level of support, outweighs the stress and frustration of the job. However, not all paid carers remain in their jobs for long. Indeed, there is a relatively high rate of staff turnover in many health and social work posts. Some workers leave the field altogether because the stress of operating with limited resources within a structurally unequal society is too great. Indeed, in 1996 a senior social worker successfully sued his employing local authority social service department for causing him to have a nervous breakdown.

For health and social care workers and carers of a friend or relative, the satisfaction derived from meeting patients', service-users' or a loved one's needs in a respectful, caring and efficient manner sustains them and makes their task worthwhile. Otherwise it would be more difficult to tolerate the related low status and often poor working environment.

Such individuals may be said to be engaged in *the privilege of caring for another.*

However much society may devalue care, it still has its intrinsic worth both for those who are employed to care, and for those who do so voluntarily or because there is no realistic alternative. Paradoxically, the personal circumstances of some carers have produced unknown resourcefulness and helped to promote personal growth within themselves.

> When you care for someone you reach a point of intimacy where you can see through their eyes and that's a privilege.
>
> I am strong – sometimes – and have become more independent and assertive.

> Actually I've grown physically and mentally stronger during the time I've been caring for my husband.
>
> (Elkington and Harrison, 1997, p.7)

For some carers there is a deepening of their relationship with the friend or relative for whom they are caring.

> I love the lady very much and so I'm happy to care for her.
>
> I never really felt as if I knew my mother very well when I was growing up. Having to care for her has helped us grow closer to one another.
>
> (Elkington and Harrison, 1997, p.7)
>
> I find that being a carer is a very positive experience. It has meant that I have been able to spend more time with my wife, and by being at home has given me the opportunity to watch my son grow up.
>
> (*Carers' Voice* (North of England), Spring 1998, p.6)

5.2 DISABLED PEOPLE

> Increasingly in recent years disabled people have come to recognize that the term 'disability' represents a complex system of social restrictions imposed on people with impairments by a highly discriminatory society. To be a disabled person in modern Britain means to be discriminated against.
>
> (Barnes, 1991, p.1)

LANGUAGE, DEFINITIONS AND TERMINOLOGY

Over the past 20 years, disabled people have become increasingly aware of how certain words and terminology act to perpetuate discrimination. 'Disabled People's International', a world-wide organization controlled and organized by disabled people, defined the key terms involved. It made a crucial distinction between *impairment* and *disability.*

- *Impairment* is the functional limitation within the individual caused by physical, mental or sensory impairment.
- *Disability* is the loss or limitation of opportunities to take part in the normal life of the community on an equal level with others due to physical, social and attitudinal barriers.

This difference in definition is illustrated by two examples:

- being unable to walk is an impairment, whereas being unable to enter a building because the entrance is up a flight of steps is a disability;
- an inability to hear is an impairment, whereas an inability to communicate clearly because appropriate technical aids are not available is a disability.

The British Council of Organizations of Disabled People (BCODP) further adds that, 'While we agree that some people have impairments it is not these impairments which "disable" us. What disables us are the barriers and attitudes which separate us from the rest of society. The fact that you can't walk is not the problem – the problem is inaccessible schools, colleges, transport, housing and discrimination in employment' (*BCODP Annual Update*, 1995, p.1).

> 'Disability' can therefore be described as the oppression which people with physical, mental or sensory impairments experience as a result of prejudice and discrimination. It is society's reaction to people with impairments that disables them. This is why the term *disabled people* is preferred to the term *people with disabilities*. The term *able-bodied* is a misnomer because it implies that *non-disabled people* do not have physical limitations, which in fact they all do. More importantly, the term 'able-bodied' distracts attention away from unhelpful social reactions, which are the true disabling agents. This preferred terminology is integral to the 'social model of disability'.
>
> (*BCODP Annual Update*, 1995, p.1)

THE SOCIAL MODEL OF DISABILITY

The traditional model of disability is known as the 'individual' or 'medical' model of disability. In Michael Oliver's words, this 'sees the problems that disabled people experience as being a direct con-

sequence of their disability' (Oliver, 1990). Thus the onus is placed on the disabled person, and the implication is that she or he has to adapt to society, to make the best of a situation and to accept the imposed limitations.

More recently, the 'social model' has become accepted (Fig. 5.2). Again, according to Michael Oliver , 'adjustment . . . is a problem for society, not for disabled individuals' (Oliver, 1990, p.23). Here the onus is on society to adapt to the needs of the disabled person and to cater for these needs as much as possible. As Colin Barnes says, the 'social model of disability . . . shifts the emphasis away from individuals with impairments towards restricting environments and disabling barriers' (Barnes, 1991, p.ix).

Tables 5.1 and 5.2 contain two sets of questions which reflect the 'individual' and 'social' models of disability, respectively. Table 5.1 is a list of questions taken from a face-to-face interview schedule used by the Office of Population Censuses and Surveys in a 1986 survey. In Table 5.2 Michael Oliver has provided an alternative list, utilizing the 'social' model of disability.

Many people, agencies and institutions, including those involved in health and social care, still use language that is no longer acceptable to disabled people. Organizations of disabled people have expressed their disappointment that even the recent Disability Discrimination Act 1995 (DDA) contains a definition of disability which equates it with impairment. The Act defines disability as 'a physical or mental impairment which has a substantial and long-term adverse effect on a person's ability to carry out normal day-to-day activities' (The Disability Discrimination Act – Definition of Disability; Minister for Disabled People, 1997, p.2).

However, there are plenty of positive indications that people and organizations are becoming more aware of language and its implications. To give just one example, the large voluntary organization working with people who have cerebral palsy changed its name from 'The Spastics Society' to the more posi-

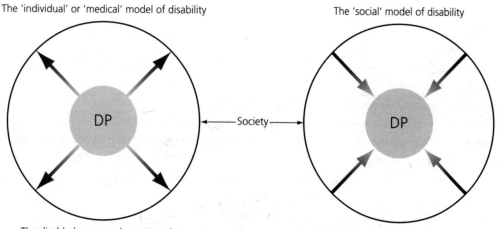

The 'individual' or 'medical' model of disability

The 'social' model of disability

The disabled person adapts to society

Society adapts to the needs of disabled people

Fig. 5.2 The 'individual' or 'medical' model of disability, compared with the 'social' model. The inner circle represents the disabled person, and the outer circle represents society.

Table 5.1 Questions used in the Office of Population Censuses and Surveys *Survey of disabled adults* (1986) reflecting the 'individual' model of disability

- Can you tell me what is wrong with you?
- What complaint causes your difficulty in holding, gripping or turning things?
- Are your difficulties in understanding people mainly due to a hearing problem?
- Do you have a scar, blemish or deformity which limits your daily activities?
- Have you attended a special school because of a long-term health problem or disability?
- Does your health problem/disability mean that you need to live with relatives or someone else who can help to look after you?
- Did you move here because of your health problem/disability?
- How difficult is it for you to get about your immediate neighbourhood on your own?
- Does your health problem/disability prevent you from going out as often or as far as you would like?
- Does your health problem/disability make it difficult for you to travel by bus?
- Does your health problem/disability affect your work in any way at present?

tive sounding 'Scope' in 1994, despite the risk that its charitable donations would decrease as a result of the public not being familiar with the new title. The renamed organization did lose funds initially, and it is working towards re-establishing a reputation for positive and creative work with disabled people under its new title.

How many disabled people are there?

The European Union estimates that one in 10 community citizens has a serious physical or mental impairment. This proportion of disabled people is the same for the world population, as well as the population of the UK. This means that just over 6 million people in this country are disabled, 4.3 million (over two-thirds) of whom are over the age of 60 years.

Table 5.2 Michael Oliver's 11 questions reflecting the 'social' model of disability

- Can you tell me what is wrong with society?
- What defects in the design of everyday equipment such as jars, bottles and tins causes you difficulty in holding, gripping or turning them?
- Are your difficulties in hearing people mainly due to their inability to communicate with you?
- Do other people's reactions to any scar, blemish or deformity you may have limit your daily activity?
- Have you attended a special school because of your education authority's policy of sending people with your health problem or disability to such places?
- Are community services so poor that you need to rely on relatives or someone else to provide you with the right level of personal assistance?
- What inadequacies in your housing caused you to move here?
- What are the environmental constraints which make it difficult for you to get about in your immediate neighbourhood?
- Are there any transport or financial problems which prevent you from going out as often or as far as you would like?
- Do poorly designed buses make it difficult for someone with your health problem/disability to use them?
- Do you have problems at work because of the physical environment or the attitudes of others?

Disabled people and deprivation

The Disability Alliance, which represents more than 100 voluntary organizations, has published material on deprivation suffered by a large proportion of disabled people. It reports that around two-thirds of disabled people (4 million people) are living at or below the poverty line. It also states that disabled people of working age are twice as likely to be living on or below the poverty line than are their non-disabled counterparts. Thus the hardship faced by most disabled people is twofold. They face practical difficulties which result from their physical impairment, and in addition they have to deal with related material hardship and deprivation.

The overwhelming dependence of disabled people upon state benefits, and the difficulties that so many of them experience in finding paid work, inevitably often lead to severe financial hardship. This is compounded by the expense associated with being a disabled person, as they may have to pay for aids to physical mobility, household adaptations, medical treatment or special diets. Although there is some state support to meet such costs, it rarely covers them in full. Consider, for example, the cost of a new basic-model wheelchair for a teenager, which is a minimum of £600. A teenager may need more than one wheelchair, depending on his or her interests. A light sports model can cost over £2000. Disabled people's experience of poverty also leads to an over-representation of disabled people in the so-called 'underclass'.

People with a physical impairment

One of the most significant features of impairment is its diversity. It may affect a person's *mobility* to the extent that she or he may need a wheelchair in order to move around, it may be a *sensory impairment* of sight, hearing or speech, or it may be *a subtle or complex neurological disorder* resulting from a stroke, spinal cord injury or epilepsy. Not all impairments are obvious – many are not visibly discernible, so it is not always apparent that a person is disabled.

The cause of impairment also varies widely. A condition may be inherited or it may be congenital (i.e. the person is born with an impairment, but it is not inherited). Accident, illness or disease may also cause impairment, and these can occur at any time in life. Ageing itself is a process that often brings with it impaired functioning as people slow down and experience a weakening of their powers.

Impairment is distributed fairly evenly in terms of class, gender and race, and it spans all ages although, as we have said, it is more common among people over 60 years of age. Not only do disabled people have to cope with the impairment itself, but they also have to deal with non-disabled people's reactions to their impairment. At best, of course, these can be helpful, sensitive and mature. At worst, they can be patronizing or prying, often motivated by voyeuristic curiosity. The 20-year-old radio programme for and about disabled people, entitled 'Does He Take Sugar?', took its title from the patronizing way in which disabled people were often addressed.

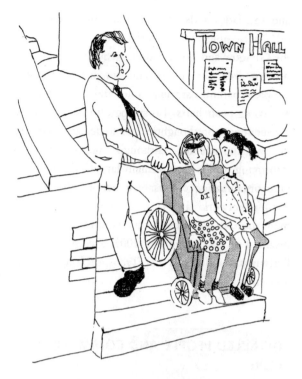

Not all public buildings are yet accessible to all people.

Mobility and access

> It's part of our culture that architects and developers are trained to build for an elite which is male, fit and aged 18–45 . . . The further you are from the stereotype, the more difficulties you have.
>
> (John Penton, architect, quoted in *Guardian*,
> 2 September 1989, p.4)

One of the chief obstacles to facilitating the integration of physically impaired people is that of 'access'. To many disabled people kerbs and steps represent an effective barrier to everyday mobility. Although all new shops and offices must now be fully accessible, other public buildings need only be accessible on the entrance floor. These may include cinemas, theatres, sports and leisure complexes. Some professional football grounds do not cater for visiting disabled supporters. Only four Premiership clubs have more than 100 wheelchair spaces. In London, our largest city, only 38 per cent of museums and 20 per cent of cinemas are currently adapted for wheelchair access (*Guardian*, 2 September 1989), and almost all of them insist that a disabled user has a non-disabled companion with him or her.

During the day of the general election, 1 May 1997, Scope carried out research into access for disabled people to 1272 polling stations in 50 different constituencies. Access for visually and hearing impaired voters was scrutinized, together with that for voters using wheelchairs. Only 6 per cent of polling stations were fully accessible to a wheelchair-user; 94 per cent had at least one access problem, and 81 per cent had two or more. The most common barrier to access was steps, while dangerous ramps, slippery floors and steep approaches presented other hazards. Scope's report, entitled *Polls Apart 2*, concludes that thousands of disabled people were disfranchised by being unable to vote. Some were even subjected to the indignity of having ballot boxes brought outside the polling station for them (*Guardian*, 16 July 1997, p.8).

Some relatively new transport systems, such as the Tyne & Wear Metro in the north-east of England

and the Docklands Light Railway in London, are fully accessible. The majority, however, including the Glasgow and London underground systems, can present great difficulties, and not just to disabled people – parents carrying babies and small children and using pushchairs also struggle to deal with the consequences of thoughtless, male design. Taxis are mostly non-adapted, although the situation is improving, while buses remain largely inaccessible. One organization of disabled people, the 'Direct Action Network' (DAN), is calling on the government to make *all* buses and trains fully accessible to disabled people by the year 2007. The group's publicity material declares that 'Transport is a right, not a privilege'.

DISABLED PEOPLE AND COMMUNITY CARE

> Historically, disabled people have been perceived as clients of social services. . . . This perception has slowly started to change.
>
> (Henry Enns, Executive Director, Disabled People's International, quoted in Barnes, 1991, p.vii)

Positive practice in social care involves fully endorsing and utilizing the 'social model of disability'. It involves working with and listening to disabled people themselves as well as organisations *of* disabled people. The ethos of community care – enabling and empowering people to live independently in their home and to take as full a part as possible in the life of their community – is congruent with the 'social model'. More than 1.2 million disabled people currently rely on home-care services provided by or purchased by local authority Social Services Departments. These services include home-helps, personal care, adaptations to the person's home and telephones.

The relationship between disabled people and local authorities has recently become troubled by a legal judgement. Under the Disabled Persons (Services, Consultation and Representation) Act 1986, Section 4, a disabled person has the right to an assessment of his or her needs, as covered by Section 2 of the Chronically Sick and Disabled Persons Act 1970 – for example, practical help in the home, help with transport to activities such as lectures, games and recreational events, adaptations to the home, holidays and provision of a telephone. However, on 20 March 1997 the House of Lords ruled in an appeal hearing by Gloucestershire County Council that the Council could take into account its own finances when assessing the needs of people who had approached it for help. This means that local authorities do not have to provide services if they do not have the resources, regardless of established need.

'Needs Must' is a coalition of over 30 organizations, set up to overturn the ruling on behalf of disabled people, older people and their carers. The organizations include Age Concern, the Carers' National Association, Mencap, MIND, RADAR and Scope. The ruling threatens the quality of life of many disabled people, and will force some into residential care because they will not be able to cope by themselves at home without the necessary support services.

Following the introduction of community care provision from April 1993, assessment became very important. As the 5-year anniversary approached, research was carried out by the Joseph Rowntree Foundation into how assessment arrangements affected disabled people and their carers. The authors of the report described the assessment process as a 'way to bring disabled people closer to purchasing decisions, empowering them and providing individualised, flexible responses to need' (*Community Care*, 11–17 December 1997, p.24). However, the research revealed very varied experiences of Social Service Departments' intervention: 'Access to assessment for most disabled people and their carers produced feelings of uncertainty, marginalization and exclusion. Most people described encounters with social services departments as confusing, fragmentary and often irrelevant to their most pressing concerns' (*Community Care*, 11–17 December 1997, p.24).

In contrast, the authors continued, 'where assessment practice was informed by a commitment to partnership with disabled people, it was well understood and highly rated'. One of their conclusions was that more disabled people should be employed at all levels in Social Services Departments. They support this view by saying that: 'Disabled people and their carers were especially responsive to disabled practitioners'.

Social Services Departments also have a role in facilitating disabled people's quality of life by liaising closely with other local authority departments, e.g. with the Housing Department to ensure that appropriate accommodation is available. In working to this end, Social Services Departments are supporting a disabled person's basic human right to live independently within her or his own community. Jenny Morris has said: 'It is clear that disabled people rely primarily on local authorities for access to the housing necessary for independent living' (Morris, 1990, p.23). However, appropriate housing is not always available within the local authority, and Social Services Departments are still having to place young people and adults 100 miles or more away from their own homes – into residential care – due to the absence of appropriate provision.

DISABLED PEOPLE AND ANTI-DISCRIMINATION LEGISLATION

Charity and Social Services are not enough to remove the discrimination that disabled people face in their societies. In Britain, the . . . charity model has become a double-edged sword. Not only has it failed to attack discriminatory practices but it has developed the myth that disabled people are well provided for.

(Henry Enns, Executive Director, Disabled People's International, quoted in Barnes, 1991, p.vii)

Services provided for disabled people through the 'mixed economy of care' would be more relevant to their needs and more accountable to them if they were supported by effective anti-discrimination legislation. There have been many attempts to introduce such law, but all of them have failed. When legislation that aimed to establish rights for disabled people was finally passed in the form of the Disability Discrimination Act 1995 (DDA), it was universally received with little enthusiasm.

The Disability Discrimination Act 1995 (DDA)

The 'Disability Alliance', which has over 100 member groups, was particularly critical of the Act: 'We believe it falls far short of the comprehensive civil rights legislation which the disability movement has campaigned for' (Paterson, 1997, p.10). The Director of the Royal Association for Disability and Rehabilitation (RADAR), Bert Massie, stated: 'It is not the Act disabled people wanted. Some argue we would be better to have no legislation at all' (*Community Care*, 22–28 February 1996, p.8). David Reubain, a disabled solicitor who has run workshops on the Act, is aware of widespread user dissatisfaction. He has been involved in drafting civil rights law for disabled people and presenting it to government. His own conclusion on the DDA is that 'It has provided some remedies for some people, but, because of the way it is so heavily qualified, it is not an effective piece of legislation and does not give comprehensive and enforceable civil rights to disabled people' (*The Lecturer* (*NATFHE*), December 1997, p.11).

However, despite the overwhelming disappointment felt by disabled people about the Act, the DDA has introduced new rights for disabled people, specifically in the following areas:

- employment;
- access to goods and services;
- selling or letting land or property.

Employment

It is now illegal for an employer to treat a disabled person less favourably than someone else because of their 'disability', unless there is good reason to do so. This applies to all aspects of employment, including recruitment, training, promotion and dismissal. A major criticism of the DDA in relation to employment is that it only applies to 4 per cent of employers – that is, those employers who employ 20 or more people. It has therefore effectively legalized discrimination for the remaining 96 per cent of employers.

The first person to win an employment case under the DDA was Barbara Tarling, a factory worker from Suffolk, whose Industrial Tribunal took place in May 1997. She had been dismissed from her job after 18 years, in January 1997, because a worsening of her physical impairment had led to what her employer claimed was a 'poor performance'. Barbara was reinstated to her job and received £1200 in compensation (*Disability Now*, June 1997, p.1).

An important reservation about the implications of cases like that of Barbara Tarling (and others) has been that she had the backing of a powerful trade union – the Transport and General Workers Union (TGWU). Other disabled people who have gone to a Tribunal with no union backing have not always been successful.

Access to goods and services

It is now against the law to refuse to serve a disabled person because of reasons relating to their impairment. For instance, it is illegal for a supermarket manager to refuse to serve someone who shops more slowly as a result of their impairment.

Furthermore, it is illegal to offer a disabled person a service which is not as good as, or is on different terms to, that provided for other people. For example, a restaurant owner cannot insist that a person with a facial disfigurement sits out of sight of other customers.

Selling or letting land or property

The Act makes it illegal for people selling or letting land or property to discriminate against disabled people. For example, a property owner (including a landlord) must not charge a disabled person a higher deposit against damages, more rent than other tenants, or a higher price for a property.

Other criticisms of the DDA

- The Act has been criticized because it is based on a limited *functional* definition of disability. Someone who is HIV-positive, but is 'symptom-free', is excluded from the Act. Similarly, someone with multiple sclerosis, if 'symptom-free', is also not covered. An exception is made for someone with Down's syndrome – although they may have only a mild learning disability, which does not impair their functioning, they have been singled out because their condition is instantly recognizable.
- The Act requires colleges of further and higher education to produce *'disability statements'* that set out what a particular college offers to disabled students in terms of access and specific facilities and resources. However, it does not stipulate minimum levels of provision in these establishments, nor does it enhance the rights of children and young people in schools.
- The Act set up a 'National Disability Council' which is regarded as being too weak in that it only has *advisory* powers and not *enforcement* powers, equivalent to the 'Equal Opportunities Commission' and the 'Commission for Racial Equality'. The Council does not even have the power to assist individuals at Industrial Tribunals.

Causes for optimism

There are three reasons to be optimistic about the future with regard to anti-discrimination legislation.

1. It is anticipated that case law will push back the boundaries of the DDA and that the role of the Trade Unions will be crucial in the process of

winning significant advances for disabled people and creating legal precedents.

2. The Labour Government set up a Ministerial task force in 1998 to recommend improvements which will strengthen the DDA and secure enforceable civil rights for disabled people.

3. The Government has also announced that it will replace the National Disability Council with a 'Disability Rights Commission' which will ensure that the law is enforced.

THE DISABLED PEOPLE'S MOVEMENT

> All over the world, disabled people are uniting to demand their rights.
>
> (Henry Enns, Executive Director, Disabled People's International, quoted in Barnes, 1991, p.vii)

A combination of disillusionment with traditional political activity and dissatisfaction with services provided *for* them, by a whole range of agencies and organizations, led to the creation of the disabled people's movement. Encouraged by movements of women and black people and the introduction of anti-discrimination legislation relating to them in the 1970s, disabled people set about forming their own organizations. In addition, Michael Oliver has identified two other specific events which provided further impetus.

- The first was the United Nations designation of 1981 as 'International Year for the Disabled'. The title itself was considered patronizing, and only after a great deal of pressure from disabled people themselves was it changed to the 'International Year of Disabled People'. As Oliver says, 'That did not stop many of the planned events from reinforcing the charitable images of disabled people'. However, disabled people set themselves the task of exploiting the opportunity that the International Year of Disabled People offered them, and formed their own national,

umbrella organization, the 'British Council of Organizations of Disabled People' (BCODP) (Oliver, 1990, p.115). From an original total of six groups, BCODP now represents over a hundred.

- The second event was a conference held in 1981, organized by 'Rehabilitation International' (RI), an organization for disabled people, at which its charter was discussed. The central aim of this was 'to take all necessary steps to ensure the fullest possible integration of, and equal participation by, disabled people in all aspects of the life of their communities' (quoted in Oliver, 1990, p.116). At the end of this conference the RI declined to turn itself into an organization of, and controlled by, disabled people. In response, 'Disabled People's International' (DPI) was formed and became the international equivalent of BCODP.

Disabled people themselves became very aware of the difference between the more traditional organizations *for* disabled people (e.g. RADAR, RNIB and Scope) and those *of* disabled people, such as BCODP. The latter type of group aims to be democratic and representative of the views of disabled people, and to promulgate the 'social model of disability'.

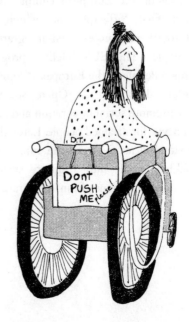

INDEPENDENT LIVING

> Independent or integrated living is a basic civil right of disabled people, empowering them to be self-reliant, to live as they choose and to participate in their communities.
>
> (Morris, 1990, p.1)

Disabled people should have the right to choose to live independently if they so wish. The pressure to empower disabled people to live independently has been gaining momentum over the past few years, to the extent that there is now an 'Independent Living Movement'.

In April 1989, at the 'Strasbourg Independent Living Conference', disabled people from 14 different countries drew up a Resolution, part of which reads: 'Independent living . . . encompasses the whole area of human activities, e.g. housing, transport, access, education, employment, economic security and political influence. We disabled people, recognizing our unique expertise, derived from our experience, must take the initiative in the planning of policies that directly affect us' (quoted in Morris, 1990, p.31). These sentiments are echoed in the Social Charter of the European Union (EU), the twelfth and final 'principle' of which states: 'Improved social and professional integration for disabled people.' The EU's 'Helios' programme ('Handicapped People in the European Community Living Independently in an Open Society') is designed to 'promote social integration and an independent lifestyle' for disabled people. Later, the programme extended its focus to the integration of young disabled people into 'ordinary systems of education' (all quotations from Hantrais, 1995, p.128).

PERSONAL ASSISTANCE

> I wanted to leave home three or four years before I actually did so. The main problem of moving was obtaining the assistance I need. Personal assistance, the help we need to sustain our daily living, isn't seen as a human right, it's seen as a privilege. This is very wrong, very tragic because it is so fundamental to us.
>
> (Richard Shaw, Personal Assistance Officer, Derbyshire Centre for Integrated Living, quoted in Morris, 1990, p.19)

In 1997, the BCODP launched the 'National Centre for Independent Living' (NCIL), which is based in London but operates country-wide. Funded by the Department of Health, one of its aims is to promote the idea of personal assistance as part of independent living. NCIL defines 'personal assistance' as 'the personal help or support a disabled person requires in order to achieve the same range of opportunities and activities as a non-disabled person, both at home and away from it. This can include day-to-day activity – dressing, cooking, reading, driving, bathing your children; and also spontaneous activity – a business trip, tidying up the garden, joining a language class or visiting old friends' (Ford *et al.*, 1997, p.5). Support schemes have been set up to help disabled people with information, advocacy, peer support and training if they wish to employ their own 'personal assistant'. These schemes can exist under a range of titles, including 'Personal Assistance Support Schemes', 'Independent Living Support Schemes', 'Self-operated Care Schemes' and 'Centres for Independent Living'.

Funding personal assistance

There are two main sources of funding:

1. Social Services Departments;
2. the Independent Living (1993) Fund.

preserve public office or simply to keep discrimination at bay. Andrew Sulivan, author, referred to a point in his own adolescence: 'In that moment, you learn the first homosexual lesson; that your survival depends on your concealment' (*Guardian*, 9 October 1995, p.2). As a result of this, the true proportion of the population who are gay is not known, but it is commonly estimated to be between 10 and 20 per cent of the population. In general, homosexuality has been forced to be expressed in secret, and this has given it a certain mystique which makes it appear a less common form of sexual orientation than it is, and this reinforces society's prejudice.

> For after all, there are millions of gays in England – and not all dress designers and ballet dancers, but practical people like civil servants, hospital workers and school teachers.
>
> (Colin MacInnes, *New Society*, 23 October 1975, p.224)

The climate of acceptance for gay people has changed in recent years thanks to the work of gay activists, gay and lesbian organizations and individuals who have been prepared to make a stand in public. In 1984 Chris Smith declared, 'My name is Chris Smith, I'm the Labour MP for Islington South and I'm gay'. In so doing he became the first openly gay MP of his generation, and has since been followed by two more male MPs and a lesbian MP, Angela Eagle, who had found 'coming out' 'personally quite difficult early on', but in 1997 felt that 'times have changed and the best option now is just to be open about it' (*Guardian*, 21 October 1997, p.4).

In contrast, within the Church of England, the only openly gay bishop, the Rt Rev. Derek Rawcliffe, was sacked for conducting same-sex blessing ceremonies in October 1996. Furthermore, it is estimated that there are over 2000 gay vicars (one in five) (*Observer*, 13 July 1997, p.1) and about 'half the church of England's 44 Diocesan bishops have knowingly licensed or ordained actively gay priests' (*Observer*, 13 July 1997, p.1). The church is not only

contravening its own teachings that 'lifelong homosexual relationships were acceptable among the laity but not the clergy', but also denying the human right of personal individual sexuality to its clergy.

LANGUAGE

Homosexual is the word used to describe the relationship between people of the same sex. 'Homo' comes from the Greek language and means 'the same', and not from the Latin meaning 'man', and is therefore applicable to both women and men. *Homophobia* describes 'the fear and resulting contempt for homosexuals' expressed by *heterosexuals* (people who are attracted by people of the opposite sex). *Heterosexism* is used, like the words racism and sexism, to describe prejudicial attitudes and actions towards homosexuals. In relatively recent times the term '*gay*' has been adopted by many homosexual women and men as a positive assertion of their identity and pride and is used instead of the more neutral word 'homosexual'. The current use of the word 'queer' by gay people shows how an instrument of oppression can be successfully hijacked and given a new meaning with positive connotations.

AREAS OF DISCRIMINATION

> We have had the Race Relations Act since 1965, a Sex Discrimination Act since 1975, and a Disabilities Act since 1995, but discrimination on the grounds of sexuality is still not barred by statute.
>
> (Martin Bowley, *Guardian*, 15 April 1997, p.17)

Age of consent

Until the passing of the Sexual Offences Act 1967, acts of homosexuality between men were illegal in England and Wales. This was later extended to both

Northern Ireland and Scotland in 1983 following separate European Court rulings. Before this date engaging in homosexual acts was a crime punishable by imprisonment, even if it took place 'between consenting adults'. Between 1967 and 1994 homosexuality between men has been legal only in private and between men over the age of 21 years. (It should be pointed out that 'in private' is defined as a private house – a hotel room, a prison or a hostel are not private in terms of the law.) At present the age of consent for gay men is 18 years. The age of consent for heterosexual sex in the UK is 16 years. (Sex between consenting females over the age of 16 years is only against the law in the armed forces.) A recent European court ruled in 1997 that to have different ages of consent for heterosexuals and homosexuals was discriminatory. The test cases, of Euan Sutherland and Chris Morris, are 'stayed' pending another age of consent in the November 1998 to July 1999 session of parliament.

The UK and Finland are the only European countries which have differing ages of consent for heterosexuals and homosexuals, as shown in Table 5.3.

'Section 28'

An additional legal restriction on the lives of gay people was introduced under Section 28, more pop-ularly known as 'Clause 28', of the Local Government Act (1988) (Fig. 5.3).

Essentially this act states that a local authority shall not 'intentionally promote homosexuality'. According to the National Association of Probation Officers (NAPO) good practice guidelines produced in May 1989, 'to contravene the Act would require a deliberate attempt to increase the prevalence of homosexuality. No local authority or probation

---

1 *A local authority shall not:*

- Intentionally promote homosexuality or publish material with the intention of promoting homosexuality

- Promote the teaching in any maintained school of the acceptability of homosexuality as a pretend family relationship

2 *Nothing in subsection (1) above shall be taken to prohibit the doing of anything for the purpose of treating or preventing the spread of disease*

It does not apply to secondary school teachers or governors who are responsible for sex education. No case has been brought against a local authority for infringement of Section 28.

Fig. 5.3 What the Act says: Section 28.

Table 5.3 Age of consent (years) for heterosexuals in Europe

Country	Male/female	Female/female	Male/male	Equal since
Belgium	16	16	16	1985
Finland	16	18	18	—
France	15	15	15	1982
Greece	15	15	15	1987
Italy	16	16	16	1889
Malta	12	12	12	1973
San Marino	14	14	14	1865
Slovenia	14	14	14	1977
Spain	12	12	12	1822
UK	16	16	18	—

Source: Independent, 15 July 1997, p. 1.

committee could introduce any measure which could change people's sexual orientation' (National Association of Probation Officers, 1989, p.5). The paper continues, 'Section 28 does not provide any legal basis for discrimination nor does it prohibit or restrict the supply of counselling, advice, support or information services to lesbians and gay men. None the less, Section 28 has inflamed prejudice and bigotry and encouraged further discrimination against lesbians and gay men in their family, working, social and personal lives' (National Association of Probation Officers, 1989, p.5).

The armed forces

Gay people are still officially banned from serving in the armed forces in case sexual orientation would affect discipline. Yet gay men and women have always served their country and continue to do so, even if their sexual orientation is not always made explicit. 'Terry Gardiner is one of a growing number of gay ex-servicemen who, after years of silence, are revealing their wartime memories to expose the "hypocrisy" of Britain's continuing ban on homosexuals in the armed forces'. He says, 'It's frankly ridiculous to suggest that gays cannot serve their country'. According to 'Outrage' '. . . the ban on homosexuals went mainly unenforced during the Second World War. Army war reports make no mention of homosexuals undermining morale. If lesbians and gay men could serve then, why can't they now?' (*Observer*, 9 November 1997, p.8).

GAY SEX OFFENCES

In a letter to the *Guardian* (9 March 1990, p.18), Peter Tatchell, a former prospective Labour MP, pointed out that more gay men are prosecuted in this country than in any other nation in Europe, and that 'the number of gay men hauled before the courts is

greater today than it was before the passage of the 1967 Sexual Offences Act which supposedly legalized male homosexuality'. He added, 'In England and Wales during 1988, 23 men over the age of 21 were imprisoned for consenting and often loving relationships with other men aged 16 to 21 years', and that 'in the year earlier, 41 gay teenagers [*sic*] aged 16 to 21 years were prosecuted for consensual homosexual acts, with one of the youths being sentenced to 12 months custody'.

However, since the early 1990s, there has been a noted improvement in the relationship between the police and the gay community, following the formation of both the London Lesbian and Gay Initiative and the Lesbian and Gay Police Association in that year. 'Nationally, prosecutions for gay offences have declined . . . and are currently running at less than half the level of 10 years ago' (*Guardian Society*, 26 November 1997, p.2).

OFFENCES AGAINST GAYS AND LESBIANS

In much the same way that proposed criminal legislation, introduced in 1998, has made racial harassment or violence a crime and is expected to outlaw race-related crime, police forces now record anti-gay and anti-lesbian assaults as a separate category of 'hate crime'. In 1997 there were 244 such cases within the first 9 months of the new recording system being in operation (*Guardian Society*, 26 November 1997, p.3).

Violence is something gays have to guard against, for in the streets of many towns and cities 'attitudes towards homosexuals are light years away from those in the trendy bars of London's Old Compton Street or Manchester's Canal Street' (*Guardian*, 30 August 1997, p.38). According to Kevin Toolis, 'queer-bashing' is prevalent but the crime remains invisible because incidents of assault are not always reported. However, the deaths of several gay men have occurred in this country as a consequence of unprovoked physical assaults. The roots of violence are endemic in society's attitude towards homosexuals.

> Homophobia does not spring from nowhere. We grow up in a society where 'poof' and 'faggot' are common insults even in the school playground. I remember being bullied in my Edinburgh comprehensive school. 'You're a fucking poof, Toolis', said my tormentor. Neither myself nor the bully knew what a 'poof' was, apart from its designation as inferior otherness. 'Tell me you're a poof or I'll bash your head in', he said. I must have been 12, but even then I knew that a beating now was far better than a capitulation to his definition of otherness and a hundred beatings to come. I said nothing and took the beating. It was a very big, virtually all-white, all-Catholic school. The only way to divide us was to invent labels, us and poofs. We did not have to look far. The vocabulary was ready for us, waiting. This schoolyard homophobia was my first introduction to the weapons of prejudice. Is it the same for today's 12 year olds?
>
> (*Guardian*, 30 August 1997, p.39)

OTHER AREAS OF DISCRIMINATION

Lesbian and gay couples are not allowed to marry and, as a consequence of this, same-sex couples are discriminated against in several other areas, including the following:

- immigration – a gay man or lesbian whose partner comes from outside the EU has no right to have that person live with them in the UK;
- pensions – many pension schemes provide for a widow's or widower's pension if the pensioner dies before his or her spouse, but in these schemes a gay or lesbian partner can never benefit;
- fringe benefits – employers provide fringe benefits in respect of a husband or wife or heterosexual partner, but refuse to apply the same

benefits to same-sex partners. Some firms have equalized these benefits in recent years, e.g. John Lewis (staff discount card);
- tax – married couples can transfer as much property as they like from one to the other without paying capital gains tax, but same-sex couples cannot do this;
- inheritance – lesbians and gay men can be thrown out of their home by their partner's family if their partner dies without leaving a will;
- adoption – a lesbian couple cannot adopt their own child in order to formalize the relationship between the child and the non-biological parent, and in cases where they do succeed in adopting, only one of them becomes the legal parent;
- next of kin – same-sex partners cannot be each other's next of kin;
- housing – lesbian and gay couples do not have the right to succeed to all council or private sector tenancies (abridged and extracted from Stonewall, 1997a).

CAUSES

Much has been written about the possible 'causes' of homosexuality, although the same question is rarely asked of heterosexuality. Heterosexuality is assumed to be the norm from which all other forms of sexuality deviate. Homosexuality is sometimes thought to be biologically determined, but society has always considered it to be a sickness and has tried to treat it as such. However, it is less common nowadays for psychiatrists and others to try to counsel gay people out of their orientation, although this was the case in the 1950s, 'when prisoners were given electric shock treatment and crude aversion therapy in an attempt to make them heterosexual' (*Times*, 28 November 1997, p.8). Others take the view that homosexuality is culturally determined – that it is acquired through social influence, and society's solution in this case is to try and limit the influence of gay culture or to apply behaviour-modification techniques in order to enable a gay person to 'unlearn' her or his sexual orientation. For others, gayness is seen as a choice made by individuals, and in this case society expects gay people to accept the consequences and to tolerate society's antagonism. There has been no satisfactory explanation as to why people are gay, and in a sense the question is irrelevant, because it is merely one form of sexual orientation. According to the British Medical Association, 'Most researchers now believe that sexual orientation is usually established before the age of puberty for both boys and girls' (*Guardian*, 8 January 1997, p.7).

'COMING OUT'

The phrase 'coming out' is used to describe the process by which homosexuals figuratively 'come out of the closet' and openly declare their sexual orientation and confront society's prejudice. 'Being out does not mean becoming flamboyant, funny, extra caring or changing one's personality. It means being positive about being gay; it means telling people; stopping people (generally men) from telling anti-gay jokes; and generally trying to educate people about what being gay means' (*Community Care Supplement*, 25 June 1987, p.6).

This description of 'coming out' was made by an 'out' gay man working in a relatively safe environment. For other gay people, 'coming out' can mean revealing one's sexual orientation only to a few close friends. There are therefore varying degrees of self-disclosure. The term 'outing' is used to describe a recent practice carried out in America, where gay groups deliberately expose a prominent person's hitherto undeclared gayness. This is done in order to lend credence to the homosexual community and to help break down the prevailing stereotypes. It is argued that the more gay men and women there are who come 'out', the more usual homosexuality will seem, and as a result there will be more positive role models with which young gays can identify.

The bestowal of a knighthood on the actor Sir Ian McKellen in 1991 marked an important breakthrough for gay people. He was the first 'out' gay person to have been granted such an honour. However, his acceptance of the knighthood was greeted with hostility among some gay people. Many were astounded that Sir Ian could accept an honour from a Government that had introduced anti-gay legislation such as 'Clause 28', and had contributed generally to the oppression of gay people in society. Others supported and applauded Sir Ian's nomination and his acceptance of his knighthood, feeling that it was a step towards society's fuller acceptance of gay people and that it highlighted the irrelevance of a person's sexual orientation when judging her or his talent.

Held back by 'the weight of society's disapproval', Sir Ian McKellen came out rather late in his life. According to him, 'Coming out is a journey. It can be accomplished quickly or slowly – in my case when I was 49'. Until then he had managed to 'dodge the assumption from strangers' about his sexuality. There was more hostility towards gays in his younger days than there is now, although negativity persists today. 'Research by the London Gay Teenage Group revealed that 11 per cent of young gay men and lesbians were told to leave by their parents when they came out' (*Roof*, September/ October 1994, p.13). Despite his struggle, Sir Ian McKellen says of his coming out, 'It was the best thing I've ever done. Better than playing Macbeth or Iago' (Sir Ian McKellen, *Face to Face*, BBC2, 1998).

RESISTANCE

In June 1969, outside the Stonewall Inn in New York, a group of gay people finally retaliated against the abuse and victimization to which they had been subjected and made a stand against police intimidation. The action taken by lesbians and gay men initially led to a riot. It also marked the beginning of the Gay Liberation movement in America, which

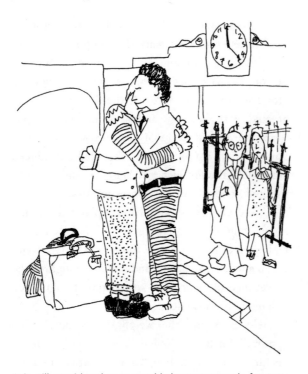

It is still considered unacceptable by many people for gay men to express their feelings openly.

has done much to improve the social standing of homosexuals in that country. Its influence was later felt in this country, where the gay movement is now established. There are several gay organizations, clubs, magazines and newspapers. However, some newsagents continue to refuse to stock gay magazines, which often merely include listings of events, news features and other articles.

The simple fact that standard gay periodicals are often not available locally to gay people serves further to marginalize them, and in a small way contributes to the insecurity and low self-esteem experienced by young gay people in particular.

SOCIAL CARE

One of the chief prejudices faced by gay people is that they are invariably seen solely in terms of their sexuality. For example, a gay social carer is seen first and foremost as being gay. All kinds of assumptions are then made about how this fact will affect his or her ability to perform the care task, and her or his other personal qualities and abilities will recede into the background.

There is plenty of evidence that Social Service Departments discriminate against homosexuals. In particular, lesbian mothers have been considered unsuitable for looking after children. For example, a contributor to a *Women in Mind* publication (Women-in Mind, 1990), stated: 'Losing custody of my child was the most devastating experience of my life so far. The Welfare Officer who made a report on us for the court told me that my daughter was one of the sanest children he had ever met – which he said must be due to the way I had brought her up – yet he still recommended that she would be better off in a "normal family" ' (Women in Mind, 1990, p.52).

Ignorance about the lives of gay and lesbian people can render social work ineffective if it is based solely on stereotypes. One woman who contacted a refuge after being abused by her lesbian partner said, 'I never felt so disparaged and utterly hopeless. The counsellor didn't have a clue what she was talking about, but she had strong stereotypes about "butch and femme relationships" ' (*Guardian*, 21 August 1996, p.2).

Gay teenagers in care are particularly vulnerable. According to the London Gay Teenage group, one in five young lesbians and gay men attempt suicide because of their sexuality (*Community Care*, 31 March 1994, p.4). It is therefore important that all young people who are being looked after by the Local Authority feel valued and able to trust caregivers during a particularly confusing time in their lives. Putting up positive images of lesbian and gay role models around the home and ensuring access to telephone numbers for support groups and information make an enormous difference to young people (and if you don't know, phone Gay Switchboard and ask). 'Staff should always challenge homophobic language and attitudes as they would any other offensive attitude. Remember, there could be a young person watching for support' (*Community Care*, 31 March 1994, p.4).

However, there is much more awareness about the needs of gay people today, and some local authorities have developed sympathetic practices. Much of this progress is a result of pioneering work undertaken by community and voluntary organizations. The Manchester Gay Centre has a successful history of supporting gay teenagers. A primary aim of the centre is to ensure that young people are able to join and meet with a peer group of other young gays. It is recognized that many young gay people are isolated within their own immediate family or among their heterosexual acquaintances, and that it is important for them to have the opportunity to discuss, argue and develop their identity with people of their own age.

It is likely that a higher proportion of teenagers who are gay are received into care compared to the rest of the population of young people of their age. This is because, in addition to other problems, so many of them have difficulties concerning their sexual orientation and disclosing it to those to whom they are close. Many parents react or are expected to react negatively to their daughter or son's disclosure, in line with society in general. Consequently, young people who grow up with the knowledge that they are gay may break away from their family at an early age and be more vulnerable to reception into care. The lack of a secure and accepting environment, isolation and/or homelessness can also increase the likelihood that these young people become involved in crime.

It would be true to say that social care – whether it is provided by field social carers, hospital social workers, probation officers or residential workers – has done very little so far to eliminate the discrimination levelled at gay and lesbian members of our society. Only in recent years has significant attention been given to their needs. Some local authority Social Services Departments are aware that lesbians and gay men have been denied social justice and have been marginalized by their policies. For example, the rights of gay people to adopt or foster children have now been acknowledged. In particular, it is especially realized that teenagers need positive role models, so young gays are now fostered with gay women or gay men.

Sexuality is still very much a taboo issue within social care. Only recently, for example, has anything been done to acknowledge the sexual rights of all clients in residential settings. In some establishments attempts are being made to enable clients to express their sexuality in the same way as the rest of the population. This positive acceptance needs to apply to gay people as well, so that they too can live full social and emotional lives. Peter Berry, a gay social worker, talks of how he regards his sexuality as a kind of 'hidden handicap'. He says, 'My biggest headache has been what is commonly called the corruption theory. This is that children should only have heterosexual models for fear that a gay social worker's homosexuality will unduly influence the child, especially as social workers are seen as models of acceptable behaviour and that a positive, adult homosexual model would be wrong' *(Community Care Supplement*, 25 June 1987, p.6). He feels that this stems from the popular misconception that gay men are more sexually attracted to children than their heterosexual counterparts. It is not only working with children that presents problems for gay men. Any client group in any social care setting 'where the client is deemed to be susceptible to undue influence is subject to particular scrutiny'. Peter Berry points out that 'gay social workers are no more likely to take advantage of clients than any other worker; rather, perhaps the opposite is true. We are aware that if we put a foot wrong, the system will come down on our heads with the weight of the public behind it' (*Community Care Supplement*, 25 June 1987, p.6).

It is likely that many heterosexual social carers will not even consider the possibility of their client being gay, since within their own lives they have not come across anyone who is openly gay. To act in this way is to flaunt basic social care principles and thus to deny the client an integral part of him- or herself. It is not only important that young gay clients have their sexual orientation acknowledged and accepted, but the same is true for adult clients. According to the London Charter for Gay and Lesbian Rights there are at least 50 000 older lesbians and gay men estimated to be living in London. The Charter points out that many of these older people 'are isolated, have kept their sexual orientation a secret or they may have been subjected to abuse from neighbours where it is known they are gay'. It is possible that the absence of children may add to an older person's feelings of isolation.

Social carers who are not gay themselves need to learn about lesbian and gay issues, their life-styles and politics, and to have a knowledge of the basic resources that are available. They need to become involved in supporting others in creating initiatives which will make the social care service more appro-priate to the needs of gay people. They also need to address all forms of discrimination, be they open or covert, personal or institutional, casual or entrenched. Finally, support should be given to gay colleagues, and every effort should be made to create a safe environment in which both client and carer can reveal their sexual identity. Care should be taken not to burden one member of the team as the unpaid expert and sole spokesperson for gay issues. This is our joint responsibility, for as Colin MacInnes pointed out some time ago, 'Sexual freedom, like social and racial freedom, is indivisible; by which I mean that heterosexuals can never be entirely free so long as homosexuals are not' (*New Society*, 23 October 1975, p.224).

5.4 GYPSIES AND TRAVELLERS

> We do not want to be regarded as curios from some forgotten era; rather we want to be seen as ordinary people and to be treated as such.
> (National Gypsy Council, in *Community Care*, 29 September 1988, p.26)

About 1000 years ago the ancestors of the Romany-speaking peoples left India and travelled along trade routes used at different times by many other migratory nations. Historical documents show that some 200 to 300 years later they arrived in eastern Europe. By the end of the fifteenth century, they had been recorded as living in the British Isles.

The Romany language has an Indian base, but words were borrowed from every country through which they travelled. The fragmented language contains hundreds of dialects. Today Romany-speaking people live throughout the world, and many have intermarried with other peoples and enjoy a large number of diverse cultures. Only a minority of Romany-speaking communities in the world remain nomadic.

Thomas Acton has made academic studies of the Romany-speaking peoples and states that 'no definition of the term "gypsy" could even begin to command universal acceptance' and he speaks of the 'illusory image of the "true" gypsy' (Acton, 1974, p.2). As far as he is concerned, 'racial purity' is as much a myth among gypsies as among any other people of the world. It is thought that the word 'gypsy' may be a corruption of the word 'Egyptian'.

There are other groups of nomadic people in our society who do not call themselves gypsies. Some have been around for hundreds of years, but others, such as the 'New Age' travellers have their origins in the 'youth movements' and counter-culture of the 1960s and 1970s. The term which finds general acceptance among all such groups (including gypsies) is 'travellers' or 'travelling people'.

Specific groupings of people are often associated with a native, 'secret' language which is private to a particular group. Those who prefer to be called 'English travellers' use what they call an 'Anglo-Romany' language. Irish travellers use the 'shelta' or 'gammon' language. The Anglo-Romany word for a non-traveller is a 'gaujo'. The language of travellers has a strong verbal rather than written tradition.

LIFE-STYLE

> We believe that respect for cultural diversity is an important part of a healthy society. The right to travel, the right to stop without fear of persecution and the right to have somewhere to stay are all fundamental rights.
>
> (Alf Dubbs, *Observer*, 13 December 1992, p.6)

Clearly there is a wide variety of life-styles among travellers. Each travelling group's life-style will depend on a number of factors, including historical and cultural traditions as well as economic status. Some travellers may be settled, either temporarily or permanently, on sites or even in ordinary housing. There is little if any truth in the image of a carefree 'life on the highways' with a pony grazing outside the caravan. Most travellers have to work extremely hard to make a living.

The majority of travellers are self-employed and are commonly involved in scrap dealing, road and path surfacing and general dealing, often in household goods such as furniture. Some travellers trade in horses, but as work horses are not utilized today they often represent a side-line or a form of capital investment. Others are involved in 'casual' agricultural work.

The development of motorized transport has changed the pace of the traditional nomadic life-style of many travellers. Very few of them now have a traditional horse-drawn wagon. Indeed, many are no longer nomadic in the strict sense. The majority live in comfortable, modern caravans with conventional facilities such as radio and television. Their leisure activities and forms of entertainment are not so very different from those of ordinary house-dwellers.

POPULATION

It is extremely difficult to say with any accuracy how many travellers there are in the UK. Numbers change all the time due to a variety of factors, but a current estimate is between 60 000 and 100 000 travellers – including Romany gypsies, Scottish, Irish and Welsh travellers, and fairground people (but not 'New Age' travellers). Counts of caravans take place from time to time. In July 1993 a Department of the Environment survey found 12 810 caravans in England. This included:

- 5 432 caravans on authorized local authority sites;
- 2 976 caravans on authorized private sites;
- 4 402 caravans on unauthorized encampments.

A total of 1190 caravans were estimated to be located in Wales (thus giving a total of 14 000 for England and Wales).

MARGINALIZATION – PUBLIC REACTION TO TRAVELLERS

Many of us may remember seeing signs displayed in the windows of some public houses which read 'No travellers'. This is a common example of the rejection of travellers by 'conventional' society. Following a court ruling in 1988 (Commission for Racial Equality v. Dutton), travellers are now protected from overt discrimination of this kind by the Race Relations Act (1976). The Commission for Racial Equality regards travellers as an ethnic minority group which must be protected against discrimination, and it has taken up several cases of alleged discrimination.

Myths and legends, often of an unhelpful nature, are still perpetuated in our society, sometimes by travellers themselves but mostly by the antagonistic sentiments voiced by non-travellers. Such sentiments are usually based on fear and suspicion and stem from ignorance of travellers' life-styles – they perpetuate prejudice and mythical stereotypes.

As recently as 1967, an official government report entitled 'Gypsies and Other Travellers' quoted a rhyme which it stated 'children still repeat':

> My mother said I never should
> Play with the gypsies in the wood.

Although it decried the thought behind the rhyme, the report stated that 'a popular legend still exists that gypsies actually steal children' (Ministry of Housing and Local Government and the Welsh Office, 1967). Legends and rhymes have traditionally been passed down orally through the centuries, and some are still believed today.

The general perception of travellers by the public is poor. One of the chief culprits in maintaining this erroneous perception is the mass media. Virtually all of the stories carried in the press about travellers are couched in terms of their being a nuisance, of illegal campsites and of travellers leaving piles of rubbish behind when they decamp. (No mention is made that this may have something to do with the fact that the local police moved them on at 6 a.m.!) The real motive underlying the antagonism may be economic. It may be driven by the fear that a travellers' site near their homes will devalue house prices, or in the case of pub landlords, that the presence of gypsies may deter other customers.

The media covers 'negative' stories about travellers, and not 'positive' ones. This is probably because ordinary members of the public rarely come into contact with travellers other than in a confrontational situation such as wanting a camp moved on. Both travellers and house-dwellers lack good shared experiences of each other. Until these occur, it is unlikely that unhelpful myths and legends will cease to be believed.

nomadic society. Our state institutions, most of which are large, bureaucratic organizations, tend to function more efficiently when they are dealing with people who can be contacted at a fixed address. At the same time, because such agencies have difficulty in contacting and working with travellers, the travellers themselves experience a great deal of hardship in coping with bureaucracy. The 'Job-seeker's Allowance', introduced in 1996, is an example of a bureaucratic obstacle faced by travellers – in order to claim this benefit and prove that they are 'actively seeking work', individuals require a fixed place to stay.

Helpful people exist in all state agencies, such as the police, health service and education departments, but it is usually the structure, rules and regulations of such bodies that cause problems in their relationships with travellers. Difficulties can arise in relation to a whole range of complex issues, such as presenting traffic documents at a police station, registering with a GP, or placing their children in a particular school. Our social agencies are not geared towards travellers' needs. Furthermore, the situation may be compounded by a low general level of literacy among travellers, as forms have to be filled in!

A government committee of enquiry into the education of children from ethnic minority groups stated in the Swann Report (Department of Education, 1985) that it was disturbed by the 'universal hostility and hatred' which was meted out to travellers. In the final section about other ethnic groups, the report stated that travellers' children were badly affected by 'racism and discrimination, myths, stereotyping and misinformation, and the inappropriateness and inflexibility of the education system'.

DEALING WITH BUREAUCRACY

Travellers face many difficulties because they remain nomadic or semi-nomadic within a non-

LOCAL SUPPORT GROUPS

Local support groups provide an immeasurable amount of help to travellers. These are just some of the issues which one local support group assists travellers with on a day-to-day basis:

- advice on rights;
- policing issues;
- DSS regulations;
- tax returns;
- education;
- crèche facilities and an under-five play-group – while their children are being cared for, the parents can seek assistance on other matters;
- youth work;
- literacy help – writing a specific letter or filling in a form;
- legal assistance, liaising with police, solicitors or probation officers;
- mail collection and dissemination – the support group acts as a permanent address when travellers are moving around the locality;
- a 'neutral' meeting place for travellers liaising with health, education and welfare services, e.g. social services, GPs, mental health services, education services or specific schools.

The 'Advice Centre' now deals with over 6000 enquiries every year from over 4000 enquirers. Travellers have participated in the running of the organization since it was established.

SITES FOR TRAVELLERS

> Gypsies, like any other people, should be able to choose whether they follow a nomadic lifestyle or whether they settle; whether they want to live on a site or in a house.
>
> (Sheffield Gypsy and Traveller Support Group, 1992)

Before the introduction of the 1968 Caravan Sites Act, the provision of sites for travellers' caravans was piecemeal and patchy. The 1968 Act was generally a progressive, liberalizing piece of legislation which represented a turning point in society's atti-

tude to travellers. It came into force from 1 April 1970, and Section 6(1) placed a duty on local authorities 'to provide adequate accommodation for gypsies residing in or resorting to their area'. Ten years later, the 1980 Local Government, Planning and Land Act empowered central government to pay 100 per cent capital grants to local authorities to enable them to provide caravan sites. Two types of site subsequently appeared – 'transit' sites for those moving on fairly quickly, and 'permanent' or 'residential' sites for those wishing to remain.

The facilities on sites varied widely. The best included an electricity supply, fresh running water, hot piped water, a bath or shower room, a weekly refuse collection, flush lavatories and public lighting. In addition, a number of private sites were established, some of them owned by travellers themselves.

Controversy has been generated as to whether or not the 1968 Caravan Sites Act fulfilled its promise. In 1992, the government published a consultation paper entitled 'Reform of the Caravan Sites Act 1968', which concluded that the Act had failed because not enough places on sites had been provided. The report gave two reasons for this.

1. The numbers of caravans had outstripped site provision.
2. Only 38 per cent of local authorities had achieved 'designation'; a local authority was 'designated' once it had provided the required amount of site provision. The fact was that 62 per cent of local authorities had therefore failed to comply with the Act.

Gypsies and their supporters felt that these conclusions were too simplistic. Their views were supported by a report published in 1991 by the Department of the Environment (DoE), entitled 'Gypsy Site Provision and Policy'. This concluded that the Act had failed because of the following:

1. a lack of political will on the part of local authorities to make provision;
2. a failure to enforce the act by the Department of the Environment;

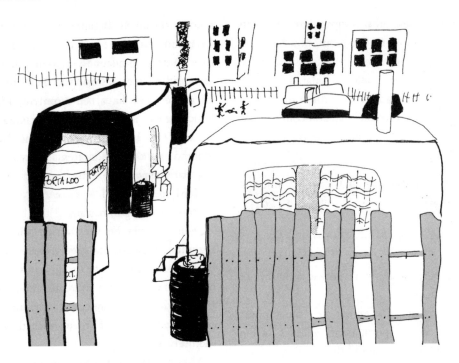

Most urban sites for travellers are far removed from the romanticized, traditional image.

3. confusion between County and District Councils over their respective roles and responsibilities concerning site provision;
4. the lack of national and regional strategies for site provision.

However, the Government ignored the Department of the Environment's findings, and instead introduced the 1994 Criminal Justice and Public Order Act. This Act relieved local authorities of their duty to provide authorized sites for travellers and abolished the 100 per cent capital grant system for their construction. However, it went much further than this. If the 1968 Act was seen as a progressive turning point with regard to society's treatment of travellers, then the 1994 Act was viewed as a turning back to intolerance. The Criminal Justice and Public Order Act was targeted at 'New Age' travellers rather than at gypsies and traditional travellers, in response to an outcry from the establishment, and some sections of the public, in relation to large gatherings, festivals and 'raves'. However, the Act has been conveniently used against *all* travellers.

The 1994 Act enables a police officer to direct *two or more people*, who have between them six or more vehicles and who she or he 'reasonably believes' to be trespassing on land with the purpose of 'residing there for any period' to leave the land and to remove any vehicles or property which they have with them. The police can do this if 'reasonable' steps have been taken by, or on behalf of, the occupier, to ask them to leave (in the case of 'common land' the local authority is the 'occupier'). Even if there are fewer than six vehicles (a caravan and the vehicle used to tow it count as two vehicles), the police can exercise this power if the occupier has asked the 'trespassers' to leave and any of them has caused 'damage' to the land or to property on it. The courts have held that walking across a field constitutes 'damage'!

If a person fails to leave the land 'as soon as reasonably practicable' or returns to it within 3 months, she or he is guilty of an offence which carries a maximum penalty of *3 months' imprisonment*.

Given that we know there has never been adequate site provision, many travellers now have nowhere to camp legally, and use of the 1994 Act has effectively *criminalized their way of life*. They are now at risk of being moved on, harassed and prosecuted. A Cardiff-based support group has estimated that local authorities have spent about £7 million in the past year on evictions of travellers. Several counties and cities have become 'no-go' areas for travellers, as councils, in co-operation with the police, have prevented them from using any council-owned open spaces. One group of travellers was recently reported to have been forced to move on through nine different counties over a 3-month period.

The immediate future for gypsies and travellers looks extremely bleak. Some are being forced to abandon their way of life and become part of the urban homeless. Many are faced with a choice between temporary 'bed-and-breakfast' accommodation or poor-quality housing if they can get it. Meanwhile, a large proportion of traveller families are sinking deeper into poverty and deprivation. Judy Hirst, who works with travellers, says: 'Growing numbers of travellers are being forced into benefit dependency, or – particularly in the case of young people – turning to petty crime' (*Community Care*, 13–19 February 1997, p.18). The situation is so repressive in this country that some families are even considering moving abroad to countries such as Ireland or Spain.

Existing sites are becoming overcrowded, while at the same time physical conditions in them deteriorate. As Margaret Tapley, a Development Officer with 'Save the Children' says: 'They're a forgotten, largely hidden community.... Things were bad enough in the past, but with local authority sites bulging at the seams, they can only get a lot worse' (*Community Care*, 13–19 February 1997, p.18).

GYPSIES AND TRAVELLERS IN EUROPE

The last few years have seen a growth in the harassment and persecution of gypsies across Europe, most particularly in Eastern Europe, although phys-ical attacks on Romanian gypsies in Germany have been substantially reported. Persecution has caused over 100 000 gypsies to flee the former socialist states of Eastern Europe and move to the West. In particular they have fled from Bulgaria, Romania and Yugoslavia and the former Czech republic. Some of the latter group arrived at Dover in 1997, claiming asylum, but were made far from welcome, both by our politicians and, more predictably, by the tabloid press.

National governments and the European Union have loudly condemned racial, ethnic and religious discrimination and violence and all that constitutes racism and 'ethnic cleansing'. In July 1992, the 'Conference on Security and Co-operation in Europe' (CSCE) at Helsinki saw European governments, including the UK, sign an affirmation which acknowledged 'the need to develop appropriate programmes addressing problems of their respective nationals belonging to Roma and other groups traditionally identified as gypsies and to *create conditions for them to have equal opportunities to participate fully in the life of society*' (Helsinki Document, Chapter 6, paragraph 35 – our emphasis).

HELP AND SUPPORT FOR TRAVELLERS

The many support groups around the country for travellers provide an invaluable source of advice and assistance. They have the further advantage of not 'stigmatizing' travellers. Contact with a social worker can in itself be a stigmatizing experience for anyone, but especially for a travelling family. However sensitive and informed social workers may be, they are usually settled house-dwellers. They are unlikely to have had experience of a travelling lifestyle, and they may well have subconscious negative feelings about the quality of life experienced in a caravan on the move. With heightened awareness of 'child abuse' in the UK and occasional attacks of public paranoia about the responsibilities of parents towards children, some of them media-induced, it is little wonder that travellers tend to regard social workers and those in authority with a certain amount of mistrust. Parents among travellers are usually well aware of the child-care powers vested in social workers.

Year-on-year cuts in local authority budgets and services have resulted in the closure of some initiatives that were set up to cater for the specific needs of travellers. This has particularly affected advice services, and specialized health and education resources. Cuts in local authority grants to gypsy and traveller support groups have also had a detrimental effect. These cuts and reductions in services have taken place at a very bad time for travellers – when they are having to cope with all the oppressive implications of the 1994 legislation.

CONCLUSION – INCREASING OPPRESSION?

> The threat which the Gypsies, as a minority, appear to represent to the larger society is largely ideological. They are seen to defy the dominant system of wage-labour and its demand for a fixed abode.
>
> (Okely, 1983, p.231)

As we have seen, the introduction of the 1994 Criminal Justice and Public Order Act, together with the associated repeal of the 1968 Caravan Sites Act, has had a profoundly negative impact on gypsies' and travellers' life-styles. Some of the effects have included eviction, harassment, enforced homelessness and prosecution. All of this has resulted in expensive pressure and demands on local authority Housing Departments, the courts, the police, the probation service and the prison system, and Social Services Departments, because of their responsibilities for children under the 1989 Children Act. This cost has to be weighed against the expense of providing for a caravan, on an authorized site supplied with water, electricity and sewage facilities. This has been estimated at £27 000 per family, which is a much lower amount than the cost of providing permanent housing for them.

The 1994 Act has considerably increased the oppression and marginalization experienced by gypsies and travellers. In order to ensure that basic, decent provision is made, the 1968 Caravan Sites Act should be restored and effectively enforced, and Central government grants for the construction of sites should be reintroduced. As the 'Penal Affairs Consortium' has said, 'the solution to the problem of unauthorized parking of caravans lies in providing an adequate number of authorised sites – not in criminalizing travellers' (*An Assessment of Part V of the Criminal Justice and Public Order Act 1994*, 1994, p.5).

5.5   PEOPLE WITH HIV/AIDS

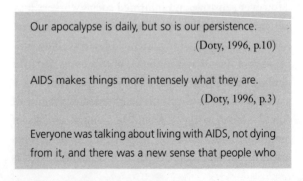

> Our apocalypse is daily, but so is our persistence.
>
> (Doty, 1996, p.10)

> AIDS makes things more intensely what they are.
>
> (Doty, 1996, p.3)

> Everyone was talking about living with AIDS, not dying from it, and there was a new sense that people who were HIV positive could live, and live well. . . . Communities of people with AIDS were offering the first shreds of hope that (people with) HIV might take charge of their condition, might view themselves as the keepers of their own health, not helpless, not – a word newly understood as dangerous, insidious – victims.
>
> (Doty, 1996, p.142)

Acquired immunodeficiency syndrome (AIDS) and infection with the causative agent – the human immunodeficiency virus (HIV) – have only relatively recently become a major public issue. Very little is known about the precise origin of the disease, why it has spread so rapidly or why some people are more susceptible to it than others. Unfortunately one thing is certain, and that is that there is to date no cure. However, anti-retroviral medication can inhibit the progression of the disease, and, along with safe-sex practices and needle-exchange policies, has contributed to the recent downturn in the numbers of people dying from the disease in Europe, America and other areas where medication is available.

NUMBERS INFECTED

In the UK in 1997 there were 1300 new cases of AIDS, 52 less than in the previous year. Although the disease is not developing as fast in this country as was forecast, it should be remembered that 10 000 people have already died of AIDS in the UK since the early to mid-1980s, and that in Inner London, HIV infection is still the leading cause of death for men between 18 and 54 years of age and the second highest after breast cancer for women of the same age range (*Guardian*, 1 December 1997, p.14).

In the developing world, however, AIDS has become an epidemic. According to the World Health Organization in early 1997:

- there are an estimated 30 million people with HIV infection or AIDS;
- 1 in 100 adults throughout the world are infected;
- 16 000 people are being infected daily;
- an estimated 2 300 000 people were expected to die of AIDS-related diseases by the end of 1997, twice as many as in 1996;
- 1 in 5 of those who die will be children, mostly infected at birth;
- the cumulative number of deaths due to HIV/AIDS is 11.7 million (the First World War claimed

the lives of 8 million soldiers) (Sources: *Observer*, 30 November 1997, p.26; *Guardian*, 1 December 1997, p.2; *Independent*, 27 November 1997, p.7).

In some countries, where information and resources are more readily available, the spread of HIV is being contained. In other, poorer countries, where there is less access to help, advice and treatment, the disease is continuing to spread at an alarming rate. This has led some observers to point to the divide between rich and poor countries:

> The poor countries are getting sicker and the rich countries are getting better – better treatment, better informed, better behaved.
>
> (*Independent*, 27 November 1997, p.7)

STIGMA

The nature or progression of HIV infection and AIDS may eventually necessitate some form of physical isolation, and this is made worse by the accompanying social isolation. Fed by ignorance and widespread, media-based scaremongering, society has shown little tolerance for people who are seen to have contributed in some way to their condition through their own life-styles. Blame is more easily apportioned than empathy. It is not surprising therefore that so many people with HIV infection are reluctant to seek help, and attempt to keep their condition secret for fear of rejection and further damage to their self-image. Some people have met with insensitivity and fear when breaking the news of their condition to members of their family:

> My parents did not know I was ill . . . I walked into their kitchen and told them. . . . A couple of days later at dinner I was given a glass of sherry that had a piece of cotton round the stem. . . . The plate was marked underneath with a cross.
>
> (*Community Care*, 8 June 1989, p.18)

I repeated the facts of my friend's illness and could hear Dad trying to take it all in. Then, about an hour later, my father rang in a distraught voice, 'Listen you shouldn't have that person staying in the house with you. I've been talking to your mother and we are both very frightened'.

(*Community Care*, 8 June 1989, p.16)

Even when it is known that a family member is HIV-positive, their condition may not be acknowledged or accepted by all of the family members. For instance, Sean, who is HIV-positive, 30 years old and gay, gave the following account:

My Dad phoned last week. He was really sweet. He asked how I was feeling. What AZT was. Do I have the courage to take it for long, etc. I wondered why he plucked up courage to phone me. It turned out Mum was away for two days.

I am going to visit my Grandma. She is 89 years old and not good at the moment. She wants her bedroom decorated after Christmas. I offered to do it for her but my parents are still insisting I am not allowed to visit her.

My Mum gave me her monthly phone call Saturday. It went 'Are you OK?'

'Yes.'

'Christmas is coming. You weren't thinking of visiting your Grandmother were you?'

'Yes.'

'Well as the rest of the grandchildren will be there, it's probably best you don't.'

'Why?'

'Er, because she thinks you're in prison so it's best left like that.'

I did not reply. She went on to say a few thing that I can't remember. And that was that.

(Quoted in *HIV/AIDS User Consultation Exercise* for Norfolk Social Services, July/August 1994, p.2)

WHAT IS AIDS/HIV?

- *Acquired* – something you have picked up not inherited.
- *Immune deficiency* – your body cannot defend itself against illness.
- *Syndrome* – the set of illnesses you get as a result.

AIDS is caused by the human immunodeficiency virus or HIV. This virus attacks the white blood cells which help to defend the body against disease. People with AIDS do not die from AIDS itself, but from some other infection or disease which their bodies cannot fight.

Antibodies are produced by the body in response to HIV. However, these antibodies do not seem to affect the virus. The antibodies can be detected in blood tests, and if they are found they will indicate that the person has been infected. However, the presence of antibodies does not automatically imply that that person will develop AIDS. Some individuals remain well, while others will move through the infection and *eventually* die of AIDS.

AIDS includes a whole range of illnesses, many of which have no medical cure. People with HIV may experience loss of vision (sometimes very rapidly), physical wasting and severe weight loss, constant fevers, persistent diarrhoea, heavy night sweats and other major physical changes. All of these symptoms advance rapidly within a short period of time. Skin cancers and cerebral atrophy also occur.

HOW IS THE DISEASE TRANSMITTED?

The established modes

The bottom line

HIV can be transmitted through sexual intercourse, sharing injecting equipment or receiving blood transfusions and other blood-related products from an infected person. It can also be transmitted from an HIV-infected mother to her baby. Alcorn and Browning (1998) have provided a detailed account.

Unsafe sex

The established and common routes are:

- unprotected anal penetration;
- unprotected vaginal penetration.

Possible but uncommon routes include the following:

- oral transmission – a very small number of cases have been reported, all of which suggest that oral transmission depends on either damaged tissue in the mouth or throat, or on ulceration of the penis;
- any sexual activities in which blood may be shared (e.g. those involving piercing, shaving, etc.);
- through blood in otherwise uncontaminated body fluids – in the mouth or rectum, or during menstruation;
- through shared sex toys, etc.

Shared injecting equipment

The established and common route is via sharing of injection equipment. Another possible but uncommon route is via needle-stick and sharps injuries.

Blood products

Possible but uncommon routes include the following:

- blood transfusions, blood products and donations (organs or skin). Since 1985 blood donations in the UK have been screened, and screening began at roughly the same time in most other countries which could afford such programmes. Organs and tissues for donation have also been screened since that time, and blood products such as Factor VIII have been heat-treated since 1984;
- surgical and other invasive procedures. Fortunately this route is very uncommon, and the risk needs to be viewed in the light of the far greater

risks routinely involved in these invasive health-care procedures;

- occupationally through blood splashes on to broken skin and needle-stick injuries;
- donations of blood, organs, tissues, semen, breast milk and bone marrow – in each of these instances a very small number of cases has been reported;
- tattooing, acupuncture, electrolysis and shaving equipment. In these cases it is assumed that infection is possible, but unlikely. A case of infection via unsterilized acupuncture needles has been reported.

Between mother and baby

Possible but uncommon routes include the following:

- through breast-feeding;
- at birth.

Impossible routes of HIV transmission

The bottom line

The virus cannot be transmitted through:

- *unbroken healthy skin*, because cells vulnerable to HIV infection do not exist on the surface of the skin;
- *breathing in* (unlike the common cold, for instance, which can be spread through sneezing), because HIV cannot be airborne. It is not present in the tiny particles of moisture that are sneezed or coughed out of someone's mouth;
- *a healthy, undamaged mouth*, because cells vulnerable to HIV infection are not present in the mouth;
- *unbroken barriers* such as a latex condom or the Femidom, because these barriers cannot be penetrated by HIV;
- *corneal transplants*, because no blood vessels are present in the cornea;
- *mosquitoes*, because although these insects suck blood, they do not regurgitate blood containing live HIV into the bodies of other victims;

- *sharing cutlery, plates or cups*, because HIV cannot be transmitted in saliva;
- *over-broad and imprecise categories* such as 'sex' or 'promiscuity' or 'drug abuse' are not themselves a risk;
- *social contact with people with HIV*, because HIV is not transmitted by touch or through the air;
- *through animal bites*, because animals do not carry HIV;
- *by caring for people with AIDS* (but remember the guidelines on universal precautions);
- *by association with blood* (e.g. donating blood in the UK);
- *by contact with small amounts of dried blood*, because HIV will not be present in sufficient quantity (all infections through blood that was not injected or transfused have occurred in cases where large quantities of blood splashed on to the broken skin of other people);
- *through swimming pools, showers or washing machines*, because HIV will be killed by the chemicals in disinfectant and detergent, or simply washed away;
- *by mouth-to-mouth resuscitation*, because HIV is not present in saliva; only if HIV is present in large quantities does it present a risk;
- *by touching objects such as telephones*, because HIV is not transmitted by touch;
- *by using the same lavatory as people with HIV*, because even if someone had bled into the lavatory, the water would immediately dilute the virus, nor would HIV be picked up from blood on the lavatory seat.

Rarely, the virus may be transmitted through:

- the lining of the mouth if there are cuts, sores, ulcers or bleeding gums;
- the nipples, if a woman is bitten by a child with bleeding gums while breast-feeding;
- the mucous membranes in the eye, if the virus is splashed there in large quantities.

PUBLICITY AND AIDS AND HIV

Much of the publicity surrounding HIV has been damaging and has contributed to the stress that is already being experienced by those who are infected. It has also added to the widespread confusion felt by the rest of the population. Harmful myths about how the disease is spread, and misleading stereotypes of the people who have the infection, have deepened the severe stigma felt by those with HIV.

The initial government advertising campaign in the late 1980s, with its doom-laden images of coffins and icebergs, did little to educate the public properly about the facts relating to HIV. A later campaign, which started in February 1990, was more effective and informative. However, misinformation has been rife. For example, in November 1989, Lord Kilbracken announced that only one person in the UK had contracted AIDS through heterosexual sex. Tabloid newspapers followed this with headlines claiming that 'normal' people did not get AIDS. In fact, according to the Health Education Authority in December 1990, 'In the UK over 600 HIV carriers had become infected through heterosexual sex' *(Observer,* 11 February 1990, p.26). Nevertheless, much media intensity has been focused on gay people, who have been blamed for the disease. This blame has facilitated the venting of other, more entrenched prejudices against gay people, and has reinforced the marginalized position that they have in society. Similarly, the reputation of black people has suffered as a result of the newspapers' claim that AIDS 'came from Africa', although Jonathan Mann, former director of the World Health Organization Global Programme on AIDS, maintains that 'on the basis of available information we believe that HIV is an old if not ancient virus of unknown geographical origin' (Global Programme on AIDS – The Global Impact of AIDS, World Health Organization Summit 1988, Barbican, London).

Oppression

In addition to coping with the physical symptoms of the infection, people with HIV need to combat social discrimination. Joshua Oppenheimer and Helena Reckitt in their book entitled *Acting on Aids; Sex, Drugs and Politics* (Oppenheimer and Reckitt, 1997), outlined in detail the extent of the discrimination experienced by many people who are HIV-positive. These authors provided illustrations of prejudice from countries throughout the European Union. Some of these examples include the following:

- HIV testing as a condition for admission to certain occupations;
- disclosure of medical information without consent;
- denial of right of access of an HIV-infected parent to their child;
- higher insurance premium rates;
- compulsory testing of Nationals from a period spent abroad;
- dismissal from work or inappropriate changes in post;
- avoidance or rejection by work colleagues
- provision of housing that is inadequate for their needs;
- protests in neighbourhoods at (or preventing) the opening of residential schemes for people with HIV;
- refusal of admission of HIV-infected children to schools;
- exaggerated or inappropriate infection-control procedures in medical settings;
- isolation of HIV-infected prisoners;
- general exclusion.

Some of these forms of discrimination were found in only one country surveyed, while others were found in several (Oppenheimer and Reckitt, 1997, p.368).

HIV and families

> Children don't get the same support as they would if their parent had a 'respectable' disease. If a child went to the corner shop and said, 'My Mum's got cancer' they'd say, 'Oh poor thing'.
>
> (*Guardian*, 26 November 1997, p.6)

Due to the stigma associated with AIDS and HIV, many infected people keep their condition secret not only from those outside but also from their own families. According to Ruth Tamplin, Director of Positive Partner Positively Children, '90 per cent of the positive mothers supported by us have not told their children about it, but often the children have sensed that something is wrong, or found out by some other route. We try to help children explore the issues and help children express their fears' (*Guardian*, 3 December 1997, p.6). She adds, 'We try to enable parents to tell their children when appropriate and at a suitable age. Frequently as children reach 9, 10 or 11 they start to pick up that there is a secret in the family and there is something that the parents are upset about. Keeping a secret puts up walls between parents and children. Children feel resentful and can't share the grief. When a parent discloses the information to a child, it enables them to support each other' (*Guardian*, 3 December 1997, p.6).

The insecurity and uncertainty generated by HIV and AIDS within the family will doubtless have an effect on the lives of all the family members, particularly the children. One HIV-positive mother who had told her son of her illness remarked, 'He gets very anxious at times, especially when I am not feeling well. I have told the teachers at the school, because he has behaviour problems. They have advised me to keep it quiet. He steals from other children, has tantrums, wets the bed and soils himself. I am sure that it is because of his fear of losing me.... Children need help with these things.... People forget about them, but my son is as much affected by HIV as I am' (*Guardian*, 3 December 1997, p.6).

The understandable reluctance of some people to share information about their own HIV status can have ramifications both for that person and for those affected by the disease. For instance, the HIV-positive person will not be able to access benefit entitlement or support from Social Services or to take up any neighbourly willingness to help. The strain on the family is then increased, and children may be forced into a caring role with inappropriate age-related responsibilities.

As well as presenting a fresh challenge to health or social care and social work, HIV serves to high-light the importance of core social work principles. The need to 'respect' and to 'value', to maintain the client's dignity and be 'non-judgemental' is under-lined by the nature of the disease. Furthermore, because of the many fundamental matters concerning the human condition that are raised by HIV, carers are being forced to examine their own attitudes with regard to death, sexuality, culture, life-style and other issues. This is absolutely necessary – otherwise how can they be of assistance to those living with HIV?

5.6   HOMELESS PEOPLE

> When you live on the pavement you soon see people from a different perspective and they do their best not to see you at all.
>
> (Midge Gillies, in Rosen, 1991, p.139)

INTRODUCTION – HOW MANY PEOPLE ARE HOMELESS?

It is impossible to know with any accuracy how many homeless people there are in the UK today. Figures about homelessness vary widely, although it is generally agreed that the problem became worse throughout the 1980s and reached a peak in 1991, estimated at 3 million people. From that year the number of homeless people began to decline.

Central government collates figures from local authorities, and the Department of the Environment (responsible for housing and homelessness in England), the Welsh Office and the Scottish Office produce statistics of the number of 'officially' or 'statutorily' homeless households (not individuals). These households are entitled to a home from either a local authority or a housing association, under relevant homelessness law. The official figures (see Table 5.4) show a year-on-year increase from 1980 until 1990. However, by 1996 numbers had decreased for the fifth year running. These official statistics represent the 'tip of the iceberg', since the true figure for homelessness is much higher. There are a number of reasons for this:

- There are single people and couples *without children* who are not included in the limited legal definition of homelessness (see below).
- There are single people and couples who live in unsuitable accommodation, which might be over-crowded or in need of repair, who are not counted as being homeless.
- There are a significant number of people, par-ticularly single people, who do not even approach their local authority for housing, but who sleep in friends' or relatives' accommodation.
- There are people who sleep 'rough' on the streets.

WHAT IS HOMELESSNESS?

Homelessness does not simply mean not having a roof over one's head – the term is more complex

Table 5.4 Local authority homeless acceptances

	Number of households																
	1980	1981	1982	1983	1984	1985	1986	1987	1988	1989	1990	1991	1992	1993	1994	1995	1996
Not held to be intentionally homeless																	
England	60 400	66 990	71 620	75 470	80 500	91 010	100 490	109 170	113 770	122 180	140 350	144 780	142 890	132 380	122 460	121 280	116 870
+ Scotland	7038	7332	8360	7770	8787	10 992	11 056	10 417	10 463	12 396	14 233	15 508	17 062	15 462	16 100	15 000	—
+ Wales	4772	4779	4896	4314	4382	4825	5262	5198	6286	7111	9226	9293	9818	10 792	9897	8638	8334
= Great Britain	72 210	79 101	84 876	87 554	93 669	106 827	116 808	124 785	130 519	141 687	163 809	169 581	169 770	158 634	148 457	144 918	125 204
Held to be intentionally homeless																	
England	2520	3020	3180	2770	3050	2970	3070	3270	3730	4500	5450	6940	6350	5660	4570	4690	5120
+ Scotland	938	773	847	808	977	980	1144	1030	1128	1271	1580	1796	2114	1827	1800	1700	—
+ Wales	674	683	715	694	617	546	703	485	532	694	737	550	452	333	396	362	815
= Great Britain	4132	4476	4742	4272	4644	4496	4917	4785	5390	6465	7767	9286	8916	7820	6766	6752	5935
All homeless acceptances																	
England	62 920	70 010	74 800	78 240	83 550	93 980	103 560	112 440	117 500	126 680	145 800	151 720	149 240	138 040	127 030	125 500	121 990
+ Scotland	7976	8105	9207	8578	9764	11 972	12 200	11 447	11 591	13 667	15 813	17 304	19 176	17 289	17 900	16 700	—
+ Wales	5446	5462	5611	5008	4999	5371	5965	5683	6818	7805	9963	9843	10 270	11 125	10 293	9001	9149
= Great Britain	76 342	83 577	89 618	91 826	98 313	111 323	121 725	129 570	135 909	148 152	171 576	178 867	178 686	166 454	155 223	151 201	131 139

Source: Department of the Environment, Scottish Office and Welsh Office.
The 1990 figures for Wales include 2000 households made homeless in Colwyn Bay by flooding in February of that year. Scottish figures are for priority need homeless and potentially homeless cases only; 1996 figures were not available at the time of compilation.

In the last year before the 1996 Housing Act changes to the 1977 homeless legislation, the numbers of homeless acceptances in England fell for the fifth year running. 1995/1996 also saw a further fall in the percentage of local authority lettings to new tenants made to homeless household, down to 28%

than that. For example, as has already been mentioned, some accommodation is unsuitable or inadequate, yet people are actually living in it. Such people may be defined as being 'homeless'.

> Homelessness itself should not be tolerated in a rich society. Instead, it is homeless people who are not tolerated.
>
> (Catherine Shelley, *Christian Socialist*, Winter 1997/1998, p.3)

The Housing Act 1996 refers to a person as being homeless 'if he or she has no accommodation available for occupation in the United Kingdom or elsewhere', or if he or she is 'threatened with homelessness if this situation is likely to arise within 28 days' (both quotes from Section 175). Yet this definition of homelessness is inadequate, because it does not include those people who are actually living in accommodation which is unsatisfactory.

'Shelter', the voluntary organization and charity founded in 1966 to 'publicise the emergency situation that exists within the housing problem, and appeal for money to carry out a rescue operation', has developed a far more satisfactory and comprehensive definition. In its publication *Homelessness –*

What's the Problem? (O'Dwyer, 1994) it states, 'To understand homelessness it is necessary to consider what is meant by a home. A home is more than just a roof over your head. It needs to be decent, secure and affordable. This means that any assessment of homelessness must recognize not just people sleeping rough but also those living in temporary accommodation: those living in poor or overcrowded conditions; those who are in mortgage arrears and under threat of repossession; and people forced to sleep on friends' floors as they have no home of their own' (O'Dwyer, 1994, p.2). Paul Balchin's subsequent definition extended Shelter's definition to include 'those sleeping in dangerous properties, and people living in violent relationships and the abused' (Balchin, 1995, p.272).

Over the past 20 years, a visible sign of homelessness has been that of people – most of them young people – sleeping rough or asking for money from passers-by, often accompanied by a dog, and frequently with a handwritten cardboard sign which says something like 'Homeless and hungry – please help!' However, we need to remember that there are many more 'hidden homeless' of all ages sleeping 'rough' or living in hostels, 'bed-and-breakfast' accommodation, 'squats' and short-life tenancies (often awaiting refurbishment or demolition).

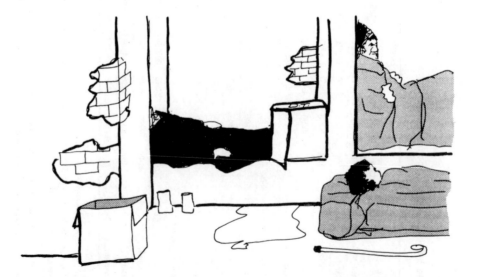

A common sight in many cities.

People are often blamed for being homeless, yet 'homelessness is a housing problem – not a people problem; it is a result of a lack of commitment by a succession of governments and this is represented in the failures of past and present housing policies. People do not become homeless as a result of their own inadequacies and failings but as a result of a housing system that has failed to provide them with a secure and affordable home' (O'Dwyer, 1994, p.2).

WHAT GROUPS OF PEOPLE ARE HOMELESS?

> The vast majority of men and women who are homeless are so because of inequality of opportunities. They have been marginalized and excluded because society has not protected them from abuse, from unemployment, from poverty. The loss of rights, due to their homelessness, means that they are, and are likely to remain, living in serious poverty.
>
> (Andy Winter, *Christian Socialist*, Winter 1997/1998, p.4)

In addition to people who are made homeless through a disaster such as a flood or fire, parents with children, pregnant women, and some people who are vulnerable due to age, disability, physical or mental ill health or an addiction to substances are the categories of people most likely to secure permanent accommodation. This is because they are most likely to be covered by housing legislation (see below). Whether or not they are covered by the law is open to a considerable amount of interpretation on the part of the local authority.

Even people who are officially recognized as homeless may spend many months or even years in what is often unsatisfactory *temporary* accommodation. Living in temporary accommodation such as 'bed and breakfast' can be a debilitating experience for individuals and families. It is impossible to put

down roots, and each day is governed by insecurity. Living in a temporary home is not only stressful and inconvenient, but it can also be stigmatizing. This is not simply because such accommodation is often situated in socially undesirable living areas, but also that one's temporary status is revealed on each occasion that an address is required by an organization or by officialdom in general. The stigma of homelessness may compound the distress of a woman who, for example, is fleeing domestic violence, or a family that is recovering after the repossession of their home.

Given the fact that so many homeless people do not fall into the official homeless category, it is not surprising that single people in particular will actually end up sleeping 'rough' on the streets of our towns and cities, and that many of these are young people. As Sheila McKechnie, an ex-director of Shelter, says, 'None of us like seeing 16-year-olds bedding down in shop doorways, queuing up for hostel places, suffering frostbite and hypothermia. But that is the reality' (*Give me Shelter*, p.11). A report by the National Inquiry into Preventing Youth Homelessness (1996) estimated that at least 246 000 young people became homeless in the UK in 1995. Furthermore, 'Centrepoint', a voluntary organization that works with young homeless people at risk, estimates that each year 50 000 young people aged 16–19 years are homeless in London alone. In 1996, they report that almost one-third (32 per cent) of the young people they admitted to shelter were 17 years of age or younger.

Former children in care

A significant proportion of young homeless people have been in the care of the local authority. Centrepoint says that this applies to 25 per cent of those who come their way, and the *Big Issue* states that 34 per cent of the people who sell their paper on the street have been in care. Less than 1 per cent of the population have been or are in care, so the proportion of care leavers who become homeless is extremely high. A number of factors contribute to this situation, including the fact that many people cannot return to their home of origin, many are unemployed, and few have received independent living training. Writing in the *Big Issue*, Ally Fogg says that this 'clearly shows the lack of transitional support. Local authorities' duty of care to a child (usually) finishes at the age of 18' (*Big Issue*, 17–23 March 1997, p.17).

Young women

For a number of reasons women may be more vulnerable to homelessness than men. For example, more men than women own their own homes or have tenancies in their name. Furthermore, the scale of women's homelessness may be less apparent than that of men. According to Jane Dibblin, 'Young women are among the most hidden and unrecognized of all homeless people'. She believes that for most of them it is 'an appalling cycle of abuse, homelessness and poverty, compounded by virtually total neglect by many service providers'. She continues, 'Very often homeless young women move from pillar to post – staying for a while on a friend's couch, someone else's floor, a spell in a bedsit or putting up with a violent boyfriend. Their level of invisibility is matched only by the level of their suffering' (Dibblin, 1991, p.9).

Maureen Rhoden adds that women face discrimination when it comes to finding a home because 'housing policies in Britain have always been based around the family'. She points out that women cannot buy housing as easily as men because they earn less on average, and because 'building societies prefer to grant mortgages to males as they are seen as more likely to have an uninterrupted pattern of employment' (Balchin, 1995, p.240). She also mentions that after a relationship breakdown fewer women than men will remain as the owner-occupier – 38 per cent compared to 50 per cent (Balchin, 1995, p.241).

The situation is worse for many black women, whom the London Housing Unit found were twice as likely as white women to experience long periods of homelessness. This fact is again often hidden, as these women tend to live with relatives and friends, and are not actually seen on the streets as homeless. Almost 50 per cent of the young people seen by Centrepoint are from black or minority ethnic communities, despite the fact that according to the 1991 census they only represented about 6 per cent of the total population. A survey on homelessness in Brent, conducted in 1986, found that African-Caribbeans were twice as likely as Asians to be homeless and three times as likely to be homeless as whites (Balchin, 1995, p.251–2). Louis Julienne draws attention to some of the problems faced by homeless black people, stating that 'Black people are likely to be faced with racial harassment and attack and are less likely to be registered with services such as GPs and dentists, therefore their health is affected' (*The Voice*, 14 April 1997, p.8).

People with mental health problems

Many of those working with homeless people report that the number of people with a mental health problem who are homeless has increased. Shelter confirms that this has intensified 'since the inadequately resourced Care in the Community programme commenced' in April 1993 (*An Introduction To Shelter*, 1996, p.2). Similarly, Charles Fraser, Director of St Mungo Community Housing Association, wrote at the end of 1996: 'We at St Mungo's (London-based) are certainly seeing more people now with mental health . . . problems than we did a couple of years ago' (*Roof*, November/ December 1996, p.19). He also draws attention to the increased proportion of homeless people who have an alcohol- or drug-related problem. He adds that 'community care doesn't seem to be working for people whose needs are complex, or who lack a community' (*Roof*, November/December 1996, p.19).

WHY DO PEOPLE BECOME HOMELESS?

The reasons for homelessness have been conventionally divided into *structural* and *immediate*. Some have already been mentioned above.

Structural reasons

The failure of community care policies would be included in structural causes, as would *repossessions* resulting from an individual's or family's inability to keep up with mortgage payments. The 'right to buy' local authority properties at 'knock-down' prices (introduced in the Housing Act 1980) and the alarming rise in house prices induced many families to purchase property, and this stretched some beyond their financial limits. In a review of the 1990s, Shelter reported that 'repossessions reached their peak in 1991, shattering the home ownership dream and highlighting the widening gap between Britain's haves and have-nots' (*30 Years of Shelter*, 1996, p.5).

A further structural cause of homelessness was the removal in 1988, by central government, of the entitlement to income support for 16- and 17-year-olds. This action created financial stress for many families and forced young people either to stay at home, often in unhappy circumstances, or to leave home and beg on the streets. Lisa Harker of the Child Poverty Action Group said of this change in young people's material circumstances, 'Great holes have been cut in social security and young people have been the first to fall through the net' (*Big Issue*, 17–23 March 1997, p.16).

The 1996 Asylum and Immigration Act also cut benefits for most refugees and asylum-seekers, forcing them into poverty and sometimes homelessness.

People who are HIV-positive are discriminated against when they want to buy their own home. Owing to the fact that they have a life-threatening condition, they are not able to take on an *endowment* mortgage (i.e. one which involves a 'life insurance'

policy), but they *may* be granted a more straight-forward *repayment* mortgage.

A final structural cause of homelessness is the dramatic reduction in the amount of '*social housing*' available. This is made up of local authority, 'council' housing, known as 'public housing', and Housing Association accommodation, known as the '*third sector*'. Almost 1.5 million council properties have been sold under the 'right-to-buy' provision since 1980, most of them being the better, more desirable public properties. The reduction in the stock of public housing has been further exacerbated by the decline in council house-building – from 41 500 housing 'starts' in 1980 to a mere 2000 in 1993. By 1989, some local authorities were no longer building any such housing, e.g. Bradford, Liverpool, Nottingham, Plymouth, Southampton and many London boroughs. During the same period there was also a decrease in the already small supply of private rented accommodation.

Immediate reasons

The two most common immediate reasons for people becoming homeless are parents or friends no longer being willing or able to accommodate them,

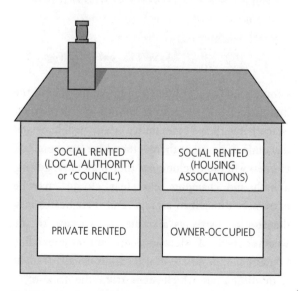

Fig. 5.4 The four different types of housing tenure in the UK.

and relationship breakdowns between partners. In 1996, research by 'Centrepoint' found that, in a study of 7 500 homeless young people, 86 per cent had been forced to leave home, rather than choosing to leave. The four most common reasons given were:

- family arguments;
- relationship breakdown ;
- overcrowding;
- physical and sexual violence (Centrepoint, 1996).

What is it like to be homeless?

The wide range of emotions experienced by people who are homeless includes feelings of fear, insecurity and dread about the future and what it will bring. As we have mentioned above, homelessness is often accompanied by other distressing experiences such as the break-up of a relationship, or being turned out by family or friends. Some people who become homeless will spend time either on the streets or in temporary accommodation.

Life on the streets

> When I first came to London I was only 16
> With a fiver in my pocket and my old dancing bag
> I went down to the dilly to check out the scene
> And I soon ended up on the old main drag.
>
> (Shane Macgowan, The Pogues)

People who become homeless are vulnerable in the first place, but attempting to live on the streets exacerbates their vulnerability. Many problems and discomforts confront them – they have nowhere safe to keep what few belongings they may have, getting a bath and changing into clean clothes may be extremely difficult to arrange, and their health may deteriorate, partly as a result of exposure to the weather, lack of decent sleep and a poor diet. Obtaining appropriate health care is usually fraught with difficulties which stem from the lack of a permanent address. Finally, homeless people are unlikely to have enough money, and attempts to beg for it may be dangerous, because of both the threat of arrest and the risk of physical attack. Black homeless people face the additional risk of racial abuse and violence.

'Rough sleepers' face loneliness and isolation. Many of them have no 'friendly face' or anyone to talk to – no companion of any kind. This can make them vulnerable to the approaches of others, to exploitation and to the potential drift into prostitution or drug misuse. A lack of control over their situation and future result in a sense of powerlessness. Lucy, who slept rough for 6 years, refers to this: 'If you're sleeping rough you can spot other people who are because they're walking round half asleep. I felt dirty, insignificant. It felt like there was nothing I could do about it; totally powerless' (Dibblin, 1991, p.33). 'Danny' is 18 years old and has lived on the streets for 2 years. He begs for money and abuses solvents as a means of release from his extremely depressing life-style. He says, 'I don't see the point in trying to get off lighter gas – no one cares about me or loves me – why on earth should I?' (*Observer*, 12 January 1997, p.10).

Life in temporary accommodation

Life on the streets is, of course, extremely uncomfortable and potentially dangerous, but being housed in temporary accommodation is far from ideal. By the end of 1996 there were 41 800 families in England alone living in this type of housing (Shelter figures).

'Temporary accommodation' can mean a number of things, including 'bed-and-breakfast hotels', women's refuges and hostels, and short-life tenancies. Rarely does it adequately meet the needs of the people using it. Temporary accommodation usually means a lack of privacy and personal space, a poor-quality physical environment and lack of decent amenities.

Black people and members of other minority ethnic groups are over-represented in temporary accommodation, and Shelter reports that, on average, they spend longer in it (O'Dwyer, 1994, p.9). This finding was corroborated by Amina Mama's study of homeless people in London, which showed that black women waited longer than white women to be rehoused. 'The observation that black women were rehoused more slowly, and in worse property, was made not only in Conservative boroughs with no policies on domestic violence, or race equality, but also in more progressive Labour boroughs' (Mama, 1989, p.111). It is not uncommon for individuals and families to spend years in 'temporary' accommodation.

Most negative publicity about this form of housing has rightly centred on the use by local authorities of 'bed-and-breakfast' hotels and guest houses. Often, because of the lack of local availability, individuals and families are forced to move a long way from their home area. Frequently a family will have to share one room, and this will mean that going outdoors is often the only way to get a break from each other. The need to keep children occupied and quiet so as not to upset other hotel guests only adds to the pressures faced by parents.

Not only is most bed-and-breakfast accommodation unsuitable, but this form of housing also represents a tragically short-sighted provision. In 1990, the National Audit Office reported that paying bed-and-breakfast charges on a long-term basis was more expensive than building new council accommodation. 'The annual cost of keeping a family in bed-and-breakfast accommodation is around £11 600 (£15 540 in London), whereas the cost of a home built to rent works out at about £8200 a year, spread over the life of the home' (*Guardian*, 23 November 1993, p.11).

CURRENT LEGISLATION RELATING TO HOMELESSNESS

The 1977 Housing (Homeless Persons) Act placed a duty on local authorities to house certain categories of people who were deemed to be in 'priority need'. Subsequently this was replaced with minor amendments by Part III of the 1985 Housing Act, and most recently by Part VII of the Housing Act 1996. The legal framework remains largely the same with regard to the groups of people that a local authority is obliged to house, with one important exception in the 1996 Act. This Act broke the automatic link, established by earlier legislation, between becoming homeless and receiving an offer of permanent accommodation in the social rented sector. It was intended to prevent certain groups of people from jumping the housing queue. However, the Labour Government has since reversed this measure and restored the status quo.

There are five areas that a local authority has to explore in order to establish whether they have a *duty* to house someone under the law.

1. The person has to prove that she or he is homeless.
2. She or he must be *eligible for assistance* in order to go on to a waiting-list, known as a 'Housing Register'. With a few exceptions, this excludes all 'asylum-seekers' (individuals claiming refugee status under the 1951 Geneva Convention, whose claim has not been finally decided – if the claim is accepted, the asylum-seeker becomes a 'refugee'; if not, she or he is simply designated a 'person from abroad').
3. A person has to be classified as being in *priority need*. There are four such categories:
   - pregnant women;
   - people with dependent children;
   - people who are vulnerable as a result of 'old age, mental illness or handicap or physical disability or other special reason' (Section 189, Housing Act 1996). The last point might include people with a serious health problem, people who are HIV-positive or those who are substance misusers;
   - people who are homeless or threatened with homelessness as a result of an emergency such as a flood or fire.
4. They must prove that they have not become homeless *intentionally*, i.e. through any fault or deliberate action of their own.

5. The local authority will ascertain whether or not an applicant has a *local connection*, or should be housed by a council elsewhere. A local connection is established if someone has lived continuously in an area for at least 6 out of the previous 12 months, or for 3 out of the last 5 years.

Once all of these areas have been explored and a person or family satisfies all conditions, then their name can be entered on the 'Housing Register'. Waiting times will vary geographically, depending on the amount of 'social housing' stock that is available and on a number of other factors, including how a particular local authority interprets the law.

Despite the existence of statutory entitlements for homeless people, they are not always granted. A research study on single homeless people conducted in Scotland, but applying to England, Wales and Scotland, was published in 1997. It examined local authority and Housing Association policies and practices, and a summary stated:

> The study found that some local authorities were failing to meet their statutory duties to single homeless people and a substantial degree of discretionary decision-making was evident. Informal 'gate-keeping' by reception and other staff could divert single applicants away from specialist officers and a full investigation of their priority need circumstances. . . . Even when single homeless people met the criteria for priority need set out in the homelessness legislation, local authorities did not necessarily accept them as statutorily homeless. Only around half of authorities said they would always, or usually, accept single homeless people who had mental health problems, learning difficulties, or were registered disabled, as being in priority need.
>
> (Anderson and Morgan, 1997)

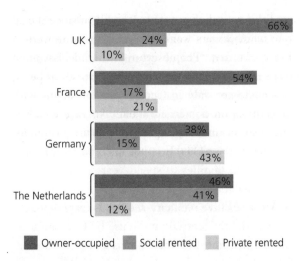

Fig. 5.5 Housing sectors in four European countries. Housing in the UK is more polarized between owner-occupation and social rented housing than in most other countries in Europe. (Reproduced from Joseph Rowntree Foundation, *Search 21*, Winter 1994, p.22, with permission)

HOMELESS PEOPLE AND SOCIAL CARE

Many people will feel that homelessness and social care or social work have little, if anything, to do with each other. Stewart and Stewart highlighted this when they wrote: 'The single homeless were not even mentioned in a book called *Social Work with Undervalued Groups*, so marginalized are both the client group and social work with them' (Stewart and Stewart, 1993, p.50).

Practice with regard to homelessness varies across the country. Social workers and probation officers may well take up a client's housing or homelessness problem as a normal part of their day-to-day work. However, housing issues are often complex, so they may refer a person on to a homelessness specialist within their own agency. Alternatively, they may liaise with staff in the local authority Housing Department.

Making links between homelessness, unemployment and poverty is crucial to understanding the *structural* constraints on people and their life situations. Taking this holistic approach will enhance the way in which carers work with clients. As Stewart and Stewart say, 'People who are homeless or trapped in bad housing may blame themselves for their circumstances and accept an "inadequate" label. Helping them to locate themselves in a structural context can increase their self-esteem and ability to cope' (Stewart and Stewart, 1993, p.147).

CAN HOMELESSNESS BE ERADICATED?

> A home needs to be secure, it should be a decent place at an affordable cost and self-contained. It ought to provide the means for you to live your own life in the way you choose. Without this you cannot really have a home in the fullest sense.
>
> (Quoted from Sheila McKechnie in the introduction to Morris, 1990, p.2)

The short answer to the question posed in the above heading is, of course, 'No'. There will always be relationship breakdowns, and families and friends will always be asking people to move out, i.e. the *immediate* causes of homelessness will remain with us. However, the high levels of homelessness and the *structural* causes of it do not need to be tolerated.

In referring specifically to youth homelessness, Sheila McKechnie writes, 'How can we live in a society that cares so little for its young that they have to beg in order to survive? How many more reports, campaigns, meetings with ministers, letters and petitions have to happen before the *crisis* facing young people is dealt with?' (In Rosen, 1991, p.11).

Ironically, Sheila McKechnie mentions the word 'crisis'. When 'Shelter' was formed over 30 years ago, its founders also spoke in terms of 'crisis'. The word is still being used in 1998, and in the intervening years it has never fallen out of currency, and yet a dictionary definition refers to a crisis as a *'sudden*

change'. Clearly the problem of homelessness is much more than a sudden event – it is a chronic situation. As has been stated, homelessness is essentially a 'housing' problem, not a 'people' problem. Solutions to the structural causes lie in politics and economics.

In recent years, some short-term measures to alleviate the most brutal effects of homelessness have been introduced, notably the 'Rough Sleepers Initiative' (RSI), started in 1990, which made money available to provide hostel spaces and create more permanent accommodation for people leaving hostels. In 1996, the RSI was extended for a further 3 years.

According to 'Shelter', the underlying cause of homelessness is the shortage of *suitable, affordable housing*. It claims that the government should increase the supply of new affordable rented housing to at least 100 000 homes a year to meet the level of housing need (O'Dwyer, 1994, p.12 [our emphasis]). Paul Balchin supports this view and also states: 'It is . . . important to increase the supply of low-cost housing by putting empty houses back into use and to embark upon new housebuilding programmes'. He adds 'the free market cannot provide solutions to Britain's substantial housing problems' (Balchin, 1995, p.278, p.286).

The election of the Labour Government in May 1997 sounded a note of optimism and hopefulness for homeless people. Apart from restoring the 1996 Housing Act 'safety net', the Secretary of State for the Environment, John Prescott, has said that local authorities will be able to spend the estimated £5 billion (in England and Wales) of capital receipts they have accrued from 'right-to-buy' sales, over a 5-year period. Housing specialists in Scotland do not feel so optimistic. As Michael Thain reported, 'Unlike England, there is no pool of available cash in Scotland. Receipts from sales of local authority stock have already been spent' (*Inside Housing*, 6 June 1997, p.18).

Gordon Brown, the Chancellor of the Exchequer, promised that councils could spend £200 million in the 1997–1998 financial year, with £700 million following in the next. This money added up to 'totals that housing chiefs estimate would allow the repair of 60 000 homes or the building of 28 000' (*Guardian*, 3 July 1997). As Shelter's *Roof* magazine declared elatedly, 'council housing is back in business!' (*Roof*, July/August 1997, p.20).

5.7 PEOPLE WITH LEARNING DISABILITIES/LEARNING DIFFICULTIES

We demand that you give us the right to make choices and decisions regarding our own lives. We are tired of people telling us what they want. Instead, let us all work together as a team. Our voice may be a new one to you, but you should better get used to hearing it.

(Barb Goode addressing the General Assembly of the United Nations in 1992; quoted in *Inside Community Care*, 29 February 1996, p.1)

SELF-ADVOCACY

The above quotation highlights the existence of self-advocacy among people with learning disabilities. Not everyone with learning difficulties is as articulate as Canadian Barb Goode, but many are developing skills and the confidence to speak up on issues that affect their lives. There are now hundreds of self-advocacy groups throughout the UK, including 'People First' and 'Skills for People'. The growth of self-advocacy symbolizes the change in attitude of many people with learning disabilities and those who work alongside them. There is now a desire to place the service-user at the centre of the services they receive – to involve them, or their advocate, in decision-making and planning in order to make available choices and opportunities for personal development.

OPPRESSION

This has not always been the case, and the enlightened professional approach to service delivery has yet to be matched by a wider society that continues to disable people with learning disabilities more severely than do their mental limitations.

In 1989, David Brandon wrote 'People with learning difficulties are among the most oppressed of all minorities. They are rejected and sentimentalized over as objects of pity, mawkishness and whimsy. There is a great danger that we may compound the overall oppression aimed at their submission. The system tries to break their spirit through enchaining them and us. We need solidarity with them, recognizing our mutual humanity.... When we work towards their gradual and eventual liberation we automatically work towards our own' (Brandon, 1989, p.96).

PUBLIC ATTITUDES AND STEREOTYPES

People with learning disabilities are oppressed in our society mainly because of public attitudes and a general discomfort with the slower pace at which some people learn and respond. This in turn has an impact on how people with learning disabilities comprehend and perform their daily living tasks. Their full integration is further hampered by the influence of myths and demeaning public stereotypes concerning people with learning disabilities, who are often confused with people who have mental health problems. The stereotypes place undue emphasis on characteristics displayed by people with a learning disability that relate to difficulties in communication. These may include unusual mannerisms and inappropriate behaviour, such as standing too close or touching too familiarly. More extreme behaviour can include sudden and violent gestures and action. Stereotypes are reinforced and perpetuated because so many members of the public do not have ordinary close contact with people with learning difficulties. Until quite recently, they may only have seen people with learning difficulties *en masse*, either being transported by Social Services, or at day centres or in hospital wards, when their collective presence may serve to emphasize any strangeness.

With the exception of those individuals who have or have had a person with a learning disability in their own family, most people in our society have had infrequent contact with people with learning difficulties. As children they rarely shared classrooms, Sunday school or other religious centres, or parks and playgrounds with them, and few now share their homes, work or social life with adults with learning disabilities, although this is becoming more common. It is not surprising, therefore, that there is so much widespread ignorance about the needs of people with learning difficulties, and so much embarrassment and apprehension among ordinary members of the public. Furthermore, the perceived social abnormality of learning disabilities is reinforced by the media, which rarely focuses on people with learning difficulties except in controversial circumstances. They are rarely featured in ordinary everyday settings.

The terms 'learning difficulties' or 'special needs' embrace a wide variety of people, ranging from those whose disability is mild and barely discernible through to those whose condition is severe and with whom communication is often extremely restricted. It should be remembered that people with learning difficulties are as unique as people without a disability. Stereotypes only obscure this individuality.

OUT OF SIGHT OUT OF MIND

Much of today's misinformation about and negativity towards people with learning disabilities has its roots in the past. From early Victorian times until the middle of this century, social provision was directed by the principle of 'out of sight, out of mind'. People with varying degrees of 'mental handicap' were incarcerated in specially built, self-contained hospitals that were often situated in remote settings far away from built-up areas. Many of these people spent the remainder of their lives in an institutional world, well separated from the rest of society. Moreover, some people with learning disabilities were 'certified' and admitted alongside mentally ill people, thus 'reinforcing prevailing stereotypes about the uniform character of madness' (National Institute for Social Work, 1988a, p.12).

In *A Price to be Born – Twenty Years in a Mental Institution* (four volumes of his life history) David Barron tells of the damaging treatment he received in different segregated settings. Figure 5.6 shows a brief extract of his life-story in its original phonetic form, which was later translated into 'proper writing and spelling' by a friend for publication. The process of compilation and subsequent publication of his life-story has enabled David Barron to deal constructively with his past: 'The books have helped me clear my system. Uncovering my story has helped keep me alive' (quoted in Brandon, 1989, pp.20–21).

CAUSES OF LEARNING DISABILITIES

It is important to distinguish briefly between learning disability and mental illness. People with a learning disability have some form of permanent brain damage. They experience difficulties in learning, the effects of which are usually noticed in the early years of life. With education and support they can be helped to overcome some of their disabilities,

ONE

MY NAME IS DAVID CENTH BARRON
i WAS BORN ON AUGUST 10TH 8/ 1925.
IN BACHELER STREET LEEDS.
MY MUTHERS NAME IS BiTRUS MAYBUL
BARRON. FORMLY CHAPMAN. MY THATHERS
NAME. IS NOT NOWN, I HAVE NAVER SEEN
MY MUM AND DAD. BUT IT IS NOT FOR
THE WONT OF TRING
I CAME OUT OF THE ORTHNIDS AT THE
AGE OF 5 YEARS. AND WAS PLAYST IN THE
CMRE OF A FOSTER MUTHER. TERND OUT
TO BE A CARDISTIKT. ONE. AT THE NOW
THE AGE OF E 11½ YEARS. I WAS
TACKON A WAY FROM MY FOSTER
MUTHER. AND PUT IN FO A MANTUL
HOSPITUL. WICH THE A FORÓTIS SAID,
WAS TO BE MY NEW HOME. AND THAT
I WOULD BE WEL LOOKT HATHTER. AND
THAT I WOULD GIT THE BEST OF
TREET. MANT. THAT WAS TO BE THE
UNDER STAYTMONT OF THE DAY AS I WAS
A BOUT TO FIND OUT. AFTEAR THE
FORMIERTIS OVE MY
HAD MISHON. AD BEEN. KONPLEETID,
THE 2 MEN WICH HAD TACKOV ME,
THERE LEFT. I WAS TACKON DAWN TO
WARD ONE. THE ATENDUNT PULD OUT
A BIG BUNCH OF KEES. UNLOCKT
THE DORE LET ME IN. WOT A SHOK,
IT WAS FOR ME AS I STOD AND LOOKT
A RAWND. WARD DORS LOCKT
BEIND ME. WINDWS WITH BARS UT
AT THAM. AND IF THAT WAS NOT BAD
IEE NUTH. I WAS TACKUN UP STARS,
AND TOLD TO STREIP OF AND FOLD AL
MY KLOWS

Fig. 5.6 Extract from *A Price to be Born* in David Barron's phonetic script. (Reproduced with kind permission of David Barron.)

sometimes to the point where their difficulty is minimal. People with a *mental illness*, on the other hand, experience a mental state emanating from stress or problems which they are no longer able to control. Their condition is often temporary, because mental illness is generally treatable or self-limiting, although relapses can and do occur. Mental illness is more common than mental handicap, and is directly encountered by an estimated one in nine members of the population at some stage in their life. Some individuals have a predisposition to mental illness. People with learning difficulties may experience

mental illness in addition to their learning disability, and some studies have shown that they are more prone to mental illness than other people.

A learning disability may be caused by a number of factors, although the exact cause is often not known. Most people are born with their disability, e.g. Down's syndrome, but some acquire the condition during their lifetime, or following a viral infection, or by sustaining brain damage through injury. There are estimated to be between 1 and 1.5 million people with a learning disability in this country. Of these, the majority have only moderate learning difficulties, and the extent to which they manage to achieve their full potential will depend, as it does with everyone, on the amount of love, stimulation and support they receive.

SPECIAL DIFFICULTIES FOR PARENTS OF CHILDREN WITH LEARNING DISABILITIES

Some families are unable to cope with the unexpected extra demands and strain created by the arrival of a child with learning difficulties. Marriages may break down, possibly resulting in either the child being received into care, or one of the parents (usually the mother) being left with sole responsibility for the child's upbringing. However, most parents react positively to their situation and strive to provide their child with all the love and attention he or she needs. In reality they have little choice. Although their task still includes many of the essential joys of child-rearing, it is often an isolating and debilitating struggle. Society's reluctance to share the responsibility means that the parents face a life-long battle without respite. This view was expressed in a letter to a newspaper which ended: 'Don't tell me that it is always difficult being a parent – will you still be paying for baby-sitters when your children are 20, 30, 40?' (A. Millerman, *Guardian*, 22 September 1989, p.11).

The same parent found herself writing again, 8 years later, to the same newspaper. It seems that little has changed:

> The new East Enders storyline about spina bifida has reopened the debate about pre-natal diagnosis and the right to life (TV review, November 28). But is it the baby alone who has the right to life? What about the parents – don't they have a right to life as well?
>
> My own twin daughters were born severely disabled 20 years ago. Since then, my life has been a constant struggle to achieve some quality of life for us all. We are mostly a society of nuclear families now, and are increasingly reliant on official services for support – but the louder I scream for help the louder comes the reply of 'no money'.
>
> Abortion should not be the only option for a disabled fetus, but nor should parents be expected to undertake years and years of back-breaking labour, and unimaginable levels of pain, without a very clear understanding of the limited amount of support available.
>
> If society continues to expect carers to cope with minimum support, abortion will remain the only solution.
>
> (A. Millerman, *Guardian*, 1 December 1997, p.9)

Those who become parents of children with learning disabilities need to make huge emotional adjustments as they endeavour to come to terms with the feelings brought about by a sense of overwhelming disappointment and loss. They may be counselled against having further children in case they produce another child with special needs. They may worry, too, about the social and emotional stresses that having a sibling with learning difficulties might place on any existing children. Parents may also experience guilt or shame at having produced a child with special needs because he or she is not seen as perfect by the rest of society. The situation is more difficult for families within some communities, where having a disabled child is seen to represent a divine punishment, and the family will have to bear that added stigma.

Having a child with learning difficulties may mean that the family will be virtually excluded from engaging in many of their hitherto cherished ac-

tivities. The following extract is from an account of how an ordinary day-to-day event served to bring home to a mother the limitations of her twin daughters, both of whom have a physical and a learning disability, and the implications for the family's future. The children were approaching their first birthday; 3 months earlier they had been diagnosed as being severely brain damaged:

> Christmas shopping had to be done. Some niceties must always be observed. I braced myself and embarked on a trip to Habitat. A harmless enough venue I thought. What confronted me there was the moment that stands out more than any other moment in the last 13 years.
>
> There, amid the glasses and the kitchenware, furniture and fancy goods, stood stark realisation. Stretching high towards the ceiling was a large display of skipping ropes. Hundreds and hundreds of them. The perfect present for a little girl. I have never known a little girl who hasn't skipped at some time in her life. It's a simple activity totally devoid of class, status, age, wealth, culture, race or religion. As I looked at them they began to represent the entire life that we would have to say goodbye to: the fell-walking that we had always loved, that would now only be possible with supreme physical effort and the help of others; the family outings that we'd dreamed of during pregnancy – trips to funfairs, zoos and the countryside, which would all now take on the proportions of a major expedition. Even nipping out to the shops was going to be a thing of the past. How could one person ever go anywhere again, on impulse, with two wheelchairs to push?
>
> The total enormity of the situation hit me in the stomach like a bag of wet cement. I sucked in my cheeks, turned around and walked out as fast as I could. I didn't cry until I reached the car.
>
> (A. Millerman, unpublished)

Parents of children with learning difficulties will need support from friends and relatives more than most families, yet they are more likely to be isolated in this respect. For various reasons, including their own embarrassment, awkwardness and ignorance, friends and neighbours may be reluctant to visit or to help out in a situation with which they are not familiar, and where they do not always feel at ease.

Social provision – ranging from financial benefits to home conversion grants, special school arrangements and respite-care facilities – is available, to a varying degree, to families with children with learning difficulties. However, such provision is often inadequate, it varies from region to region and is not always available from birth, and strict eligibility criteria exclude some families. White, middle-class parents may be more skilled at matching the criteria and more articulate in their appeal for services.

There is some evidence that the needs of ethnic minority families in particular are not being met by service providers. It has been said of Asian adults with learning disabilities that they 'experience double discrimination: stigma because of their learning disability and racism because of their ethnicity' (*Community Care*, 10–16 July 1997, p.31). In one study it was shown that only 17 per cent of carers felt that services were satisfactory, and 31 per cent were dissatisfied. The main reasons given were lack of awareness about what was available, lack of interpreting services or staff who could speak appropriate languages, culturally inappropriate services, and racial discrimination within the services (*Community Care*, 10–16 July 1997, p.31). The article pointed out that, with appropriate support, 'Asian carers, like any other group of carers, can provide a fulfilling life for themselves and their families. The challenge to the service is to make this fulfilment a reality' (*Community Care*, 10–16 July 1997, p.31).

As children grow older the difficulties for their parents increase. The children become physically more difficult to manage, and they may need extra support in coping with the changes brought about by puberty and adolescence. While they are at school they are cared for during the day. However, when they get beyond *school age*, the responsibility for full-time care goes back to the parents. In some cases residential care is necessary but for many families this is not appropriate. The Wagner Report (National Institute for Social Work, 1988b), *Residential Care – A Positive Choice,* and other reports published since, recommend that 'Education and training for people with *mental handicap* should aim at enabling them to live with minimum support in ordinary housing' (National Institute for Social Work, 1988b, p.7). Until appropriate provision is made for all people with learning difficulties, parents will continue to be plagued by their major concern, namely 'Who is going to look after them when I'm gone?'

SOCIAL PROVISION FOR PEOPLE WITH LEARNING DIFFICULTIES

Children and young people

Children and young people with special needs have a statutory right to education from the age of 2 years until they are 19 years old. Since the 1981 Education Act, every young person who is considered to have special needs, including those with learning difficulties, has a right to be made the subject of professional assessment and to have a statement drawn up outlining his or her needs. Furthermore, in order to encourage integration, children and young adults with learning difficulties should, where possible, have their education provided within mainstream education. The principle of *integration* has its detractors, who feel that children and young people with learning difficulties may miss the specialized support which is found only in special schools, and may experience a sense of failure in the larger mainstream schools. However, it is argued that children with learning difficulties will benefit from experiencing ordinary schooling, albeit with special support, and an opportunity to grow up and make friends with ordinary children. Children without special needs will also benefit from exposure to people with learning difficulties from an early age.

Adults

As already mentioned, once people with learning difficulties have left school their parents face the most testing times. Education is statutory, but once it is over people with learning disabilities are not automatically entitled to support. The Disabled Persons Act 1986 recommends, but does not insist, that local authorities should define need and provide for it. People with learning disabilities are entitled to support under the National Assistance Act 1948, the Chronically Sick and Disabled Persons Act 1970 and, of course, may be assessed under the provision of the National Health Service and Community Care Act 1990 and provided with a package of care as appropriate. Those who care for them are also entitled to a separate assessment under the Carers Recognition Act 1995, which was implemented in April 1996.

Example of a community-care package

Imaginative and personally tailored care packages may be devised in order to meet a person's individual needs. Figure 5.7 shows a weekly timetable of activities arranged in order to support Graham, a young man with Asperger's syndrome (a form of autism) to live in his own flat within the community.

Graham does not like crowds or meeting new people. He likes to walk, but chooses to do this either when it gets dark or at quiet times of the day. He has spent some of his adult life in hospital and in residential establishments, but has lived the majority of it at home with his parents, who carried out many of his daily living tasks for him. Consequently, he is still developing independence skills.

Graham does not like to receive any visitors before 11 a.m., by which time he has completed his routine and has washed, shaved and had his breakfast. He needs routine, and the timetable has been devised with this in mind It also aims to provide him with stimulation and variety and a chance to develop independent living skills. Graham and his advocate, Bill, were involved in planning the care package with the social worker who meets with Graham each week to offer support and monitor progress.

Periodically, all of the paid workers and Graham's advocate meet to discuss and plan on his behalf. Graham and his parents – with whom Graham has a strained relationship – attend for part of the meeting. One issue considered at the meeting was Graham's imminent return to the church social club a week on Friday, to which he was looking forward. He was coming to the end of a 3-month ban following a violent outburst there. He enjoys this

Mon	Tues	Weds	Thurs	Fri	Sat	Sun
2–4 p.m. Claire Cleaning	12–1 p.m. Joanne Counselling 6–8 p.m. Social centre	12–2 p.m. Gulshen Cooking	1–3 p.m. Andy Walking	4–5 p.m. Don Social worker 6–8 p.m. Church social club fortnightly	12–4 p.m. Andy Walking	1–2 p.m. Lunch with parents

Fig. 5.7 A weekly timetable of activities arranged in order to support a young man with Asperger's syndrome.

social centre where he has an evening meal and plays draughts. He feels safe at the social club and can always retreat to a seat in the corner if he feels agitated, perhaps if it becomes too busy or crowded, although the numbers attending regularly are quite small. He was banned for a short period in order to give him an opportunity to appreciate the consequences of his violence and to learn to take responsibility by controlling it. More recently he also lost his temper with Andy, one of his support workers, when he was unsettled by a passer-by and her small barking dog. He has since apologized to Andy and the matter has been satisfactorily resolved.

The outcome of the last meeting was that the social worker should plan a supported holiday with Graham. A more long-term aim was for Graham to do some of his own shopping. At the moment this is done by his parents, who bring the shopping to his house in his absence each Tuesday lunchtime. Despite his difficulties, Graham is coping with living on his own. He pays his own bills, prepares much of his own food and is involved in planning his care and support. He gets lonely from time to time, in the same way that many people who live by themselves do, but he is developing skills and gaining independence. Each month he collects money door to door for a charity, from local people who have got to know him. He may always need support to maintain himself in his own flat. The less satisfactory and probably more expensive alternative would be either residential or hospital care. At present he is being supported so that he can manage independently in the community.

Philosophies of care

For years services have been moving away from the model of 'total care' towards one which promotes skills training and independence. This shift results from the recognition that old ways were adding to people's handicap by increasing dependency and perceived deviance from others.

(Brandon, 1989, p.9)

As has already been stated, philosophies concerning the care of people with learning disabilities have moved on in recent years. Care is very much more than containment. In the 1960s the seemingly straightforward concept of *normalization* was developed in Scandinavia by Bengt Nirje, who defined it as 'making available to all mentally retarded people patterns of life and conditions of everyday living which are as close as possible to the regular circumstances and ways of life of society'. The principle of normalization was taken further by Professor Wolfensberger, who sought to improve the lives of people with learning disabilities and to combat their devalued status by advocating a service that was as close to 'normal' as possible. Defining what was normal was then and always has been problematic. *Social role valorization theory (SRV)* has superseded normalization and is an influence on current practice. In simple terms, it emphasizes the need to validate individuals and encourage them to obtain and maintain positive social roles. SRV supports the principle of *integration*, whereby people with learning disabilities are encouraged to integrate in everyday settings in order to widen their basic choices and responsibilities.

O'Brien's *five accomplishments* form a standard around which services may be measured. The simple statements have been incorporated into many organizations' practice guidelines and some Local Authority Community Care plans. The five accomplishments are as follows.

- *Dignity and respect* – people with learning disabilities have the right to be treated with respect and dignity. They should be offered services which are based on their individual circumstances, choices and expectations, they should participate in decision-making and be given information, they have the right of refusal and complaint through self-advocacy and advocacy, and they should be involved in developing and evaluating the services that they receive. People should have services which are appropriate to their age that they will be proud of.

- *Community presence* – people with a learning disability are part of the community and must not be separated from it. They should have equal opportunities in having easy access to shops, leisure and recreation facilities, housing, education, employment, health services and social services.
- *Community participation* – people with a learning disability must be able to develop a full range of personal relationships, to be involved with others as friends, relatives, colleagues, consumers and citizens, and to have sexual relationships and options to include marriage and parenting.
- *Choice* – people with learning disabilities have a right to make choices and decisions about their daily lives and activities, and to be enabled to make choices and decisions with support and information about options, responsibilities and consequences. People with a learning difficulty have the right to services which promote the taking of risks and the holding of personal opinions.
- *Competence* – people with a learning disability will have opportunities to develop skills throughout their lives by building on their skills and abilities in a variety of settings and by a variety of means to enable them to be involved in the community.

Citizen advocacy, self-advocacy and circles of support

People with learning disabilities vary in their capabilities, and some are profoundly impaired and incapable of self-advocacy. It is therefore necessary that people with severe and complex needs are represented by an advocate. The use of advocacy within the service to people with a learning disability is well established. An *advocate* will endeavour to communicate the wishes, needs and expectations of the service-user to all concerned in that person's care. He or she will befriend the service-user, attend planning meetings and reviews, write letters and make telephone calls in order to ensure that the service is effective (in the case illustrated earlier, Bill

would have performed these tasks in consultation with and on behalf of Graham).

Much of the impetus for change in service delivery has come from users themselves, particularly since the advent of *self-advocacy*. Richard Malin of Herts People First says, 'We want to be more involved in our services . . . to have a more powerful say in our lives . . . for people with learning difficulties to be more independent in themselves, like an ordinary citizen in society, to have their own rights' (quoted in Simons, 1995, p.132).

Richard belongs to 'People First' – a self-advocacy organization which represents the views of people with learning disabilities. Part of their role is to voice the view of service-users and to make information accessible to them. The illustration shown in Fig. 5.8 is taken from *Oi! It's My Assessment. Why Not Listen To Me!*

As has already been mentioned, self-advocacy is not possible for everyone who has a learning disability, owing to the severity of their mental impairment. For such people, and also for those who are more able, *circles of support* represent a new way of working. Frequently circles of support may be established when a crisis or transitional point has been reached, such as leaving school or moving from an institutional setting. 'The circle is a way of bringing together a number of people who care about the person sufficiently to want to act collectively on his or her behalf. Everyone is there at the specific request of the "focus" person, invited as an equal to enable the person to dream and to achieve those dreams. The members may be friends, family members, lovers, colleagues and neighbours' (Mandy Neville, *Inside Community Care*, 29 February 1996, p.4).

The National Health Service and Community Care Act 1990 has done much to promote the support of people with learning disabilities living in the community. 'There is now a *supported living movement* – a loose coalition of service staff, users and carers all with interest in and commitment to developing new ways of supporting people' (*Inside Community Care*, 29 February 1996, p.2). Many day-centres are

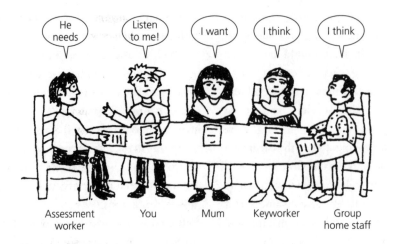

Fig. 5.8 The assessment meeting.

changing their role and have become less building-based, operating as resource centres or as a landing-pad from which service-users with the support of day-centre workers may use ordinary community facilities. For instance, individuals or small groups may go shopping, use the leisure centre or attend a well-woman or well-man centre.

Some authorities have devolved the day-centre staff, who now work alongside users in ordinary everyday settings, perhaps in college or work settings. There are many examples of constructive and creative work being carried out with people with learning disabilities that contrast starkly with the legacy of the past. It would appear that, within the caring professions, people with learning disabilities are more commonly being valued and respected as individuals.

5.8   LONE-PARENT FAMILIES

> Single parents – for which read women on their own – do not destroy communities. They shore them up.
>
> (*Community Care*, 12–18 June 1997, p.17)

Single-parent families are not a social problem. However, they are often regarded as such by policy-makers and the general public alike. The negative image of lone-parent families stems in part from the long associated stigma of immorality that has been attached to unmarried mothers and their children. Earlier this century women who became pregnant outside marriage were often classified as 'moral defectives' and admitted to mental hospitals. Since then other myths and prejudices have evolved concerning one-parent families, including young women deliberately becoming pregnant in order to obtain council housing, idle mothers living off maintenance and fatherless teenagers turning to drugs. Single mothers are often assumed to be permissive and therefore, it is thought, they are unable to discipline their children properly, while lone fathers are thought to be unable to react emotionally towards their children.

Sue Slipman, Director of the National Council For One-Parent Families (NCFOPF), formerly the National Council for the Unmarried Mother and Her Child, writing in the National Council's Annual Report (1988), stated: 'The spectre of immorality, so potentially alive at our foundation (in 1918) still haunts the official and popular imagination, re-affirming the myth of one-parent family life. There can be few areas of public policy-making so dominated by prejudice and ignorance and so little informed by fact' (National Council For One-Parent Families, 1988, p.5). The idea that lone-parent families are a problem-ridden alternative to the 'normal' two-parent family is harmful and creates difficulties for those who are members of lone-parent families. It is more accurate to view single parents and their children as belonging to one of several existing and legitimate family forms, and one which, following the increase in numbers over the past 20 years, is here to stay.

PROPORTION OF THE POPULATION

Single-parent families are on the increase. In 1971 there were just over 500 000 families headed by a lone parent, whereas today there are over 1.51 million. Figures produced in 1998 (Fig. 5.9) showed that one-parent families represented 22 per cent of all those households with dependent children, and that one child in five is in a family unit headed by

a lone parent. Ninety-one per cent of these families are headed by women. Very few Asian families (less than 5 per cent) were headed by lone parents, but the family form was common among people of West Indian or Guyanese origin (around 32 per cent).

WHO ARE THE SINGLE PARENTS?

While it is true to say that an increasing number of women are deliberately choosing to bring up children on their own, they are still very much in the minority. Some women decide to have children and bring them up by themselves because they want to be independent of a relationship with a man. Often they have had negative experiences of men. Other women who want to be mothers may be part of a lesbian relationship, and they are therefore able to form a different type of two-parent family. However, the majority of people who become single parents do not attain their status by choice – it tends to be thrust upon them by a traumatic event, such as death, divorce or separation. As is shown in Fig. 5.10, most single parents were married at one stage (this

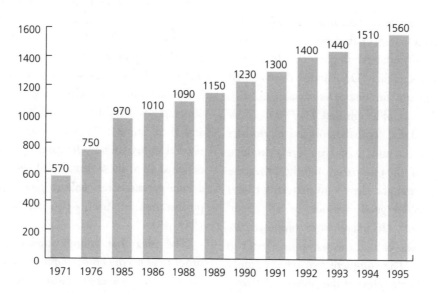

Fig. 5.9 Numbers (in thousands) of lone parent families in the UK. (Reproduced from *Population Trends, spring 1998*. Office of Population Censuses and Surveys.)

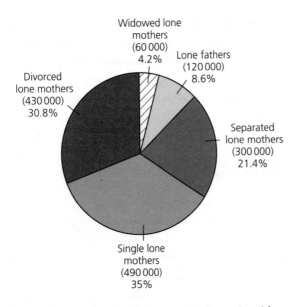

Widowed lone
mothers
(60 000)
4.2%

Lone fathers
(120 000)
8.6%

Divorced
lone mothers
(430 000)
30.8%

Separated
lone mothers
(300 000)
21.4%

Single lone
mothers
(490 000)
35%

Fig. 5.10 Marital status of lone parents. (Reproduced from *Population Trends 1994*. Office of Population Censuses and Surveys.)

figure does not include those lone parents who were in cohabiting relationships).

PREJUDICE

Myths, negative media reports and other prejudices concerning single parents have been created and do little to foster an understanding of the difficulties that many of them face. Dr Rhodes Boyson MP aroused no sympathy for lone parents when, in 1987, he published his pamphlet entitled *The Defence of the Family*. He alleged that 'football hooliganism, riotings and muggings in the middle of cities are a product, in a large case, of the one-parent family, where the father is not present and there's no pattern for boys of what controlled good manners is all about' (Boyson, 1987, p.2). His views were supported by one member of the public who wrote in a letter to the *Daily Express*, 'The complete two-parent family with built-in self-discipline is the norm and always will be. Circumstances will always produce exceptions to the rule and these must have an equal place

in society, but they must never be accepted as "normal" ' (*Daily Express*, 25 April 1987).

In the early 1990s other politicians and the media inflamed the moral panic about the growing number of one-parent families and defined them as a social problem. First, the then Prime Minister, Margaret Thatcher, emphasized 'individual responsibility' prior to the introduction of the Child Support Bill. This Bill led to the creation of the controversial Child Support Agency which has the responsibility of tracing, assessing and collecting financial contributions from both parents, more commonly the child's putative father. Peter Lilley's famous 'little-list' speech given to the Conservative Party Conference in 1992 targeted 'young girls who get pregnant just to jump the housing queue'. A year later John Redwood continued the attack on young mothers, this time in Cardiff, equating them with family breakdown.

These rather extreme views of one-parent families are based on a number of misconceptions. The first is that all single parents are female, whereas in fact there are over 120 000 lone fathers. Secondly, it has been suggested that all lone parents choose their single status but, as we have seen, the majority were formerly married or in a relationship. Thirdly, it has been suggested that children of lone parents get into trouble more frequently than children of two-parent families *because* they are members of one-parent families. There is no research to support this view. In fact, according to Penny Letts of the National Council For One-Parent Families, 'In over 60 years of working first with unmarried mothers, and then, since 1973, with single parents of any marital status, we have found that ' "There is no evidence at all to show that a child being brought up by a lone parent is less able to grow up into a whole person than one from a two-person home" ' (Letts, 1983, p.7).

The idea that young women get pregnant in order to jump the housing queue has been described as one of society's most mischievous myths. According to research carried out by psychologist Emma Clark, 'Far from housing being the first consideration, it was probably the last thing on their minds. No one has thought pregnancy or motherhood is a passport to guaranteed housing or income. Often when I raised the question it was greeted with derision or disbelief. It seemed laughable or tragic to them that anyone would use a baby in this way. They had got pregnant because of a complex variety of circumstances – just like women of any age' (quoted in Dibblin, 1991, p.88).

More recently it has been pointed out that 'even in the long run, children who have experienced family breakdown may do less well at school, further education and the labour market and have poorer health than those whose parents stay together' and 'children from multiply deprived backgrounds are more prone to delinquent behaviour' but 'it is too simplistic to associate lone parenthood with delinquent outcomes for children' (Scare in the community. Britain in moral panic. *Community Care*, 1995, p.27).

Instead, the authors go on to say: 'It is increasingly agreed that the key influence in children's upbringing is how they are cared for – and how consistently – by their parents and their relationship with them. Inadequate parenting by poorly skilled parents – rather than growing up in a lone-parent household – is the main problem (*Community Care*, 1995, p.27).

It is tempting to assume that children from one-parent families miss out in the absence of one parent and therefore lack an appropriate role model. However, it is argued that depending on a child's surroundings, good role models may be provided by other people in the family network such as grandparents, friends or other people close to the family. Love, consistency and security are what children need, and this *can* be provided by one person. Indeed, it is clear that many two-parent families fail to provide children with the love and care which they need. Some people feel that there are positive benefits for children of lone parents. A single parent, writing in *Bringing Up Children On Your Own* (McNeil-Taylor, 1985), claims a distinct advantage to single parenthood: 'When you're on your own with your kids, something happens to you – you can give yourself entirely to them. If there are two adults in a family it is split down the middle with the adults in one camp and the kids in the other, but

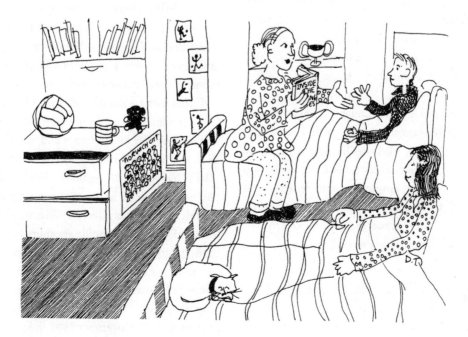

Lone parents are often able to spend more time with their children than their counterparts in two-parent families.

when you are a single parent you and your kids are all part of the one unit' (McNeil-Taylor, 1985, p.141). Another parent stated in a letter to the *Guardian* on 31 January 1990: 'Single parents live for their children. In a lot of ways they get more attention than children from two-parent families.' The writer further added, 'I think there is less chance of them becoming juvenile delinquents'.

Lone parents differ in every case, just as all individuals differ. What they have in common is the sole responsibility for their children and a strong likelihood that they will experience social deprivation and live on or around the margins of our society. Poverty is experienced by the majority of one-parent families.

FINANCIAL HARDSHIP

Most single parents of small children are not free to work, either full-time or part-time. In order to do so they would have to earn substantial amounts of money to cover the cost of child care, meet the extra costs of going to work and make up for the loss of any state benefit. Some parents are able to work part-time, but a characteristic of part-time work is that it is low paid and rarely offers the benefits of full-time employment such as maternity leave, pension schemes and annual holidays. Part-time employees are also more vulnerable to redundancy. Single parents of older children are more able to find work, but employment is again likely to be part-time. Lone parents often experience discrimination in the job market where some employers are reluctant to employ parents with sole child-care responsibilities. Consequently, single parents are often forced to take jobs below their qualification or skill level.

EUROPE

The UK has the highest proportion of lone parents in Europe except for Denmark, but unlike their Euro-pean counterparts, lone parents in the UK are less likely to be in paid work. For example, in France, 82 per cent of lone mothers are employed, compared to 41 per cent in the UK (Daycare Trust, 1997, p.2). The shortage of affordable child-care in the UK is a key factor because lone mothers have to pay child-care costs out of only one wage packet. Consequently, the majority of one-parent families rely exclusively on state benefits and so experience a feeling of fixed dependency. There is evidence that many more would like to work but are hampered from doing so by the lack of available, inexpensive, good-quality child care and other financial policies that would make finding work outside the home viable.

WELFARE TO WORK

In 1997 the Government introduced its 'Welfare to Work' scheme, aimed at helping single parents with school-aged children. The government offered counselling and advice and introduced a number of after-school clubs in all areas. The scheme claimed some initial success, with many single parents successfully obtaining jobs. However, Liz Sewell, Chief Executive of Gingerbread, said that the absence of child-care facilities was limiting progress: 'At the moment there is not enough child care to go round and what there is is too expensive'. She added, 'If the Government does not implement a national strategy that delivers for lone parents and allows them to go back to work, then this scheme is not going to work' (*Daily Telegraph*, 24 January 1997, p.12). Single parent Carmen Fielding, who managed to find work but felt that this was adversely affecting her son, said: 'It is unfair to force single mothers out to work by reducing their benefits and I do not see how providing more after-school clubs is going to improve things. They will have to be free and operate for longer hours and during school holidays' (*Independent*, 27 November 1997, p.5).

The absence of adequate state-funded child-care provision, the difficulties that lone parents experience in obtaining well-paid work, and the enforced reliance of so many on state benefits means that the majority of single parents and their families face permanent financial hardship. One in two children living in the poorest households is part of a lone-parent family, and the financial hardships experienced by so many lone parents result in their being less able to take part in life-enhancing activities. They are less able to afford to be involved in leisure pursuits, to enjoy public entertainment or to go on holidays, whereas such activities tend to be taken for granted by the rest of society.

Although this also depends on their social network, a report produced by the Rowntree Foundation showed that families were socially and materially better off, regardless of income, if they had grandparents to support them (*Guardian Society*, 10 September 1997, p.6).

HOUSING AND LIVING STANDARDS

Housing is another area where single parents and their families often experience difficulties and hardship. Approximately 6 out of 10 single mothers live in local authority housing (National Council For One-Parent Families, 1990). Since the 1980 Housing Act, the availability of public housing has been reduced; much of the better housing has been bought by tenants exercising their right to buy. This has left only the more dilapidated and less desirable properties which councils have been unable to restore due to a lack of financial resources. Because of their desperate plight, some lone parents are forced to accept accommodation in 'hard-to-let' properties, or they are put up temporarily in hotels or hostels while they wait for more permanent accommodation. Lone mothers are particularly vulnerable to homelessness – some may be turned out of their home and some may find it necessary to seek refuge from male violence.

STIGMA

Apart from experiencing material disadvantages, single parents and their children suffer the stigma of being viewed as an incomplete family and therefore inadequate. Single fathers may not be considered capable parents, single mothers may be branded as failures because they have been unable to keep their man (the assumed goal for all women!), and doubt may be cast on their ability to guide and discipline children properly on their own.

Martin Hughes, who featured in a television programme called *Someone Like Me* (BBC, 18 March 1990), talked about his family experience since the death of his wife 3 years previously. He and his children struggled to survive, first on his redundancy pay and then on state benefit. He was unable to get a job as well paid as the one he had voluntarily given up to care for his sick wife, and he felt that society had treated him like 'the dregs of the tea-pot'.

Lesbian single parents arouse twice the disapproval, on account of both their single status and their sexual identity. Often they are reluctant to seek help from the authorities because of the disapproval and hostility to which they fear they may be subjected.

LONE FATHERS

Nine per cent of lone-parent households are headed by a male and, according to one of them, Tony Gordon, his task is made more difficult by the sexism he encounters: 'I discovered that just as there remains a substantial group of men who believe that women are not really competent in "male" jobs – and who resent it when they are – a substantial number of women both resent it and feel threatened when they see men take on the main child-rearing role. I have stumbled upon a culture found in children's books, in school circulars, in the different treatment by (mainly) women teachers and mothers of boys and girls, and in much of the school-gate chatter. I call this culture "Mummery" '. He goes on to say: 'One manifestation of mummery is the assumption in children's books that the main care is and should be the mother's,' adding, 'I have never encountered a literary representation of the single father'. It is Tony Gordon's opinion that men are just as capable as women of carrying out the prime caring role. He says: 'The ability to be a good parent is no more an attribute of gender than is driving a car. Some people are good at it, some aren't. Some prefer to do a lot of it, some don't. The skills are not gender specific but common to us all. All the technological aspects can be learned' (*Guardian*, 29 October 1997, p.10).

ISOLATION

Single parents are more likely than parents with partners to experience loneliness and isolation. Since the great majority of single parents do not work outside the home, they not only miss out financially, but they also lack the social and psychological rewards that a job could bring, such as regular contact with adults, a feeling of belonging and being needed, independence, stimulation and the achievement of career goals. As previously stated, general poverty prevents lone parents from playing a full role within society. Practical difficulties such as finding and paying for a baby-sitter may prove prohibitive. Single mothers are more likely to be isolated than lone fathers because it is more difficult for them to go out unaccompanied. The streets are often dangerous after dark, and in many social settings a single woman would feel conspicuously uncomfortable on her own. 'Like every other single parent there are a lot of negatives in my life. I get lonely, I get depressed, I feel sad when I see couples and feel superfluous at social gatherings.' Many parents lose confidence as a result of their isolation. Self-help groups such as Gingerbread have done much to highlight the position of one-parent families and to provide a focus for support and a chance to share their readily identifiable problems.

CHILDREN

As stated previously, there is no evidence that children of lone parents suffer emotionally or psychologically because they are brought up by one parent. One parent is fully capable of providing the love and security that children need. Indeed, a one-parent family where there is concern for each member is infinitely preferable to a two-parent household characterized by discord and violence. However, many children from one-parent families do suffer from the consequences of fixed poverty. Being part of a family with a low income precludes single-parent children from enjoying school-related activities. They are not always able to afford school trips abroad, necessary sports equipment, music lessons, or their own computer at home. Their education and life-chances are correspondingly adversely affected.

Furthermore, it must be remembered that 80 per cent of one-parent families are formed as a result of marital breakdown caused by death, divorce or separation, and any one of these events is likely to have a traumatic effect on a child or children of the relationship. Despite the immediate relief that children may feel following the break-up of parents who do not love one another, they are often left with confused feelings and divided loyalties. Children require time to adjust appropriately to the loss or absence of a parent.

The following are key findings of the Citizens' Commission into the Future of the Welfare State on Lone Parents 1997 (as outlined in *Community Care*, 19–25 June 1997, p.27):

- many feel trapped in the welfare system and want a way out of it;
- most would like to work, but in decent jobs that take them out of the poverty trap;

- finding and paying for suitable child care is a major obstacle to getting back to work;
- benefit levels are viewed as grossly inadequate for raising a family;
- many have scathing comments to make about the Child Support Agency, which penalizes them if they refuse to give the name of their former partner;
- many feel degraded by the experience of being on benefit because of public attitudes towards single parents;
- they feel that the work they do in raising their children is undervalued by society;

- they are not asking for something for nothing. They have paid for welfare through direct and indirect taxation and their unpaid work as carers.

Poverty is the main problem faced by single parents and their families. The great majority of lone parents are women, and often a huge drop in the family's standard of living is experienced when it is the father who leaves a family. Some families start out headed by lone parents. Whatever their origin, it is true to say that the discrimination that lone parents experience and the regard in which they are held are closely related to the unequal position of women in general in our society.

5.9   PEOPLE WITH MENTAL HEALTH PROBLEMS

> Mental disorders and vulnerabilities are extremely common and touch every family in the land at some time in our lives.
>
> (Royal College of Psychiatrists, 1997, p.6)

INTRODUCTION – WHAT ARE 'MENTAL HEALTH PROBLEMS'?

We are all likely to experience mental health problems at some time in our lives, either directly or through a relative or friend. If these problems are mild, individuals will carry on with their lives without any particular upheaval or disruption, and we must accept that a certain amount of sadness, stress or anxiety is simply part of day-to-day life.

However, if feelings or experiences become overwhelming and interfere with our daily functioning, we may need to seek professional help. The most common types of mental health problem are anxiety and depression, and they are often experienced together. Anxiety can range widely from feel-

ing mildly anxious about an impending event to severe panic attacks, irrational fear or phobia and obsessive or ritualistic behaviour which seems to be out of control. Likewise, depression can vary from feeling 'down' to experiencing delusions or hallucinations, or even becoming suicidal.

More severe mental health problems may involve:

- profound mood swings – manic-depressive disorder describes a shift in mood from elation to depression, usually interspersed with periods of relative stability;
- disintegration of the normal functioning of the mind – thoughts, feelings and memories no longer function in a congruent way. Instead, experience becomes confusing and bewildering, and reality and fantasy are intertwined. Mental health problems such as these are usually referred to as a group of conditions called schizophrenia.

As people grow older, a minority may experience the onset of dementia. This is a general term for a number of brain disorders which involve an irreversible decline in mental functioning. Dementia particularly affects the ability to think, reason and remember. About 50 per cent of those who have dementia have a form of it known as Alzheimer's disease (named after a German neurologist).

Neurosis and psychosis

A good deal of the language concerning mental health problems has now changed. Until recently, the term 'mental illness' was commonly used to refer to 'mental health problems'. It is now felt that the term is too negative and that it has connotations of stigma and marginalization. Furthermore, mental illness was traditionally categorized as either a *neurosis* or a *psychosis*, classifications which are less commonly used today.

- A neurosis or neurotic illness was the least serious of the two. It referred to an exaggerated mood or emotional state, and it was most commonly used to refer to anxiety and depression. The term became so broad and vague that it fell into disfavour with mental health workers.
- A psychosis or psychotic illness was more profound and affected a person's everyday functioning. It seriously distorted a person's ability to distinguish between what was real and what was imaginary – it might involve hearing voices, developing delusions or experiencing vivid perceptional hallucinations. Common forms of psychotic disorders were 'manic-depression' and schizophrenia. Many professionals, in particular clinical psychologists, have questioned the usefulness of the term 'psychosis' and its meanings, and no longer use it.

It has been recognized that such diagnostic terms can have a detrimental, 'labelling' or stigmatizing effect on the lives of the people to whom they are applied.

WHAT CAUSES MENTAL HEALTH PROBLEMS TO OCCUR?

- *Life events* – most mental health problems occur as a result of events that happen to people and the difficulty they have in coping with them. A bereavement or any other loss, such as that of a job, may trigger different responses in different people. Some will cope well and not be unduly affected, while others will be profoundly affected by depression, anxiety, or both. The event and its aftermath can interfere with the individual's 'normal' or usual functioning.
- *Physical ill health* – often a physical condition will trigger a mental health problem. For example, a long physical illness may result in the onset of depression, prolonged stress at home or at work may aggravate conditions such as stomach ulcers and skin complaints, or a young person, worried about her or his weight and physical shape, may develop anorexia nervosa or other eating disorders.
- *Biochemical disturbances* are a common cause of mental health problems, particularly the more severe disorders. Brain chemistry is the basis of mental health as well as illness.
- *Heredity* is now accepted as being a significant factor in determining the vulnerability of an individual to developing severe mental health problems. However, the specific genetic mechanisms which operate are not yet clear, and much research is being conducted currently to clarify them.
- *Deprivation* contributes to mental health problems. Poverty, unemployment, poor and overcrowded housing and a lack of community resources and facilities can all lead to loneliness and isolation. In some deprived areas the admission rates to hospitals for mental health problems are three times higher than the national average.
- *Gender* – women are more likely to have mental health problems than men. This is partly because they are less likely to be in interesting and stimu-

lating jobs than men and they are more likely to experience the stress and strain of caring for children, particularly as lone parents. Overall, they suffer disproportionately from the effects of social deprivation and the resultant social exclusion. It is not surprising, therefore, that women are statistically more likely to be admitted to a psychiatric hospital than men.

- *Life-style* plays a large part in determining mental health. Our society has become increasingly materialistic and competitive, and for most people the pace of life has accelerated. As a result, people are subject to higher levels of stress, which are evident in the increased incidence of mental health problems.

HOW MANY PEOPLE EXPERIENCE MENTAL HEALTH PROBLEMS?

Mental health problems that are severe enough to require some kind of professional intervention are as common as heart disease and three times more common than cancer. More than one person in ten will seek help for a mental health problem at some time in his or her life.

STIGMA AND DISCRIMINATION

> For people who use mental health services, the stigma and discrimination can be worse than the original problem.
>
> (Sayce, 1997, p.2)

The Labour Force Survey 1995 reported that users of mental health services have higher rates of unemployment than any other group of disabled people or people with long-term physical health problems. Indeed, only 21 per cent of people with long-term mental health problems are either working or seeking paid work.

Not surprisingly, the stigma surrounding mental ill health often has a detrimental effect on a person's chances of obtaining a job or gaining promotion. Society's negative perceptions of mental health force a service-user to be reluctant to 'come out' about her or his history or experiences, and deters some people from seeking help from mental health professionals in the first place.

NIMBY

'Schizophrenics go home' was a slogan used by a group of residents in Bromley, Kent, when in 1996 they opposed the setting up of a mental health project in their neighbourhood. Presumably 'home' for those protesters meant an institution a long way away from Bromley. Such 'NIMBY' ('not in my back yard') sentiments, based on ignorance of mental health issues, are fuelled by a hostile media.

Media images

Research by the Glasgow University Media Group discovered that two-thirds of news and current affairs coverage of mental health issues made a link between mental ill health and violence (Philo *et al.*, 1993). This was despite the fact that there has been no increase in the numbers of murders committed by people with mental health problems in the last 20 years, while the incidence of murder generally has more than doubled. The stereotypical relationship is so firmly established that most people are reluctant to accept the fact that people with mental health problems are statistically no more likely to commit a violent offence than anyone else.

The media generally tend to portray an item on mental health as a 'bad news' story. Tabloid newspapers use similar negative words and phrases to those we might hear as terms of abuse in a children's playground. The Sunday tabloids were the worst offenders according to research commissioned by the Health Education Authority, which found that 45 per cent of mental health items used pejorative terms such as 'loony', 'psycho', 'nutter' and 'maniac' (Friedli and Scherzer, 1996).

Cinema films may also contribute to the build-up of prejudicial fears. Most horror movies, for example classic films such as *Psycho* and *The Silence of the Lambs*, depict people with severe mental health problems as 'dangerous monsters', and so help to confirm existing fears and prejudices.

Concern about the poor quality of media coverage of mental health issues led five leading national charities to set up 'Mediawatch' in August 1997. The five groups are:

- the Mental After-Care Association (MACA);
- the Manic-Depression Fellowship;
- the Mental Health Foundation;
- MIND;
- the National Schizophrenia Fellowship.

The project intends to monitor media coverage, challenge negative portrayals and poor use of language and to make constructive comments on storylines in radio and television series and 'soap operas'. 'Mediawatch' wants as many people as possible to be involved, in order to 'help to improve the general public's awareness of the issues and understanding of the real facts' (*Challenge the Media*, Mediawatch, 1997).

In 1997, MIND launched a separate, broader campaign aimed at the media and institutions outside the media and entitled 'Respect: time to end discrimination on mental health grounds'. It called for a 'fair deal' for people with mental health problems in three ways – in the public eye, as employees and as citizens. As part of its campaign it intends to increase public awareness of the fact that mental health service-users are entitled to rights defined in the Disability Discrimination Act (DDA) 1995.

The following year, the Royal College of Psychiatrists, in a similar vein, launched a 5-year campaign 'to increase public awareness of mental disorders and vulnerabilities and reduce the stigma and discrimination relating to them'. The campaign is called 'Every Family in the Land', and the goal is 'to bring about a change of public attitudes'. It will focus on eight specific 'mental disorders' which the Campaign will deal with in pairs. These are:

- depression/anxiety;
- schizophrenia/personality disorder;
- addiction/eating disorders;
- learning disability/dementia.

The Royal College of Psychiatrists has identified the following specific groups which it aims to target or work in collaboration with:

- the general public;
- central government, the health service and other statutory bodies;
- educational organizations;
- employers;
- ethnic minority groups;
- the media.

HELP FOR PEOPLE WITH MENTAL HEALTH PROBLEMS

A wide range of interventions is available to people with mental health problems, ranging from so-called 'talking therapies' such as counselling and psychotherapy through to the more drastic 'physical treatments' such as electroconvulsive therapy (ECT) and psychosurgery.

Medication is commonly used to treat people with mental health problems, but there is some concern about over-reliance on this form of therapy. In fact, 25 per cent of all medication prescribed on the NHS is for the alleviation of mental health problems. Although the quality of these drugs is constantly being improved, not all of the harmful side-effects have yet been eradicated.

Treatments are not, of course, mutually exclusive, and various combinations will occur. For example, in treating mental health problems such as anxiety and depression, medication and 'talking therapies' are very often used side by side. Figure 5.11 indicates the range of available interventions.

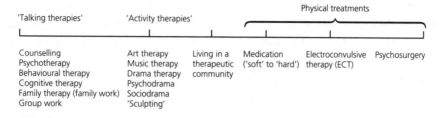

Fig. 5.11 The range of mental health interventions. Note that some 'physical treatments' will take place in a hospital setting.

It would be wrong to assume that all of these interventions are freely available to everyone. For instance, the 'talking treatments' are not widely offered to NHS patients. There are often long waiting-lists for counselling through the NHS, and most people make their own arrangements to see a counsellor privately. Furthermore, there are geographical variations in available treatment. For example, only one-third of GP practices have a counsellor attached to them.

SERVICES FOR PEOPLE WITH MENTAL HEALTH PROBLEMS

Services are provided by a range of different kinds of agencies within the 'mixed economy of care'. The two major statutory providers are the National Health Service and local authority Social Services Departments. Voluntary organizations and private bodies also contribute, and a growing service-user movement including groups such as 'Survivors Speak Out' and a number of black service-user groups are actively involved.

Two systems operate in statutory mental health services today and which of the two applies to a particular service-user is largely dependent upon whether the National Health Service or the local authority is funding the care provided.

1. *Care management* is operated principally by Social Services Departments, following the National Health Service and Community Care Act 1990. They have a duty to assess a person's needs, decide on her or his eligibility for services and, if eligible, draw up a package of community care. The care manager who oversees the care provided may involve specialist mental health social workers, known as 'approved social workers' (ASWs), or other social workers, and health service staff authorized by the local authority. The Social Services Department may also commission a voluntary organization, such as Mind, to provide hostel accommodation.

2. *The care programme approach (CPA)* has operated under the aegis of the National Health Service since 1991, when 'community care' arrangements commenced in the health service. (Note that local authority Social Services Departments did not have fully operational community care arrangements until 2 years later, in April 1993.) About £4.2 billion is spent each year by the National Health Service on mental health services, including payments for in-patient care, out-patient care, drugs and community health care. This is significantly more than the amount spent by local authorities, which is about £1.7 billion.

The care programme approach is in place in a growing number of areas, but there is still some progress to be made. Under the care programme approach a mental health service-user has a formal, individualized plan of care, similar to a local authority 'care package'. Regular reviews take place in order to monitor progress, and a named key-worker is allocated. A survey carried out by the Community Psychiatric Nurses Association in 1996 discovered that 80 per cent of service-users on the care programme approach had a community psychiatric nurse (CPN) as their key-worker. This makes sense, because the CPN usually has the most frequent contact, much of it being relaxed and informal. Key-working is a demanding role, and the professional bodies involved recommend that a key-worker should have a caseload of no more than 15 service-users at any one time. However, at present key-workers can have caseloads of up to 50 in many inner-city areas.

The CPA is generally regarded as an improvement in practice, with yet further potential for future development. Geraldine Mahon says of the approach, 'it can promote the empowerment of service users and carers and give them choices about the care they want' (*Community Care*, 28 August – 3 September 1997, p.3). Dave Middle also mentions the CPA's potential for empowerment: 'The CPA.. allows the service-user and all agencies involved in a care package to meet regularly. This brings clarity and crucially empowers service users by increasing their opportunities to feel in control' (*Community Care*, 28 August–3 September 1997, p.4).

Mental health professionals from within the National Health Service, local authorities and the independent sector have pressed for care management and the care programme approach to be operated together as a simple system, and this has happened in a growing number of areas. They agree that a single system would enhance continuity of care, aid co-ordination of services, and reduce confusion and duplication.

COMMUNITY MENTAL HEALTH TEAMS

The growth of the care programme approach has taken place hand in hand with an increase in multidisciplinary 'community mental health teams'. Such teams usually attempt to involve the service-user as much as possible in her or his own care, and include her or him in planning and review meetings. Such teams use a 'needs-led assessment approach' which concentrates on a service-user's expressed needs, rather than on either a 'diagnosis (or illness) -led approach' (e.g. 'Richard is manic-depressive, he requires medication') or a 'service-led approach' (e.g. 'Melanie seems suitable for a women's group; I'll refer her').

Members of community mental health teams include workers from a wide range of disciplines and training backgrounds. A typical team (see Fig. 5.13) might include a consultant psychiatrist, possibly one or two junior psychiatrists, occupational therapists, community psychiatric nurses, clinical psychologists, a psychology technician (a psychologist in training) and social workers. A team might also include a specialist worker such as an art therapist, drama therapist or speech therapist.

The 'care programme approach' says that those covered by the CPA can *expect*:

- an assessment of health and social care needs;
- a written care plan to meet those needs;
- to be involved in drawing up the care plan;
- a regular review of the care plan;
- to have a named keyworker who is responsible for care.

NOTE: The Charter differentiates between:

rights – which all users of mental health services will receive all the time; *and*

expectations – which are 'standards of service which the NHS is aiming to achieve'.

If 'exceptional circumstances' mean that these standards are not met, then the reasons for this *should* be explained to the service user

Fig. 5.12 The Mental Health Services Patient's Charter includes the 'care programme approach'.

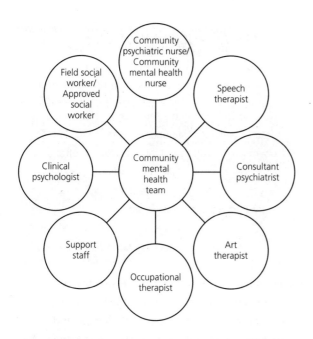

Fig. 5.13 Potential members of a Community Mental Health Team. Good communication is clearly of great importance.

COMMUNITY CARE

> Talk of crisis isn't helpful; care in the community does work. But the stark reality is that there is an urgent need to make it work better.
>
> (Lucy Burns, *Community Care*, 30 November – 6 December 1995, Supplement p.1)

The state became involved in the care of the 'mentally ill' as long ago as 1808, with the County Asylum Act. This rather crudely provided for 'care in the maintenance of lunatics'. Gradually, asylums to accommodate 'mentally ill people' were built throughout the country. They were large, barracks-like buildings, both in their external appearance and in their internal planning and organization. One hundred and twenty-two years later, the Mental Treatment Act 1930 replaced the term 'lunatic asylum' with 'mental hospital', and slowly conditions in these institutions improved. However, incarceration

in a mental hospital still meant, as it does today, disruption of someone's usual social life, a break in family relationships, separation from home and familiar things, loss of employment (sometimes permanently), and having to face social stigma upon returning to the community.

The number of beds in psychiatric hospitals began to decrease in the mid-1950s. In 1959, the first Cabinet-level politician to enunciate the policy of 'community care' was Minister of Health Derek Walker-Smith, who criticized the state of the asylums, and whose government introduced the liberalizing 'Mental Health Act' of the same year. Later, in 1963, a subsequent Health Minister, Enoch Powell, made a now famous speech about the asylums. They were, he said, 'isolated, majestic, imperious, brooded over by the gigantic water-tower and chimney combined, rising unmistakable and daunting out of the countryside' (*Independent*, 21 February 1996, p.5). He also called for their closure.

The peak number of 'psychiatric beds' was reached in 1954, when it stood at about 144 600. The figure has subsequently gradually reduced, the decrease accelerating during the 1960s. Today, it is much lower, at around 35 000, since most people with mental health problems are now treated outside hospital, in the community.

Community care has proved popular with people across the political spectrum, chiefly because it is considered a more creative and humane way of supporting individuals. According to Suman Fernando, 'Community care is not about applying institutional models in the community; it is about different ways of thinking about people with mental health problems living in the community.... Developing community care is not an academic exercise – it is political action concerning real people' (Fernando, 1995, p.196).

However, not everyone has been in favour of this development. Disquiet built up in the early 1990s because it was felt that there were now not enough beds for people with severe mental health problems. Concern was further fuelled by the publicity surrounding a small number of cases in which people with mental health problems attacked, and in some cases killed, other individuals while living in the community. These cases received widespread publicity, especially in the tabloid press.

Moves have since been made to slow down, if not reverse, the psychiatric hospital closure programme. However, it is felt by many that such measures are too late, and that more hospital places are needed. Some estimate that at least 5 000 additional places need to be provided for the most 'disturbed patients' in some 400 'new residential homes', with 24-hour nursing care.

The Labour Government shares the previous administration's belated concern about people with mental health problems. In September 1997 it announced that the closure of the remaining 40 long-stay psychiatric hospitals had been 'put on hold' and that an 'independent reference group' would be set up to review the position. This group consists of representatives from 26 mental health organizations, and its task is to ensure that adequate services are in place in the community before any patient is released from a long-stay hospital. It is to be hoped that these moves will restore some of the public's lost confidence in 'care in the community'. Most people agree with the *policy*, and feel that it is the lack of *resources* that has sabotaged its full and successful implementation.

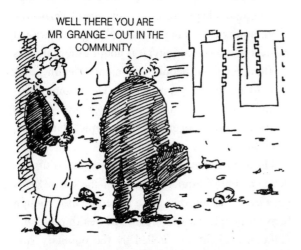

(Reproduced from *Care Weekly*, 31 May 1990.)

THE SERVICE-USER MOVEMENT

> the psychiatric system, as currently established, does too little to help people retain control of their lives through periods of emotional distress and does far too much to frustrate their subsequent efforts to regain self-control. Whatever power I may now have over my life, I have, to a large extent, won in spite of rather than because of psychiatry.
>
> ('Peter Campbell's Story', from Brackx and Grimshaw 1989, p.12)

The above quote denigrates the psychiatric system for the way it breaks down rather than empowers users. However, many areas of health and social care have in recent years seen a burgeoning service-user movement. In relation to mental health issues, self-help groups have been formed, such as 'Depression Alliance' and 'Survivors Speak Out', and support and advice organizations such as the 'Manic-Depression Fellowship' (primarily for users) and the 'National Schizophrenia Fellowship' (NSF) (primarily for relatives and carers) have also been set up. In addition, in response to the special problems experienced by black people with regard to mental health services, a black user movement has started to emerge. 'NAFSIYAT' is a London-based organization which provides advice and support for black people with mental health problems. All of these groups have sought to empower the individual and to place her or him at the centre of the service.

BLACK PEOPLE AND MENTAL HEALTH PROBLEMS

For some time there has been growing research evidence that African-Caribbean and African people are over-represented in psychiatric institutions. They are most likely (together with Irish people) to be detained in locked psychiatric wards, most likely to be given higher doses of medication than other groups of people, and are more likely than any other ethnic group to be diagnosed as having 'schizophrenia'. It is felt that these results are the consequence of institutionalized racism.

It is well documented that black people experience disadvantage and racism in the education system, in employment, in housing and other areas of life, and where this occurs it will also have an impact on their mental health. This situation is exacerbated when black people come up against a lack of understanding of cultural differences within the mental health system.

'MIND' published a report entitled *Raised voices* in September 1997, which gave African-Caribbean and African people a chance to express their own experiences of mental health services. Some of the findings were as follows:

- 58 per cent had experienced general discrimination in society because of their ethnic origin;
- 36 per cent felt that no mental health professional with whom they had had contact had been aware of their ethnic origin and culture when considering treatment options;
- 36 per cent expressed dissatisfaction with the care and treatment they had received (Wilson and Francis, 1997).

There is now much more awareness about the problems faced by black people within the area of mental health. For instance, Paul Boateng, a junior health minister, has recently publicly acknowledged the 'double stigma' that confronts black people with mental health problems. Suman Fernando, a consultant psychiatrist and Mental Health Act Commissioner (the Commission has the task of ensuring that the Mental Health Act is correctly applied within hospital settings), has stressed that there is an 'urgent need for the incorporation of anti-racist measures in all aspects of (mental health) work – in training professionals, in developing their modes of assessment, and in their interventions' (Fernando, 1995, p.208). He continues, 'The ideal is that eventually all services will be accessible to and appro-

priate for all ethnic groups – multi-ethnic services for a multi-ethnic society' (Fernando, 1995, p.214).

CONCLUSION

> Instead of a seamless service, we've got a service that's coming apart at the seams.
> (Gary Hogman, National Schizophrenia Fellowship, *Community Care*, 22–28 February 1996, p.17).

Much good practice takes place daily in the delivery of mental health services. The introduction of community mental health teams and the care programme approach have generally been acknowledged as representing sound improvements. Furthermore, medication is now more effective and many harmful side-effects have been eliminated or reduced. There also appears to be a greater awareness and understanding of mental health issues on the part of the general public.

However, there is much that still needs to be done on a number of fronts.

- In common with all areas of health and social care, resources are urgently needed. Both the previous government and the present administration have acknowledged this, and each has committed extra finance to mental health. However, it is clear that more is still needed. Several recent official reports on the treatment of people with severe mental health problems (the cases of Christopher Clunis, Kenneth Grey and Stephen Laudat) have a common theme, namely a call for more resources. Two-thirds of mental health expenditure in England and Wales still goes to hospital-based services, although half of the hospitals have closed, and those that remaining are operating well below capacity. Funds saved by the closure of long-stay psychiatric hospitals have not been spent on community care, but have gone into other areas of health care instead.

- Communication between professionals in health and social care and between the statutory and voluntary sectors has improved, and this trend needs to continue. There have been some instances where consultant psychiatrists, in particular, have appeared too distant from other workers and service-users. They have also been accused of sometimes being out of touch with new developments.

- The recent suggestion of joint pre-qualifying training of nurses and social workers in mental health issues has been welcomed. It is expected that the anti-racist components of training will be strengthened.

- It would be beneficial if certain interventions that have proved successful were made more readily available. For instance, psychotherapy needs to be more readily available for people experiencing depression, and 'family work' needs to be extended to more people who have been diagnosed as having schizophrenia, because there is evidence demonstrating that it is often effective in preventing relapse.

- Homeless people who have mental health problems, and who may also have a history of substance misuse, clearly need more support. Research carried out by the University of York in 1991 on homeless people found that 'rough sleepers' had 11 times the frequency of mental health problems found in the general population, while those living in hostels or 'bed-and-breakfast' accommodation had 8 times the frequency of mental health problems. Depression and anxiety were substantially more common among homeless people than in the rest of the population (*Search* Issue No. 21, Winter 1994, p.31).

- The Mental Health Services Patient's Charter needs to be strengthened. It uses the two terms '*rights*' and '*expectations*', the latter being 'standards of service which the NHS is aiming to achieve' (p.2). Expectations clearly outnumber rights, and this situation needs to be reversed. As Philip Timms, Senior Lecturer in Community Psychiatry, Guy's and St Thomas's United Medical and Dental Schools, London, has said, 'Rights without the resources needed to provide for them boil down to the right to complain and nothing else' (unpublished communication, 9 March 1998).

- The statutory mental health services have begun to listen to and work more closely with user groups, and the service providers have increasingly moved away from 'diagnosis-led' and 'service-led' assessments, and towards 'needs-led' assessments. This trend needs to continue so that services cater more appropriately for individuals, women, black people and members of other minority groups in our society.

5.10 OFFENDERS AND PRISONERS

> there can be no criminal justice without social justice.
>
> (Maurice Vanstone, *Probation Journal*, September 1997, p.130)

INTRODUCTION

Many people believe that, unlike many other social groups dealt with in this chapter, offenders and prisoners have directly contributed to their marginalized position in society – in short, that they have brought it on themselves. To a certain extent this is true. Committing crime is wrong – whatever else it is, it is antisocial and should be punished. Society needs to send a message to offenders that it will not tolerate crime and that a certain amount of stigma will attach to those who commit it.

However, it is important that people who commit offences are diverted from further offending. Punishment should include some provision for help and advice to enable offenders to live more constructively in the future. The Probation and Prison services exist in order to do just this, both in the community and in custody.

As a civilized, advanced society we should treat offenders humanely, otherwise how can people be encouraged to behave *well*, if we treat them *badly*? As Drakeford and Vanstone write,'people in trouble with the Law are part of, rather than just apart from, our shared society' (Rescuing the social, *Probation Journal*, April 1996, p.18).

Imprisonment represents perhaps the ultimate form of *social exclusion*. We lock certain people away for a number of reasons, including the fact that they may pose a serious threat to society. However, it should be remembered that offenders are sent to prison *as* a punishment and not *for* punishment.

- The Prison Service's 'Statement of Purpose' states that 'Our duty is to look after them with humanity and help them lead law-abiding and useful lives in custody and after release'.
- The 'Values' of the service remind us that 'Their punishment is deprivation of liberty and they are entitled to certain recognized standards while in prison'.
- The 'Goals' mention that prisoners should live in 'decent conditions' and prisons should 'provide positive regimes which help prisoners address their offending behaviour and allow them as full and responsible a life as possible'.

THE SOCIAL CONTEXT OF OFFENDERS

> Probation Service clients are, characteristically, caught up in that nexus of. . .unemployment, poor housing and vulnerability to illness which are the product of living in enduring poverty.
>
> (Rescuing the social. *Probation Journal*, April 1996, pp.18–19)

If we examine the social and economic circumstances of offenders, together with the quality of their family backgrounds and relationships, certain patterns emerge. In research conducted in Kent by the Probation Service and published in 1996, 857 offenders were studied, all of whom had been solely supervised by the Kent Service. Some of the findings were as follows:

- 75 per cent of the sample were unemployed;
- 60 per cent had accommodation problems;
- 42 per cent had relationship problems linked to their offending;
- 35 per cent had an alcohol-related problem;
- 34 per cent had a drug-related problem.

UNEMPLOYMENT

Of all the factors that are considered to have an influence on the development of crime, the factor of overwhelming significance is *unemployment*. In 1992, the Cleveland Probation Service reported that 84 per cent of offenders with whom it was working were unemployed, and that only one in ten offenders who were eligible for work were in full-time employment. At the time, Roger Statham, Cleveland's Chief Probation Officer, said: 'Finding people jobs has been a traditional part of the probation service's attempts at the rehabilitation of offenders. This task is becoming increasingly hopeless for probation officers' (*Probation Matters*, December 1992, p.1).

Unemployment is debilitating. Apart from debt and other financial difficulties, it can create the obvious day-to-day inability to provide a decent material quality of life. In a summary of research conducted by Stewart and Stewart into the social circumstances of young offenders published in 1993, we read: 'What is revealed is routine poverty, chronic multiple debts, theft as a survival measure and dependence upon mail-order catalogues for purchasing day-to-day necessities' (*Association of Chief Officers of Probation Journal*, February 1993, pp. iv–v). The authors also reported that young offenders had become 'complete outsiders. They have no access to funds, education or jobs' (*Association of Chief Officers of Probation Journal*, February 1993, p.ii).

It would be false to claim that there is a simple causal relationship between unemployment and crime. However, there is a correlation. As David Dickinson writes, 'There are...strong reasons why unemployment may lead to crime. Unemployment brings a raft of negative features with criminogenic potential: loss of status, boredom, alienation and the erosion of social values, and, possibly of most importance, loss of income' (*New Statesman and Society*, 14 January 1994, p.21).

In April 1994, the *Independent* newspaper revealed that the Home Office itself admitted there was a link between unemployment and crime. The paper referred to a leaked internal document which commented on a review of 397 research studies on young offenders, conducted both here and abroad. The document was quoted as saying that the 'single most effective form of intervention (in reducing crime) was the provision of employment to offenders' (*Independent*, 8 April 1994, p.1).

Unemployment greatly increases the chance of further offending. In carrying out the 'Kent Reconviction Study', Mark Oldfield reported that unemployment problems alone 'increase the odds of further offending by almost 2' (*Probation Journal*, March 1997, p.5).

It is well established that once someone has a 'criminal record', it becomes far more difficult for them to obtain work. There is therefore the increased likelihood of a 'downward spiral' into further crime, as the individual has, in a sense, 'nothing to lose'. Without work, there is no real incentive or investment in 'going straight'.

SUBSTANCE MISUSE

Substance misuse appears to have played an increasingly prominent part in the commission of crime in recent years. According to surveys, every other male and every third female aged 14 – 25 years admit that they have used drugs. Alcohol misuse also appears to be on the increase among young people, and to be a factor in the crime rate. Apart from offences directly related to the possession or supply of drugs, the government estimates that one in five acquisitive crimes may be committed by a person who is dependent on hard drugs (National Association for the Care and Resettlement of Offenders, 1997, p.3). In the early 1990s, when 'crack' cocaine began to be readily available in this country, senior policemen believed its increasing use was mainly responsible for a dramatic rise in crimes of violence. One young man who was arrested in London in 1992 'admitted a £400 a day "crack" habit, fed by 20 armed robberies', and this was not thought to be uncommon at that time.

OFFENDERS WITH MENTAL HEALTH PROBLEMS

Inevitably, many people with a mental health problem end up in the criminal justice system having committed an offence. If their condition is acknowledged, they may be referred to as 'mentally disordered offenders' or 'mentally disturbed offenders'. However, the criminal justice system is not equipped to cater for their needs, and according to experts it frequently does them harm. For instance, prisoners receive little if any help for their psychiatric condition and, as a result, they experience a deterioration in their mental health. In research published by the 'Penal Affairs Consortium' in February 1998, it was estimated that 20 per cent of convicted prisoners and 25 per cent of remand prisoners had mental health problems.

The government has accepted that this situation needs attention. Circular 66/90, issued in 1990 by the Home Office, stated: 'It is government policy that wherever possible mentally disordered persons should receive care and treatment from the health and social services.... Careful consideration should be given to whether prosecution is required by the public interest.' This circular led to the setting up of *Court Diversion Schemes*, which aim to divert mentally disordered offenders away from the criminal justice process. However, these schemes are not available everywhere and are often inadequately resourced. They may even be unknown to some agencies.

Specialists working in this field believe that there should be more 'diversion at the point of arrest' schemes, rather than those that come into operation later, when an offender appears in court. They also believe that each scheme should be able to draw on a full range of professionals, including:

- a probation officer;
- an approved social worker who could facilitate a mental health assessment for admission to a hospital or secure unit;
- a community psychiatric nurse who would link with local hospitals and other agencies.

YOUTH CRIME AND YOUTH JUSTICE

It is well known that most crime is committed by young men. Every year in this country over half of all known offenders are aged under 21 years and about one-third are under 17 years of age. For certain specific offences, the proportion of young offenders is even higher than is shown by statistics. For instance:

- 7 out of 10 burglaries are committed by those under 21 years old;
- the 'peak age' for shoplifting is 14 to 16 years;
- the 'peak age' for assault, damage to property and drug-related offences is between 17 and 20 years.

It is also recognized that most young offenders grow out of crime as they mature and take on more commitments and responsibilities.

In recent years there has been growing public and media concern about a relatively small number of persistent young offenders, the majority of whom are male, who have caused a considerable amount of distress to local neighbourhoods and communities. In responding to this concern, the government has introduced new measures to deal with youth crime. At the end of 1997, it published a White Paper on youth justice entitled 'No More Excuses', in which it announced a number of new measures, including the setting up of multi-agency '*Youth Offending Teams*' (YOTs), each headed by a manager. The purpose of these teams is to plan and supervise community intervention for young offenders. The first Youth Offending Teams were to be pilot-tested in 1998 and then will be set up throughout England and Wales between April 1999 and March 2000. Each team will consist of at least one local authority social worker, a probation officer, a police officer, a person nominated by the health authority and a person put forward by the chief education officer. The work of the teams is to be monitored at national level by a new Youth Justice Board. To facilitate the work of the Board, local authorities are required to provide audits which identify the number of offenders aged 10–17 years in their area.

BLACK PEOPLE AS OFFENDERS

Black people are more likely to be criminalized, more likely to end up in custody and less likely to be given community sentences such as community service or probation than are white people. National figures on 'stop and search', carried out by the police, show that black people are up to five times more likely to experience this procedure than white people.

As early as 1981, the Commission for Racial Equality discovered a tendency for probation officers to recommend probation proportionally less often for black offenders, and this action contributed to a higher representation of black people in the prison system. It is believed that this is partly due to a lack of confidence on the part of white officers when working with black clients. Research by Whitehouse discovered the widespread use of 'cultural stereotypes' in probation reports. This finding later contributed to the setting up of 'gate-keeping' procedures, whereby all officers have their reports monitored for racist terminology or viewpoints.

There is still ample evidence of the existence of *institutionalized racism* throughout the criminal justice system. However, many positive initiatives have taken place to remedy this situation.

- There has been a determined attempt to recruit more black staff into the Probation Service. In 1995, 7.6 per cent of the work-force were black, which is a higher proportion than that of black people in society (5.5 per cent). However, black staff remain under-represented at all levels of management.
- Certain projects have been set up to cater exclusively for the needs of black probation clients. A growing number of probation offices now run 'black-only provision' schemes as part of their rehabilitative programme, giving black offenders the chance to explore their experiences, to focus on their offending and to be empowered to solve their own problems. Many of these initiatives appear to have been successful.
- One example is 'The Cave' project in Birmingham which has focused specifically on the needs of African-Caribbean and Asian offenders. It is a multifaceted centre providing a valuable community resource, including a range of creative arts, along with more conventional probation intervention. Part of its success

appears to be in reinforming the users' black identity in a positive way.

Drawing on work by Bandana Ahmed, Peter Raynor and his colleagues have produced a number of 'indicators of effectiveness' when working with black people. These include:

- 'the extent to which black people have equal access to community-based sentences which do not reinforce social control but assist rehabilitation. This will necessitate the monitoring of sentencing outcomes for black offenders reported on by probation officers;
- the degree to which black people view the services offered by the probation service as relevant to their needs and problems;
- the extent to which staff and (probation) committee training is effective in promoting antiracist attitudes and actions' (Rayner *et al.*, 1994, p.81). It should be remembered that anti-discriminatory practice requires constant vigilance with regard to our thoughts, attitudes and use of language, and how these affect practice.

RACIST OFFENCES

In a welcome development, the Home Secretary, Jack Straw, announced at the Labour Party Conference in October 1997 tougher sentences for racially motivated crimes. Evidence of racial hostility is to be regarded by courts as an 'aggravating factor' when sentencing. The 'Crime and Disorder Bill' published at the end of 1997 included a requirement that courts must, when imposing a prison sentence, add up to 2 years for crimes with a component of *racial harassment* or *racial violence*.

OFFENDERS IN CUSTODIAL INSTITUTIONS

Nobody now regards imprisonment, in itself, as an effective means of reform for most prisoners.

(Government White Paper, Home Office, 1990, p.6.)

If prison worked to deter crime, jails would be empty and crime would fall.

(Roger Graef, *Independent*, 12 October 1995, p.4)

A RISING PRISON POPULATION

Since 1993, the UK prison population has increased at a much faster rate than previously, and by October 1997 it stood at a record level of 63 000. Overcrowding had become a major problem in the prison system. In the same year, the Home Office published 'Projections of Long-Term Trends in the Prison Population to 2005' (Home Office Statistical Bulletin 7/97). This forecast a rise in the population to 74 500, including a rise in the number of women in prison to 3 500, up from the current figure of 2 300.

Overcrowding increases stress and tension among prisoners as too many people are forced to live too close to others. This situation is exacerbated when there is a dearth of available prison officers, which leads to prisoners being locked up in their cells for too long each day. This in turn often results in activities and 'association' (i.e. mixing with other prisoners) being curtailed. As Stephen Shaw, Director of the Prison Reforms Trust, says, it means that 'prisons end up as nothing more than human warehouses' (*Guardian*, 8 July 1997, p.6).

Category A

Prisoners who are regarded as 'top security'; their escape would be highly dangerous to the public. Category A prisoners are not classified by Local Prisons, but by the headquarters of the Prison Service

Category B

Prisoners who are not 'top security', but who are regarded as a threat to society should they escape

Category C

Prisoners who cannot be trusted in 'open' prison conditions, but who are not considered to be serious potential escapees

Category D

Prisoners who can be trusted to serve in 'open' prison

Note: Escapees (or 'E's) are prisoners who have either attempted to escape, or who have done so but have subsequently been recaptured. They wear yellow patches on their prison uniform, and as a result are sometimes referred to colloquially as 'patches'.

Fig. 5.14 There are four different categories of prisoner.

THE FINANCIAL AND HUMAN COST OF CUSTODY

Imprisonment is...an expensive way of making bad people worse.

(Government White Paper: *Crime, Justice and Protecting the Public*, 1990, p.6)

Currently, it costs British taxpayers an average of £25 000 per year to keep a prisoner in custody. By contrast, the average annual cost of a probation order is £2 230 and that of a community service order is £1 670. Different types of prison vary widely in their cost. For example, each prisoner in a top-security dispersal prison costs an average of £31 400 per year, whereas a place in a male open prison costs less than half that amount, at £13 800.

Sending someone to prison represents the most extreme form of *social exclusion* in the UK today. However, doing so does not merely deprive an individual of her or his liberty – it often has a number of other damaging consequences.

- It cuts a prisoner off from her or his family – prisoners are often incarcerated a long distance from their home area.
- It can turn an unaccomplished offender into a more sophisticated one, hence the frequently heard description of custodial institutions as '*academies of crime*'.
- There is now widespread concern about *drugs* in prison. One prison governor recently described his institution as being 'awash with cannabis' (*Independent*, 30 March 1995, Section 2, p.1). Roger Graef writes: 'It is an open secret that drugs are easier to obtain in most prisons than on the street. Drugs help inmates to do their time' (*Independent*, 12 October 1995, p.4). Furthermore, there is frequently an escalation of drug use by people in prison so that it is now possible to find a released prisoner has developed a 'hard' drug (opiate) addiction whilst 'inside'.

It makes life on release very difficult as poverty, homelessness, poor job prospects and fractured family relationships frequently greet the released prisoner. Research carried out by the University of York investigated what happened to prisoners after release, and found that less than 50 per cent of respondents were able to return to their previous accommodation. In 1997, the government reduced from 1 year to 13 weeks the period over which Housing Benefit could be paid to prisoners to help them retain their homes. The National Association of Probation Officers estimates that, because of this measure, at least 4 000 prisoners lose their tenancies each year. Ex-offenders are now more vulnerable and at greater risk of committing further offences (*Probation Journal*, June 1997, p.102).

LIFE 'INSIDE'

In 1990, Tessa Blackstone echoed the words of many observers throughout history when she described prisons thus: 'Britain's prisons are institutions of which we should be ashamed. They are absurdly expensive, yet scandalously inhumane. For the most part they are in old or decrepit buildings, but even where the buildings are new they are often badly designed. They absorb large amounts of manpower, yet typically lock inmates in their cells for many hours a day. They are overcrowded and unhygienic. They enforce idleness and encourage helplessness. They certainly punish; they hardly reform' (Blackstone, 1990, p.1). Oscar Wilde, who was sentenced to 2 years' imprisonment with 'hard labour' in 1895, had this to say about prisons:

> This too I know – and wise it were
> If each could know the same –
> That every prison that men build
> Is built with bricks of shame
> And bound with bars lest Christ should see
> How men their brothers maim.
>
> (from *The Ballad of Reading Gaol*)

We should remind ourselves that, as stated earlier, people are sent to prison *as* punishment, not *for* punishment. As the Howard League for Penal Reform says, 'The loss of freedom is the purpose of imprisonment. But in prison, people not only lose their liberty but they can lose their right to privacy, to communication, to personal possessions and to basic human rights' (Howard League for Penal Reform, 1994, p.2). Nothing is achieved by keeping prisoners in poor physical conditions, and doing so will dehumanize not only the inmates but also the prison officers who work with them.

As well as frequently having to live in poor physical conditions, prisoners are often under-stimulated. Routines are often dull and monotonous, and cutbacks have led to fewer educational classes and less meaningful work. The amount of time that prisoners spend with their fellow inmates has also been reduced as budgets have tightened. A remand prisoner awaiting trial or sentence may be regularly locked in her or his cell for up to 23 hours a day. This applies more often at weekends when staffing ratios are reduced. This lack of stimulation provides fertile ground for substance abuse.

As we have said, prisoners have limited contact with their partners and families. The usual pattern of visits is one every 28 days (and daily for remand prisoners). This obviously puts an enormous strain on relationships. In The Netherlands, Sweden and some parts of North America, a prisoner is allowed to have a physical relationship with their spouse. In Canada, 'extended family visits' mean a prisoner can spend a weekend in a caravan or 'pre-fab' within the prison fence, with their partner and family. None of this happens in British prisons, although some long-term prisoners here are considering applying to the European courts in order to gain their 'conjugal rights'.

WOMEN IN PRISON

> The Prison Service still (does) not seem to recognize that the needs of female prisoners are different from their male counterparts.
>
> (*National Association of Probation Officers News*, March 1997, p.3)

Women who are receiving a first custodial sentence tend to have fewer previous convictions than men at the corresponding point in their criminal careers. It is believed that this is partly because probation officers may be recommending women for a probation order too readily. Women certainly miss out on other sentencing options which would allow them to remain in the community. For example, in 1995 only 8 per cent of Community Service Orders were given to women. One reason for this may be the lack

of child-care facilities for women, which prevents them from undertaking this option.

As a society we send too many women to jail, and it is estimated that only about one-third of them need to be locked up for reasons of public safety. Furthermore, two-thirds of women who are remanded in custody eventually receive a non-custodial sentence. In the 1960s it was predicted that imprisonment for women would be gradually phased out. In fact it has greatly increased, and continues to do so.

Of the women in prison, about 70 per cent have dependent children. It is now widely acknowledged that prison is the wrong place for pregnant women and mothers, and this is currently under review. In 1996, 64 babies were born in prison. Some of these will remain with their mothers in one of the four 'Mother and Baby Units'. The other babies will be separated from their mothers after about 1 year and either be looked after by members of the family or by the Social Services Department.

In January 1997, the case of a woman prisoner in Holloway hit the newspaper headlines when it was discovered that she had been manacled to the bed for 10 hours while in labour. The fact that the procedure still took place, and the pain, distress and humiliation inflicted on the woman shocked the nation. It was later revealed that she had suffered 'post-traumatic stress disorder' within a month of the birth of her daughter.

BLACK PEOPLE IN PRISON

Black people have been over-represented in custodial institutions for a long time. At present, about 18 per cent of the prison population are from an ethnic minority (compared to 5.5 per cent in the general population). They still form a minority group inside prison and are particularly vulnerable to racial attacks. Research carried out at Oxford University in 1994 made the following findings:

- about 25 per cent of black prisoners and almost as many Asian prisoners claimed that they had been racially abused by staff;
- about 20 per cent of prison officers had experienced incidents of racial harassment between prisoners; 10 per cent had experienced violence between prisoners which had a racial aspect;
- there was a gap between the low number of 'racial incidents' recorded by the Prison Service and the high number actually reported;
- many prisoners have failed to report examples of racial harassment or violence because they believed there was nothing to be gained by doing so (National Association for the Care and Resettlement of Offenders, 1995, pp.21–2).

SEX-OFFENDERS

Sex-offenders in prison are a special category of prisoner and may need to be protected from other inmates by being categorized by 'Rule 43' (Fig. 5.15).

It is generally acknowledged that sex-offenders are very difficult to divert from further offending. In the past, most prisoners serving sentences for sex-related offences have been left to stagnate 'inside', with no meaningful attempts being made to help them. Now, however, a '*sex offender treatment programme*' (SOTP) has been developed and it is the Prison Service's aim to make this available to all relevant inmates who wish to take part in the programme. By 31 March 1997, 2 247 prisoners had completed the course. Staffing the programme is a co-operative arrangement which draws on prison and probation officers and psychologists. Prisoners applying to join the programme undergo an assessment which considers each individual's suitability, and the relevance of the programme to their needs. After release from prison, home probation officers continue with the rehabilitation work.

HMP Wayland in Norfolk, a prison for adult males, has a 'Sex Offender Treatment Unit' which contains about 130 prisoners, most of whom are tak-

Rule 43 of Prison Rules (Rule 46 in Young Offender Institutions) is implemented when:

- a vulnerable prisoner needs protection, either temporarily or permanently. Most request segregation. This will commonly be because of the sensitive nature of their offence, e.g. sexual offences against children (these prisoners are known as 'nonces' ('nonsense cases') in prisoners' parlance) or because of who they are, e.g. a police officer involved in corruption;
- a prisoner is regarded as a threat to the maintenance of 'good order and discipline' (referred to by prison staff as 'GOAD' prisoners). 'GOAD prisoners' are usually segregated against their will.

What we might call 'solitary confinement' gives the 'Rule 43' prisoner a poorer quality of life. Certain 'wings' in some prisons are allocated exclusively to such inmates.

Approximately 2000 prisoners are currently on Rule 43, 87 per cent of whom are there for their own protection.

Fig. 5.15 'Rule 43'.

ing part in the programme. Based on a 'cognitive-behavioural approach', the course involves a personal examination, by the offender, of the process of the offence(s) and the effects on his victim(s). Participants are encouraged to think about how they reached the decisions that led to them offending, and how they might be able to reduce the risk of further offending in the future. Mike Fowler, one of the (probation) course tutors involved, says that SOTP 'enables the offender to directly address and challenge his thinking and behaviour, working on the premise that he is responsible for his actions and is capable of control and change'.

CURRENT DEVELOPMENTS IN IMPRISONMENT

> We must get away from this idea that prison is the only real punishment.
>
> (Mary Tuck, *New Statesman and Society*, 8 April 1994)

The chances of being sent to prison are greater in the UK than in any other European country; 93 people are imprisoned per 100 000 members of the population. In France this figure is 81 per 100 000, and in The Netherlands it is only 44 per 100 000. Many critics of the criminal justice system claim that we should, and could, reduce the numbers of people in prison. For instance, community sentences should be used more often, and we should stop jailing fine defaulters. If there were fewer people inside prison this would enable a more positive intervention in prisoners' lives, through education, training, work and the use of social work and counselling skills, since the ratio of staff to inmates would be lower. Using these approaches more intensively would afford prisoners a greater chance of leading more law-abiding, constructive lives on release. This, in turn, would help to create a safer society for us all.

Home-leave and temporary-release arrangements should be liberalized to allow for the establishing of better family relationships and improved plans for release. An innovative experiment in Whitemoor high-security prison for men serving long sentences is trying to help those taking part to become more involved in parenting their children. Jointly run by the local probation service and a regional charity, it consists of a 6-week programme, which is followed up by individual counselling. The participants are made aware of their children's needs and difficulties, and are encouraged to take a greater part in their lives.

CONCLUSION

> The mood and temper of the public in regard to the treatment of crime and criminals is one of the most unfailing tests of the civilization of any country.
>
> (Winston Churchill, speaking in the House of Commons, 1910)

We shall never eradicate crime in our society, but there are three important things we *can* do.

- We can *prevent* some crime from happening. Every time we prevent a crime we prevent someone from becoming a *victim*. Part of prevention is improved security or 'target hardening', another important element is being vigilant and observant in our local communities, and a third is providing more positive alternatives to crime, especially in the form of jobs, so that more people can lead law-abiding lives. The Crime and Disorder Bill published at the end of 1997 places a duty on local authorities to develop and implement crime prevention strategies and to enhance community safety. In doing this, they must co-operate with other agencies such as the police and probation services.

- As a society we have a responsibility to provide sensitive and relevant support for the victims of crime. This can be practical help or support in the form of counselling, which may be provided either informally by a community network, or more formally by probation officers

- We can also work constructively with offenders, in order to divert them from further offending. In the community the Probation Service is at the forefront of this work, while in custodial

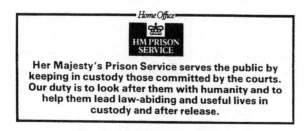

Her Majesty's Prison Service serves the public by keeping in custody those committed by the courts. Our duty is to look after them with humanity and to help them lead law-abiding and useful lives in custody and after release.

Fig. 5.16 HM Prison Logo and Mission Statement

institutions a combination of Prison Service and Probation Service staff have the responsibility. In working with offenders, *anti-discriminatory practice* is not only a *moral imperative*, it is also a *legal requirement*. Section 95 of the Criminal Justice Act 1991 places a duty on all those working in the criminal justice system to '*avoid discrimination*'. The Probation Service initially responded by setting up systems of '*gate-keeping*', whereby reports for the courts were scrutinized by colleagues for discriminating language or attitudes. This supervisory practice has now been taken

over by management as a more general 'quality-control' measure.

Offenders and prisoners are marginalized and socially excluded. If all we do is punish them, and we do not help them by confronting them and helping to change their social circumstances, then we will not successfully divert them from committing more crime in the future. A civilized, so-called 'developed' country like the UK should treat those who break its legal code humanely and with dignity, and be confident about their ability to change.

5.11 OLDER PEOPLE

Age is no barrier if you've got the energy. I got up at 6 o'clock yesterday and went to bed at midnight, after spending an hour on the diary. I enjoy very good health. I've got a happy family and a very interesting job. If I'd known what fun it was to be 70 I'd have done it years ago.

(Tony Benn MP, *Guardian*, 11 April 1997, p.17)

Elderly members of our society form an increasing proportion of the population, yet they remain largely on the periphery, unable in many cases to enjoy the benefits of a developed society to which they have all made a contribution. There are, of course, many examples of older people living full and active lives well into their eighties and even nineties, but for those suffering ill health and/or financial hardship, old age is a struggle often spent in isolation.

In other societies, notably in the East in countries such as India and China, and even in many European countries, elders have a more important functional role, particularly within the family, but also within wider society in general. They are respected for their age and are afforded responsibility and recognition, whereas in the UK, old age is

seen primarily as a problem. Of course, there are certain difficulties associated with old age, including the likelihood of physical impairment and the possibility of mental deterioration, but these health issues are very much compounded by society's attitude towards its elders.

The ageing process starts at birth and slowly begins to accelerate when we are in our late twenties, when the first physical signs such as greying hair or facial lines begin to show, and early aches and pains start to establish themselves. However, most of us become accustomed to having to live with a gradual diminishing physical capacity, and by the time we reach old age we are psychologically adjusted to cope.

With regard to the mental state of older people, it is estimated that about 20 per cent of people over the age of 75 years suffer from some form of senility – a disease involving degeneration of the brain cells which often manifests as confused behaviour. Correspondingly, this means that around 80 per cent of the elderly population are as alert as ever. Despite this fact, elders are still generally stereotyped as confused geriatrics.

The mass media bear some responsibility for generating and maintaining society's attitudes to older people. On television and radio, and in newspapers and magazines, elders are often portrayed as figures of fun – as harmless, confused, powerless human beings who are usually irascible, awkward and set in their ways. Rarely are they associated with serious issues unless they happen to be celebrities, or are asked to perform important roles in dramas or to feature centrally in other settings. The world of advertising is obsessed with images centred around youth, good looks and conspicuous 'success'; older people are almost entirely absent, except when they are needed to endorse pension schemes or insurance packages. News stories about older people tend to focus on them as victims, highlighting the occasions when they are robbed or attacked in their own homes. This in itself helps to convey an unnecessary feeling of insecurity to elders who are, in fact, statistically the least likely age group to be mugged or robbed.

An experiment conducted in New York over a 3-year period highlights the fact that elders within society are handicapped not so much by their physical disabilities as by the attitudes and psychological barriers that are set up by other people. Pat Moore, a social scientist and researcher in her thirties, disguised herself as an elderly woman and roamed the streets of New York. She experienced 'being a young mind in an old shell' and became 'so intimidated by the attitudes of others [she started to move aside to let people pass and began to say [to herself] "After all, old ladies have plenty of time don't they?"]'. During the experiment she would, as her normal self, go into the same social situations she had been in as 'old Pat', only to find she was treated more courteously and on a more equal footing by the same people who had abused and patronized her earlier *(Guardian,* 1 August 1989, p.17).

In the UK, colloquial terms such as 'old dear', 'old codger' and even 'pensioner' convey images of passivity and frailty. Within the health service elders are commonly mislabelled as geriatric even when the illnesses they happen to be suffering from may affect anybody and have nothing specifically to do with old age! The terms and words that we com-

monly use in association with elders help to perpetuate the stereotyped image of their dependency and perceived uselessness, and so deny their human validity. It is more respectful to refer to elders as 'older people', yet they are commonly labelled '*the* elderly' by official organizations, including the government, alongside '*the* homeless' and '*the* unemployed', and so are lumped together as if they were a distinct homogenous group.

POPULATION

According to official figures, in 1996:

- there were 9.2 million people over the age of 65 years in the UK, representing nearly 16 per cent of the total population;
- those over 75 years old numbered 4.1 million;
- those over 85 years old numbered 1.8 million;
- it is estimated that this potentially more vulnerable age group is likely to reach 2.0 million by the year 2006;
- in 1994 there were 8 000 people aged 100 years or over in the UK (Age Concern, 1996);
- in Europe, the proportion of older people within the population is similar. At the beginning of 1990, people aged 60 years or and over represented about one in five members of the population. This is projected to rise to one in four by the year 2020 (Hantrais, 1995, p.130).

Income

- Since few people of pensionable age are economically active, the majority are dependent on their fixed incomes for survival. These fixed incomes often reflect a person's class position and life-long social status. Consequently, more women, retired manual workers and people from ethnic minorities experience old age in or on the margins of poverty. For those people who retire following many years of high earnings with related benefits such as membership of occupational pension schemes, job security, incremental pay rises, opportunities to save and property ownership, the risk of state dependency is minimal. For those who have worked in low-paid occupations, have experienced periods of unemployment and have been unable to save, retirement is a time of economic hardship, and some experience inequalities in living standards more starkly than at any other time in their lives. The UK's pensioners survive on the lowest pensions in Europe, and for those without any additional financial resources everyday life remains a struggle.

- In 1993, 51 per cent of pensioner households depended on state pensions and benefit for at least 75 per cent of their income.
- In 1995, 1 781 000 people aged 60 years or over were receiving income support because they had no other income.

It is clear that our society values those people who are still working, because they contribute to the wealth of the nation more than those who do not work now, even if they have done so in the past. In this way elders share a common status with others who are unemployed. In retirement, people lack the legitimacy and purpose attributed to those who work. Low incomes are seen as one of the several inevitable consequences of old age to which older people are expected to adjust. It is recognized that they are likely to suffer from hypothermia and social isolation, but these sufferings are attributed to their age and not to the fact that as older people they may have insufficient incomes to heat or light their homes properly, or to pay for telephone calls or travel.

Women represent nearly two-thirds of the older population, and are more likely than men to be poor pensioners. Most men earn both state and occupational pensions, and some have or are building up personal pensions, whereas women are more likely to depend on the state pension as their main support in old age. Furthermore, 'Women's occupational pensions were less than half of men's average occupational pensions' (Equal Opportunities Commission Factsheet, *Income, pensions and finance*, 1997, p.3). This inequality can be seen to be a consequence of women's average lower earnings throughout their lives, their interrupted work patterns and their longer life-span.

LIVING CONDITIONS AND QUALITY-OF-LIFE INDICATORS

Lack of money is a major problem faced by many older people, and in some cases the effects of this are worsened by the living conditions that many of them have to endure.

- In 1991, in England, 12.4 per cent of single people aged 60 years or over lived in the worst dwellings, compared to 7.6 per cent of older couples.
- The poorest conditions are experienced by single older people over 60 years of age living in the private rented sector, who occupied 46 per cent of the worst houses in 1991, compared to 34 per cent in 1986.
- Older couples occupied 32 per cent of the worst private rented housing, about the same as in 1986.
- This situation exacerbates still further the trials of those older people who live in isolation and suffer from loneliness.
- Again this is primarily a female issue, as 59 per cent of those over the age of 75 years who live alone are women.
- They are less likely than the rest of the population to have basic conveniences. In 1994/1995, of pensioners living alone and mainly dependent on state pensions:
- 73.6 per cent had central heating, compared to 84.3 per cent of all households;
- 9.9 per cent had a car, compared to 69 per cent of all households;
- 59 per cent had a washing machine, compared to 89 per cent of all households (Age concern, 1996).

Health, social work and social care provision

Support services exist for older people, and are now provided by a variety of organizations. Statutory support is provided by Social Services Departments (Social Work Departments in Scotland) and the National Health Service. Services are also provided by the many voluntary organizations who specialize in working with older people, such as Age Concern, Pensioners' Link and Help the Aged. These organizations, alongside other non-statutory organizations, are responsible for much of the innovatory and developmental work that is being done to help elders. There has been a spectacular increase in the number of private companies providing care following Government incentives during the 1980s and 1990s and the terms of the NHS and Community Care Act 1990, which urged Local Authorities to stimulate a 'mixed economy of care'. 'In mid-1986 there were fewer than 190 000 places in private and voluntary homes. By the middle of last year (1995) there were 440 000' (*Guardian Society*, 16 October 1996, p.2).

Provision ranges from full-time residential care, in either a care home or a nursing home, to short-stay or respite care and day-care or domiciliary care. Home-based care may include services such as meals-on-wheels, home care, personal care laundry, transport and volunteer visiting schemes. Most older people are cared for in their own homes by relatives; very often this is the spouse alone, who may also be elderly. The help they receive will depend on the resources that are available. Since the Carers (Recognition) Act 1996, carers have been entitled to have their own needs assessed.

Despite the many instances of good practice in various social care settings within both the state-run and independent sectors the needs of the elderly population are not being met. Indeed, the general disregard for older people by the public sector amounts to *institutional ageism*, where older people are denied the services that are provided as a right for younger members of society. It is expected that old people will be ill and suffer a higher level of social deprivation.

The policy of 'community care', aimed at maintaining people in the community and outside residential establishments, has been described as being a 'nightmare' for old people, who constitute the largest group of service-users (Walker, 1994, p.1). Walker points out that only those people who are assessed as having a 'need' are eligible for permanent care, and that 'choice' of accommodation is restricted to existing vacancies within prescribed cost levels. There are few alternatives to residential care, so day-care, respite-care, sheltered housing and neighbourhood-support schemes are subject to high demand and long waiting-lists.

The availability of services depends on local resources and the demographic profile of the population. For this reason people may have to go outside their local authority in order to have their needs (particularly residential care needs) met.

Comparisons with Europe provide an illustration of a more effective relationship between the family and the state in providing care for older people. 'Denmark has the most developed home care provision in Europe, with three times as many home carers as in the UK. In Denmark, as a result, more than two-thirds of older people receiving care are getting help from the social services, compared with only a quarter in the UK. In contrast, just over two-fifths of Danish older people are helped by their families, compared to three-fifths in the UK (Walker, 1994, p.1). The responsibility for care in this country rests mainly with the family – effectively with its female members.

Now that care is being provided within a 'mixed economy', there is concern about the quality of care being offered. Although there continue to be high standards on offer within both the public and independent sectors, instances of poor practice are regularly being uncovered. One carer cited an example of an agency care worker 'Who used the flannel on my wife's face after using the same flannel on her bottom' (*Guardian*, 18 June 1997, p.3), and went on to stress the effect that inadequate support services were having on him: 'I love my wife dearly, but today's carer is rapidly becoming tomorrow's patient'.

Within the residential sector, too, there is concern about the standard of care being offered. Many homes are unstimulating and do not meet the residents' need for independence and fulfilment.

Furthermore, a survey carried out by the Alzheimer's Disease Society in May 1997 discovered that one in 10 carers of people with the disease say that their relatives have been mistreated in residential or nursing homes. The mistreatment included restraint, rough handling, neglect of personal hygiene, poor standards of feeding and lack of stimulation. Furthermore, it is estimated that this represents only 'the tip of the iceberg' (*Guardian*, 18 June 1997, p.3).

The attention and resources of the local authority Social Services Departments (and Social Work Departments in Scotland) have focused mainly on other client groups – notably families with young children and people with serious mental health problems, where the departments have a pronounced statutory responsibility. Legislation concerning older people has either not been implemented, or has been ignored because it is too costly to deliver. In general, work with elders has been viewed negatively by social workers, who may view older people in a stereotyped manner as being without the potential for change. Social workers have often ignored the great age differences of people over 65 years and the tremendous variety of needs which exist even between relatively young elderly people and those who are very old. Instead, there has been a tendency to see elders as a homogenous group for whom creative enabling intervention is not really possible. This attitude is reflected in those Social Service Departments where work with older people is undertaken mainly by unqualified staff or social work assistants, and whose homes and day centres lack stimulation and imagination.

The low priority given to elders by Social Service Departments has had an adverse effect on those who care for their relatives, who have had to continue without support. The growing numbers of black elders have also suffered from inadequate services which have lacked sensitivity and appropriateness. Assumptions that ethnic groups such as the Chinese and Asians do not need help because of support

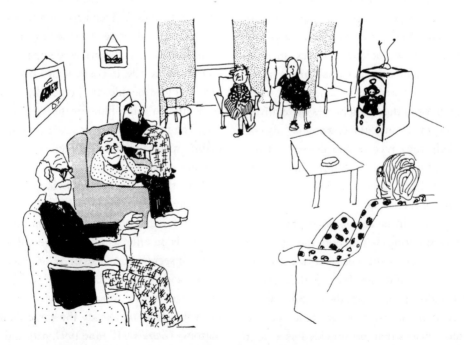

The traditional image of residential care – a thing of the past?

from their extended families have proved unfounded. Linguistic and cultural differences have meant that the uptake of services for many ethnic minorities has been poor. Black elders have tended to look to the voluntary agencies or self-help for social provision.

A similar situation exists within the National Health Service, where less prestige is associated with working with elders and their routine requirements are therefore given a low priority. For example, long waiting-lists are common for operations such as hip replacements, despite the enhanced quality of life that this normally totally successful operation brings. Furthermore, older people are not seen as a priority for other general services such as counselling or occupational therapy, and consequently illness, depression and confusion often go untreated because they are considered normal and therefore to be expected in old age.

Older people who are disproportionately dependent on the health service do not have their needs met, and face inherent, ageist attitudes in both hospital and community settings. Work with elders is often unpopular and can be considered to be unrewarding. Correspondingly, investment and research into geriatric medicine are less likely to be funded than proposals from more prestigious health disciplines.

The fact that the health services in general are not geared to meet the needs of elderly people has been commented on by Allison Norman (1985):

> Individual practitioners from the various professions are often excellent, but overall the tendency is to grudge the time, trouble and resources needed to give elderly people genuinely equal treatment. Many GPs take little interest in their elderly patients, and may indeed take them off their list if they need too much help. The acute wards of hospitals are often not geared to maintain elderly patients' physical and mental functioning at optimum level, so that the trauma of admission for treatment or an operation can be compounded by unnecessary confusion, incontinence and immobilization. Geriatric and long-stay wards are usually in the oldest sections of the hospital building and are often relegated to another site away from the facilities and consultant supervision. The prestige of working with the elderly is low, and it is one indication of racism in the National Health Service that from consultants to nursing auxiliaries – an unusually large proportion of this workforce is of Afro-Caribbean and Asian origin. For elderly people living in the inner cities, the position is even worse. As the Black Report has shown, health services of all kinds are inadequate and overstressed, and here again, if a choice has to be made in the allocation of resources, the elderly will lose out.
>
> (Norman, 1985, p.3)

The way in which elders are treated by the caring services highlights their oppressed position within society. If investment in our older people is viewed as short term and regarded as being less important, and resentment is felt about the need to use scarce resources on people who have already 'had their lives', society will continue to deny enormous human potential by focusing on a chronological milestone.

Discrimination against older people represents a psychological distancing from a position which we will all reach provided that we live that long. At that stage we shall not relish being subject to the effects of ageism, since we shall remain intrinsically the same but older versions of ourselves. As Mary Sarton reminds us in her novel, *As We are Now*:

> Old age is really a disguise that no one but the old see through. I feel exactly as I always did, as young inside as when I was 21, but the outward shell conceals the real me – sometimes even from itself – and betrays that person deep down inside. . . I sometimes think I feel things *more* intensely not less.
>
> (Sarton, 1992, p.80)

Despite the existence of established clients' rights, and compliments/complaints procedures in most caring establishments, some older people may not wish to make use of them as they regard themselves stereotypically as being beyond normal social involvement. In the better care and nursing establishments, older people's needs are met and their rights are maintained within service delivery.

Good homes offer residents the opportunity to extend themselves and to participate in as many areas of life as possible – for instance, to develop relationships (including sexual ones), to participate in regular residents-only forums or meetings, and to take part in a range of internally run activity groups and have access to relevant activities outside the home. Some older people will be happy with regular accompanied outings to the local park, shops, pub or religious centre. Others may not want or may be unable to venture beyond the grounds of the home. However, for many older people there is the need to maintain old interests and to develop new ones – to go to art galleries, theatres and other places of interest and excitement. There are several examples where care-workers have successfully arranged for a resident who has dementia to visit the opera or to attend a concert. In such cases, the care-workers have carefully planned the outing with the resident

and accompanied them on the day. In other instances, carers have supported residents' wishes to go on holiday or to travel and stay with relatives. In 1997, British Airways, as part of its celebrations, organized a free trans-Atlantic flight for centenarians only, and easily filled the plane.

In cases where care-workers or carers, in the myriad of seemingly insignificant ways in which they may be involved, look to extend, value and enable an older person, whether in a residential setting or in their own home, then they treat that person with due respect. They leave the older person to 'rage against the dying of the light' in their own individual manner.

> Do not go gentle into that good night,
> Old age should burn and rave at the close of day;
> Rage, rage against the dying of the light.
>
> (Dylan Thomas 1953: Do Not Go Gentle Into that Good Night. In *Collected Poems*. J.M. Dent. Reprinted by permission of David Higham Associates.)

5.12　ASYLUM-SEEKERS AND REFUGEES

> Asylum-seekers are made a useful scapegoat for those who wish to appeal only to other people's self-interest or who promote a narrow nationalism. The reception given to those applying for asylum is an illuminating indicator of the state of a society's moral health.
>
> (Cardinal Basil Hume, *Exile: Newsletter of the Refugee Council*, September/October 1996, No. 94, p.4).

Refugees have fled their own lands and sought to settle in another country throughout history. Some countries, notably America, Australia and Canada, have been heavily dependent on the contribution of immigrants for their nation's development. In others, such as Britain, the role of the immigrant has been

less pronounced due to the restrictions it has placed on people wanting to live here and coming from countries abroad. Before 1905 and the passing of the Aliens Act there were no restrictions on entry. Non-British subjects (aliens) were subject to the technicality of a royal prerogative that is, they could be refused entry or expelled only on the decision of a monarch. 'The Act applied to boats with more than 20 people and to those travelling steering class who could be excluded if "undesirable" – unable to support themselves and their dependants' (Joint Council for the Welfare of Immigrants, 1997b, p.5).

Later, between 1962 and 1971, the concept of British Citizenship was redefined to the exclusion of many, mainly black people within the British Empire, making settlement in Britain more difficult for some and impossible for others. All Western countries now have restricted entry requirements for those who are not nationals, with a variety of complex needs criteria which have to be met by all those wishing to settle permanently. The UK in particular now has very stringent immigration controls which have been variously charged as being unfair, unnecessarily lengthy and damaging to individuals and their families.

DEFINITION OF AN ASYLUM-SEEKER AND A REFUGEE

The 1951 UN Convention Relating to the Status of Refugees defines a *refugee* as someone who has a *well-founded fear of being persecuted* for reasons of race, religion, nationality, membership of a particular social group or political opinion, and who cannot expect protection in her or his own country. A refugee is a person who has been accepted for asylum (Commission for Racial Equality, 1997g). Asylum is another word for 'refugee status'. An '*asylum-seeker*' is someone who is requesting asylum or refugee status in the UK, whose application has not yet been decided (Joint Council for the Welfare of Immigrants, 1997b, p.310).

There are a number of refugees throughout the world. The United Nations High Commission for Refugees (UNHCR) recognized 18 million people world-wide as refugees in 1992, with an additional 20 million being displaced within their own countries. Most refugees try to settle in an adjacent country in order to minimize disruption and, if possible, to maintain safe links with all that is familiar to them. The majority of refugees originate in the less-developed countries of the world. Consequently, 'It is the poorest countries which carry the major responsibility of trying to contain and support those affected by natural disasters, war and political upheavals. The West takes in about 10 per cent of them' (*Community Care*, 14–20 August 1997, p.16).

In 1992, the UNHCR recorded some 4 million refugees in Europe, almost four times the previous year's count. However, it has since become more difficult for non-Europeans to settle in Europe, as the member states have co-ordinated policies prioritizing arrangements for people from European Union countries at the expense of people from outside the EU. The nickname *'Fortress Europe'* has emerged to reflect current policies.

The exact number of resident refugees in the UK is not known. Between 1984 and 1995 there were approximately 226 000 applications for asylum, and around 61 000 of these (amounting to about 90 000, including dependants) were granted exceptional leave to remain. 'If all these people were still living in the UK they would amount to 1:600 or 0.2 per cent of the population, which is a lower proportion than in most other European countries' (Commission for Racial Equality, 1997h).

APPLICATIONS FOR ASYLUM

The Home Office may make one of three decisions in response to an application for asylum.

- It may grant *asylum or refugee status* to the individual, initially for a period of 4 years, after which time they may apply for indefinite leave to remain (settlement).
- It may grant '*exceptional leave to remain*' *(ELR)* in the UK for a specific period. This may be given to people to whom the Home Office has refused refugee status but does not think it is safe for them to return for the time being. This provision may be extended to others with compassionate reasons for needing to remain. It is entirely outside the immigration rules and at the discretion of the Home Office. Those granted ELR may apply for settlement after 7 years with that status.
- The Home Office may *refuse the application* (in the 18 months before 1993, 47 per cent of applicants were refused, compared to 78 per cent in the following 15 months (Commission for Racial Equality, 1997h).

As can be seen from Table 5.5, the number of decisions on asylum has generally increased, as has the proportion of those who have been refused. In 1996 the 2 240 people who were granted refugee status represented just 6 per cent of the decisions made. Those granted exceptional leave to remain (5055 in total) represented less than 15 per cent; the substantial majority (nearly 80 per cent) were refused both asylum and exceptional leave to remain.

Although the number of asylum decisions made in the UK increased in 1996, the number of actual applications for asylum decreased compared to the year before. This matched the trend in Western Europe, where asylum applications dropped by an average of 15 per cent. Germany and The Netherlands, the two countries which together with the UK that attract the highest proportion of asylum-seeking applications, received a smaller number of applications. Sweden, France and Italy also recorded significant falls. Europe is now characterized by freedom of movement of individuals within the member states and increased exclusion of people from other countries.

DELAYS

According to the Refugee Council 'Average waiting times for decisions from 1985–1990 were between 12 and 17 months'. This is in part due to the complexity of the process. 'The asylum-determination process has been for the past five years subjected to the most rapid, and convoluted, procedural changes. The twists and turns have frustrated representatives and denied justice to applicants' (Joint Council for the Welfare of Immigrants, 1997c, p.13). Furthermore, in 1997 there were '55 695 persons awaiting decisions on their asylum applications, while another 20 455 were awaiting appeals concerning the refusal of asylum' (Joint Council for the Welfare of Immigrants, 1997c, p.15).

The stress of waiting is compounded by insecurity. The process is often a long one, made worse by the uncertainty surrounding the outcome: 'The reason for refusal can seem utterly arbitrary, based on personal whim' (David Rose, *Observer*, 29 October 1995, p.16).

GOVERNMENT POLICY

In 1996 the Government withdrew the right of benefit from people who did not apply for asylum on their arrival at port, and for all those who were appealing against refusal of their asylum application. This action made many asylum-seekers destitute and reliant on charity and the work and support of others. In effect they were made victims once more. Local authorities where the refugees resided were faced with the cost and responsibility of providing non-monetary support. The local authorities were forbidden to provide cash, except where appropriate, under the Children Act 1989, and could only

Table 5.5 'Unwelcome to Britain': decisions on applications received for asylum in the UK, excluding dependants, in 1990–1996

Year	Total decisions	Refugee status	Exceptional leave to remain	Refusal
1990	4025	920	2400	705
1992	34 900	1115	15 325	18 465
1994	20 990	825	3660	16 500
1996	38 960	2240	5055	31 670

Column 3, recognized as refugee and granted asylum; column 4, not recognized as refugee but granted asylum; column 5, total refusal.

Source: Home Office Statistical Bulletin, 22 May 1997, Table 1.2, Asylum status UK 1996.

provide services in kind. For one Inner London borough at least, this meant providing refugees already accommodated by them (outside the borough, where housing costs were lower) with food supplies contained within a cardboard box. For the refugees, who are banned from taking up paid work, it meant the initial humiliation of having to request food from Social Services and the accompanying indignity of having to call at the office in order to collect their regular groceries. They were reliant, too, on their social worker for the taxi fare back to their outer London address, as this was the only way to transport themselves and the food. Another Authority was forced to provide full-board to refugees, deskilling and undermining their confidence and independence in the process. Thus the asylum-seekers were not permitted much control over even fundamental areas of their lives, such as the food they eat. Commenting on the importance of the basic issue of food to refugees, Helen Bamber points out that 'Food has a symbolic meaning to asylum-seekers, many of whom have been in prison. It is used in prison as punishment. Being in control of food, even if it is not adequate, is very important. Choice is about dignity, it confirms that they are survivors' (*Community Care*, 6–12 November 1997, p.25).

The local Social Services budgets have been adversely affected by these expedient yet inefficient and humiliating forms of service provision. Similarly, Kent Social Services bore the major cost of providing for refugees arriving in Dover from the Czech and Slovak Republics in late 1997. Refugees are a national responsibility. They should not be left solely to those local authorities in which our airports and international rail termini are situated. At present Newham Council has 1 500 asylum-seekers, while Havering has only 20 (*Community Care*, 12 November 1997, p.25).

NEEDS

Allison Fenney, Social Services Adviser to the Refugee Council, says: 'the problems are immense

and social services departments have had to respond in a totally unplanned way for a service outside their remit. People do have other needs, such as mental and physical disabilities brought on by torture, for example. But it is difficult to respond to them or even see them – when the immediate need is for food and shelter. People have to be pretty desperate to get a service now' (*Community Care*, 16–22 October 1997, p.17).

Refugees need a range of support. Primarily they need housing, and assistance with sorting out immigration difficulties and finding employment, where they are allowed to work. However, as some have witnessed atrocities by officials in their own country, they may have difficulty in dealing directly with officialdom in this country. Some voluntary organizations are using established refugees to enable newly arrived refugees to overcome their problems. The emphasis, so far as is possible, is on empowerment rather than on hand-outs which do not provide real long-term help. However, the standard of services fluctuates according to the resources available.

Daloni Carlisle points out that services to refugees can be improved by the following:

- making links with voluntary organizations and community groups;
- employing skilled refugees in mainstream services;
- not ignoring social needs and problems such as social isolation;
- developing services that enable refugees to help themselves (*Community Care*, 16–22 October 1997, p.17).

THE MEDIA

'25 000 say kick out the Gypsies' – Sun readers voted by 18:1 in favour of booting-out asylum-seeking gypsies yesterday. A total of 24 823 called our You The Jury hotline in favour of expelling them. Just 1377 said they should stay.

(*Sun*, 24 October 1997, p.3)

The headline at the end of p.207 appeared the day after several hundred Slovak and Czech refugees arrived in the UK. Not all of them stayed for long, and some, fleeing physical abuse and oppression in their own country, applied for asylum. Tabloid newspapers referred to 'the Dover Deluge' and inflated the figures and spoke of the 'thousands of Gypsies' or 'tide', whom they referred to as 'bogus asylum-seekers' here to 'milk the benefits system'. A climate of fear was created and the National Front took the opportunity to mount a demonstration in Dover. Thus the refugees were threatened with the very force from which they were trying to escape – that is, the threat of racial violence. According to Hana Sylova, a Czech academic, in their own country Slovak and Czech gypsies only wanted a life free from routine persecution: 'Even when they try to integrate, the Czechs just reject them. Since the end of Communism, racial violence has soared. In the past five years, 28 Czech Romanies have been murdered in racial attacks and 450 seriously injured. Meanwhile unemployment among gypsies has risen to 70 per cent compared to the national rate of only 4 per cent' (*Daily Telegraph*, 21 October 1997, p.9).

Of course there are people who make false claims for asylum, just as there are people who make false claims on their income tax returns for expenditure not incurred, or for dependants who do not exist. All claims need to be investigated properly. However, the fear of the bogus asylum-seeker has been used to perpetuate a tighter policy on refugee controls, the rationale for which goes something like this. A large number of applicants are not being accepted for asylum, their claims are bogus, therefore there is a need to enforce more stringent entry requirements. This in turn results in more applicants being refused, more claims being seen as bogus, and the need for more restrictive entry criteria again being justified, and so it goes on. In the process a rather unsympathetic image of the refugee is created – that of an undeserving interloper bent on exploiting the resources of the host country. Yet, in contrast 'A Home Office survey of 263 refugees published in 1995 found that two-thirds had been employed in their own country, 25 per cent had university degrees, and 30 per cent had professional backgrounds' (Carey-Wood *et al.*, 1995).

VICTIMS OF TORTURE

As previously mentioned, many people who seek asylum may also have been tortured in their own country. They need special help both in adjusting to their current circumstances and in dealing with what has happened to them in the past. A specialist organization, the Medical Foundation for the Care of Victims of Torture, was set up in 1986 and has since provided help for over 11 000 people who have variously been abused, tortured and disabled. Recently it has needed to pour its energies into basic survival programmes at the expense of specialist psychological counselling, due to the lack of basic services.

All refugees need to be listened to and understood when they come to settle in this country. They need their past acknowledged and validated so that they can fully adapt to their new life-style. After the Second World War, around 2 000 survivors of the Nazi concentration camps came to begin a new life in Britain only to meet, in many instances, with hatred and indifference. They were also expected to assimilate quietly. 'The Englishman attaches very great importance to modesty, understatement in speech rather than overstatement and quietness of dress and manner'. 'At best they faced blank incomprehension about their experiences, at worst indifference. And ignorance: a woman at a cocktail party who noticed my mother's Auschwitz tattoo on her arm asked if it was her telephone number'. 'Many did want to speak about the trauma from which they had just emerged, but found no one ready to hear them, so they talked to their children, who became the keepers of their stories' (*Guardian*, 25 June 1996, p.3).

DETENTION AND ENFORCEMENT

> I didn't just do it (attempt suicide) to get out of the detention centre. But everything has a limit and the authorities are just under-estimating my life. To have been trying so long to save myself but I am still not safe.... I feel I have lost everything – if I lose my health too.
>
> (Joint Council for the Welfare of Immigrants, 1997c, p.9)

There are many uncharged and unconvicted asylum-seekers kept in secure accommodation. In 1997, of the 778 asylum-seekers held in detention, 279 were in prison, 84 were in police cells and 415 were in detention centres. Amnesty International described detention as 'arbitrary and inefficient' and said that the average duration of detention was lengthening rather than decreasing. A number of establishments, notably Rochester Prison, saw the refugees take hunger strike action during 1997, in protest against the lack of legal safeguards and uncertainty surrounding Immigration Act detention. They were successful in publicizing their plight.

Enforcement of deportation and removal figures show an 'upward trend, with action being initiated against 20 900 persons in 1996, more than 5 000 more than in the year previously' (Joint Council for the Welfare of Immigrants, 1997c, p.9). In some cases these decisions have the effect of dividing families as do the long delays and hardships that continue to stem from other points during the slow, over-complex, often arbitrary and unfair asylum-seeking process.

Yasmin Ali Brown remembers the experience of her own countrywomen and men who were thrown out of Uganda in the 1970s by the country's despotic president, Idi Amin. She says, 'We still weep when we remember those times and no amount of money or success can make us forget that indignity and that loss of a homeland. What you don't do is depend on people. You try to regain your self-respect by working insanely hard, by educating your children and thereby conquering adversity' (*Community Care*, 14 August 1997, p.16). Refugees are ordinary people, many of whom have had extraordinary experiences and have known great pain and loss. They should not be faced with more unnecessary hardship when they are striving to put down roots in a strange and foreign land. A booklet entitled *The New Asylum and Immigration Proposals – A Reflection on the Morality of the New Regulations*, produced by the Joint Council for the Welfare of Immigrants (1997a), quotes the words of Mahatma Gandhi in order to contrast the Government's policy of denying benefits to asylum-seekers and point to the spirit in which asylum-seekers ought to be supported. 'Recall the face of the poorest, most helpless person you have seen, and ask yourself if the step you contemplate is going to be of any use to that person. Will that person gain anything by it? Will it restore that person to control over their life and destiny?'. These sentiments have since been matched by those of the late Rabbi Hugo Gryn: 'I believe that loving the stranger is the mark of a civilised society. As we are approaching the end of this complicated century, it is imperative that we proclaim that asylum issues are an index of our spiritual and moral civilisation' (*Community Care*, 14–20 October 1997, p.14).

5.13 UNEMPLOYED PEOPLE

Unemployment is the single most serious challenge facing European member states today.

(European Commission Background Report – European Social Policy, 1993, p.3)

You cannot be sure of anything these days, certainly not of a job for life.

(Michael Ignatieff, *20–20 – A View of the Century*, BBC Radio 4, June 1997)

At 3 p.m. on Sunday 3 May 1987, more than 350 000 people linked hands to form human chains in many of our large cities, including Liverpool, London, Leeds, Nottingham and Birmingham. The campaign 'Hands Across Britain' planned this event to emphasize the fact that there were more than 3 million people unemployed in this country at the time, and that this situation did not have to be inevitable. It was hoped that this action would heighten public concern about the issue of unemployment, just as the 'Jarrow Crusade' and other 'hunger marches' of 1936 had done over 50 years earlier.

In the 1960s, Harold Macmillan, Conservative Prime Minister, voiced the opinion shared by all post-war governments until the 1980s, that the British people would not return to office any government which allowed unemployment to go above the 1 million mark. It would seem that, by 1987, this country had lost its concern for people out of work and accepted the inevitability of large-scale unemployment.

SOME EFFECTS OF UNEMPLOYMENT

A man who set himself ablaze in his car just yards from 10 Downing Street yesterday left a suicide note saying 'too young to retire, too old to live', in a protest about unemployment.

Mr Derek Bainbridge, 43, from Workshop, Notts, had been out of work for three years.

Police, who found petrol cans in the shell of the burnt-out car, stressed that Mrs Thatcher, who was in No. 10 at the time of the incident, was not in any danger.

(*Daily Telegraph*, 17 February 1988, p.6)

Unemployment can have a very destructive effect on individuals, families, neighbourhoods, communities and even whole regions. Unemployed people may experience stress, despair, a lack of purpose, and low self-esteem that can result in a range of physical and mental health problems. Moreover, unemployment is usually accompanied by poverty and material deprivation. For some people, the lack of meaning in their lives can lead them to seek solace in self-destructive forms of behaviour. Shaun Quirk, himself unemployed, has written: 'Unemployment creates problems like drug addiction, alcoholism, solvent abuse, prostitution, begging and homelessness...unemployed people are the army of the forgotten, unwanted and abandoned' (*CAP Voicebox No. 11*, September 1996, p.3). Kevin, who is also unemployed, refers to the isolation he feels: 'Unemployment is hell: it is being surrounded by the good things of life and having no access to them. You are not desirable: other people do not want to be tainted by the stifling dead-endedness of your existence. Your life implodes; you become isolated' (*CAP Voices*, 1995, p.1).

When unemployment stems from the closure of large-scale, heavy or manufacturing industry, whole neighbourhoods and communities can suffer the knock-on effects. There are fewer people in the area with money to spend, local shops and businesses are forced to close down, and this in turn puts more people out of work. A spiralling sense of despondency may devolop, the physical environment becomes run down, houses, shops and offices are boarded up, and a general air of dereliction is created. It then appears that nobody cares about the community or neighbourhood.

Absence of work can lead directly to *marginalization* and *social exclusion*, as unemployed people are denied full integration with their communities and are effectively trapped in their own homes by poverty.

Traditionally, poverty has affected certain groups of people, notably those past retirement age, disabled people who are unable to earn a living and, more recently, single parents without access to adequate child care. However, '*new poverty*' affects a wider range of individuals due to the effects created by changing work patterns and a corresponding increase in unemployment. Now almost everyone is vulnerable to unemployment. A reflection of this situation is the people in their late twenties who have not worked since leaving school, and people in their thirties, forties and fifties who are made redundant and face a struggle to get back into paid work, and who are regarded as 'commonplace'.

HOW MANY PEOPLE ARE UNEMPLOYED?

In August 1997, the official government unemployment figure in the UK was 1 550 000 when seasonally adjusted, which was the lowest figure for 17 years. In the same month, the total for the 15 countries of the European Union was 18 million, so the problem of unemployment is not exclusive to the UK. However, it is a more serious issue in this country than in most European countries. According to the Employment Policy Institute's (EPI) published statistical research, the UK had a larger number of families with children in which no one was in paid work than any other European country except Spain and Ireland. This figure (20.6 per cent) represents just over a fifth of all families with children. In Germany and France about 8 per cent of families have no 'breadwinner'. The EPI report concluded:

'Our (British) children are increasingly, and unusually across Europe and elsewhere, growing up in families with no one in work' (*Observer*, 20 April 1997, p.4). Some people are sceptical about the accuracy of the UK figures. During the 18 years of Conservative Government, 32 changes were made to the way in which the number of people out of paid work was calculated.

The cumulative effect of these 32 modifications was to reduce the official unemployment figure to that which was in reality only a *claimant count* – that is, it exclusively referred to those who could register for and receive benefit. Many other people, estimated in 1997 at over 2 million, were seeking work but were not included in the official figures. The Labour Government has since committed itself to reviewing how the numbers of unemployed people are measured, in order to make the figures more truly representative.

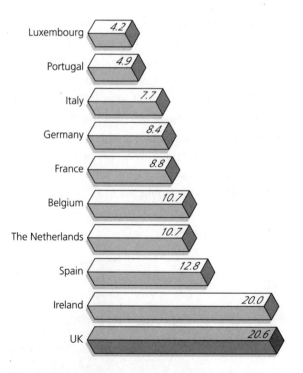

Fig. 5.17 Workless homes: EU households with children but no workers (expressed as a percentage of all homes with children). (Source: *Guardian*, 16 April 1997, p.13. *Guardian* is the copyright holder.)

THE CHANGING PATTERN OF WORK

In many countries across the world, especially those with so-called 'advanced' economies like our own, there have been profound changes in employment and patterns of work which began around 20 years ago, and have accelerated, particularly in the last 5 years. Some of these changes are permanent, while others may not be.

In the UK, the early changes in employment reflected the decline in heavy and manufacturing industries and a growth in service industries (Fig. 5.18). In essence, there has been a fall in 'blue-collar' jobs and a rise in 'white-collar' occupations, leading to a loss of full-time work for many men, and to more women going to work. Accompanying these changes there has been a large increase in part-time work, with almost one-third of all employees now working part-time.

Not only have there been changes in the nature of work, but there has also been a shrinkage in the work-force, as fewer people are required to carry out paid work. This partly reflects rapid changes in technology. Between the general elections of 1992 and 1997 there was a decrease of over 0.5 million jobs. Any increase in part-time jobs has not made up for the overall reduction in full-time positions. Of the new jobs created during this 5-year period, only 38 per cent were for permanent full-time employees.

The decline in the number of unskilled and semi-skilled jobs, mainly carried out by males, has had particular consequences for young men, who now find it difficult to obtain work straight from school without a qualification. It has also made life more difficult for older men without qualifications, some of whom have become long-term unemployed. Technological advancement has put more pressure on young people to gain academic and vocational qualifications. It has also put more pressure on older employees to retrain and learn new skills.

Related to these changes there has been a dramatic rise in job insecurity. The Conservative Government presided over a massive increase in unemployment from the early 1980s. As a deliberate plank of their 'monetarist' economic policies, they encouraged unemployment as a method of reducing inflation. It could be said that the increase in unemployment and the corresponding insecurity felt by those in work created a more pliant work-force that was less able to oppose a decline in working 'conditions of service' and wages. A large pool of unemployed people meant a more 'flexible' work-force.

There has also been a *casualization of work*, whereby a 'job for life' has become a thing of the past. This process has included an increase in the number of *temporary contracts* or *fixed-term contracts*, and has even seen the introduction of *nil-hours contracts*, which have no regular guaranteed hours of work.

Meanwhile, the real value of wages has been pushed down, partly through the abolition of the

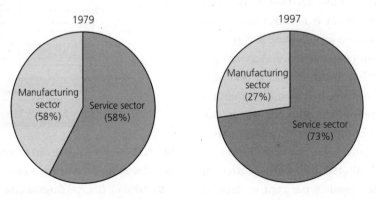

Fig. 5.18 The decline in manufacturing jobs.

Wages Councils in August 1993. These were originally set up by Winston Churchill in 1909 in order to protect low-paid workers. In the last year of operation, they covered 2.5 million workers in vocational areas such as hotels and catering, shops, hairdressing and clothing manufacture – all traditionally low-paid occupations. Combined research conducted by the 'Low Pay Network' and the 'Campaign Against Poverty', published in 1994, discovered that 17 per cent of jobs were already being paid at below the old Wages Council rate.

The diminishing power and influence of the Trade Unions over the past 20 years has also fuelled insecurity at work. Workers in the UK now have substantially fewer rights than workers in other European countries. There is as yet no *minimum wage* in this country, and workers here do not even have the right to paid holidays or paid bank holidays. Before 1979, workers could claim *unfair dismissal* if they had worked for an employer for more than 6 months. After extending this period to 1 year, the Government later doubled it to 2 years, so today a worker dismissed within this period has no redress.

As we have said, 'jobs for life' *may* be a thing of the past. There has been a reduction in the *average* length of employment in one job. In 1975 this was 8 years 2 months for men, and 4 years for women. By 1995 the figure had dropped to 6 years 1 month for men, but there was a slight increase for women to 4 years 4 months. Looking back over this century, Patricia Hewitt MP points to a reversal of the relationship between men and women and work outside the home:

> men born in the early part of this century... worked for virtually the whole of their adult lives. They started when they were 14 and they worked, most of them, until they dropped dead. . . . Men growing up towards the end of the century . . . will spend a decade of their lives less in employment than their grandfathers did and that's a startling change. Now for women, it's a rather different pattern. Women growing up towards the end of this century are likely to spend a decade

> and a half more in employment than women did who were born at the beginning.
> (*20–20 A View of the Century*, BBC Radio 4, June 1997)

THE VALUE OF WORK

> Work is . . . the most effective solution to poverty and the key to achieving social inclusion.
> (Carey Oppenheim, *Community Care*, 31 July 1997, p.15)

Work provides an income, but it also has other benefits, including a reason to get up in the morning, interest and stimulation, self-esteem and a sense of belonging, and an opportunity to meet people, make friends and form other social contacts.

Will Hutton writes about the more profound qualities that work should ideally bring to all of our lives: 'the most important indicator of individual well-being is to work in ways that allow you to feel that you are acting on the world in the best way that you can. To work is to earn an income, certainly; but it is to acquire skills, to win friends, to gain status, to assert your very existence. Enforced idleness is numbing; it is no coincidence that the highest rates of suicide are among the unemployed' (Hutton, 1997, p.34).

DISCRIMINATION AND WORK

A number of groups of people face discrimination both in applying for jobs and whilst in work. We shall focus on three of them, namely women, black people and older people.

Women

> Women make up more than half the population and tend to live longer, yet they account for over half the registered unemployed in the European Community and often have lower paid jobs. Less women are actively engaged in employment in Europe (66 per cent) than in the USA or Japan (72 per cent)'
>
> (European Commission, 1996, p.11).

Women represent over 44 per cent of employed people in this country, and the proportion of women in paid work is increasing. In the UK, 71 per cent of women are either in a job or looking for work. Most of the women who are new to the labour force are mothers with young children, and the majority have children under five. Indeed, over 50 per cent of all women with children under five either have or are seeking paid employment. The fact that the average age at which women have their first child is now higher than ever (28 years) means that they now have a better chance of establishing themselves in work during the years after leaving school. They are also in a better position to return more speedily to the labour market after having one or more children.

Having said this, women face many negative effects of discrimination in relation to work. We have already mentioned that a large proportion of recently created jobs have been part-time, low skilled and low paid, and that the majority of these have been taken up by women.

The gap between men's and women's average earnings is gradually narrowing, but women's average earnings are still only 75 per cent of those of men. Furthermore:

- women are twice as likely as men to be low paid;
- 2.3 million people earn less than £3.50 an hour and 75 per cent of them are women;
- 800 000 women earn less than £2.50 an hour; women working at home, e.g. in clothing manufacture (so-called 'home-workers'), can earn as

little as 50 pence per hour (Church Action on Poverty, 1996).

There are long-held stereotypes of women's role in society – for example, that women's real 'place' is in the home, that their true role is to care for and service others, and that women only really work for 'pin money', i.e. to 'top up' a partner's income and buy luxury items. More recently, however, these assumptions have been challenged by the need of many households to have both partners in paid work, and by a call for equal opportunities.

Yet equal opportunities policies have so far only had a superficial effect on women's progress at work, particularly in relation to promotion. In almost all vocational areas women are over-represented in low-status roles, yet under-represented in middle and higher management. This situation is particularly true for Social Services Departments (Social Work Departments in Scotland) and the Probation Service.

Ethnic minorities

> Most blacks and Asians are not poised to take on high-flying jobs in the upper echelons of government and business: they are concentrated at the very bottom of the economic, social and professional heap.
>
> (*Guardian*, 22 July 1997, p.16)

There is plenty of evidence that black people are discriminated against in the workplace, and in many ways their circumstances are similar to those of women – they are concentrated in low-paid occupations and are under-represented in positions of seniority. In addition, all ethnic minority groups experience higher rates of unemployment than white people.

Unemployment in 1993 for ethnic minority groups was 20.9 per cent, compared to 9.6 per cent for the white population. The highest rates of unemployment were among the Pakistani/ Bangladeshi group, at 30 per cent, and the African-

Caribbean community, at 28 per cent. Within each of the main ethnic minority groups the highest rates of unemployment were among 16- to 24-year olds.

The difference between the unemployment rates of white and ethnic minority groups cannot be explained by differences in qualifications. At each level of qualification, the proportion of unemployed people was higher among ethnic minorities than it was among white people (Equal Opportunities Review, No. 56, July 1994, p.26).

Older people

> The extent of discrimination against older people is causing deep concern. With all other significant causes of discrimination now regulated by law, there is a risk that age discrimination may be seen as the one that doesn't matter. But for those it affects, the waste, frustration and indignity are acute.
>
> (Richard Worsley, *Guardian*, 2 March 1996, p.6)

In relation to work, age discrimination is not illegal in this country. An employer can place a job advertisement which states, for example, 'People over 40 need not apply' or 'Applicants under 30 will be particularly welcome'. This situation relates not only to recruiting staff, but also refers to promotion, training and selection for redundancy. As industries and organizations have 'downsized', growing numbers of people in their forties and fifties have been consigned to redundancy with little if any prospect of gaining future employment, let alone at the same pay and conditions.

Structural ageism is based on certain myths – that older workers cannot retrain or learn new skills, that they are inflexible, and that they lack energy and have less to offer than younger people. This stereotype undervalues the maturity, experience, skill and loyalty which age can bring. The workforce should include people of all ages if it is to be balanced and fully effective.

A number of initiatives around the country prove that the public feel strongly about age dis-crimination. One of these is the *POPE project* ('people of previous experience') in Bradford. Established in 1993, it exists to provide support for older people in finding employment. Training and counselling are offered free of charge so that new skills can be learned and negative experiences of rejection by potential employers can be dealt with in a positive way.

MEDIA IMAGES OF UNEMPLOYED PEOPLE

> The problem is that far too many...people would rather be unemployed. They'd rather beg, they'd rather lean and sponge on others, they'd rather anything than take on work which they choose to see as not 'a proper job'.
>
> (Professor David Marsland, *Daily Mail*, 19 January 1990, p.9).

As the above quotation demonstrates, in a society where fewer jobs are available than previously, unemployed people continue to be stigmatized by the media, which 'blames the victim'. Terms like 'scroungers' and 'shirkers' have commonly been used in order to whip up a 'moral panic' against those who are unemployed.

Undoubtedly, a small number of people do not want to seek paid work. However, there are two very important reasons why most people need to find paid employment.

1. The level of benefits is too low to support that which most people consider to be a decent standard of living. There is plenty of evidence that benefit levels do not even allow for a balanced, nutritious diet, let alone new clothes, a holiday or a car. As has already been mentioned, the constant struggle to survive can damage people's morale and mental health.

2. The sanctions applied to people who do not take up job offers, even inappropriate ones, have

become increasingly punitive. For instance, if a person leaves work or refuses a job offer without 'good reason', he or she can be disqualified from receiving the 'Jobseeker's Allowance' for up to 6 months (26 weeks).

The 'Jobseeker's Agreement', which the claimant has to sign, sets out the agreed tasks that the claimant should undertake in the pursuit of work. The Employment Service may stipulate a change in a person's appearance or behaviour in order to make them 'more employable'. Two women in receipt of the Jobseeker's Allowance describe their experience of the Employment Service. Carol, a 'supply teacher', says: 'I was treated in such a way that I have been made ill. I have suffered constant anxiety and lost whole nights of sleep as a result of the tactics directed against me. Sadly, the staff are just carrying out orders.' Pam says: 'Then there is the humiliation of signing on, the fear of the inquisition as to whether one is doing sufficient to search for the non-existent work. ...This all leads to terrible depression and anger. There is no dignity or self-respect, no control over your own life, you must do what the DSS say or lose your benefits' (both quotes from Church Action on Poverty, 1997, p.2).

There have been a growing number of cases of people being disqualified from benefit on unfair grounds. One man lost his Jobseeker's Allowance and received no benefit for 2 weeks because he was deemed to have voluntarily resigned from his job. In fact, he had resigned because he said he could not cope with night work, heavy manual labour and 3 hours of travelling each day. He was left with no money for food or electricity (*Observer*, 20 April 1997, p.9).

A woman was denied benefit for leaving a bar job 'voluntarily', after she had been physically attacked three times. She said that the Benefits Agency staff had told her that this was an 'occupational hazard' (*Observer*, 20 April 1997, p.9).

CONCLUSION

An important report, entitled *The Churches Enquiry into Unemployment and the Future of Work*, was published on 8 April 1997, having been commissioned by the Council of Churches for Britain and Ireland. It stated that real unemployment was twice as high as official figures, suggesting and challenging the defeatism of those who believed that 'good work' for everyone was a thing of the past. According to the report, 'full employment' should still be a policy priority and unemployment should primarily be tackled by creating jobs. Unemployment has become institutionalized in this country and accepted by many both in and out of power as inevitable. The Churches' report insisted that most unemployed people are not 'work-shy'. It went on to attack the support provided by the benefits system, saying, 'We do not believe that the level of benefits paid in Britain today is generally adequate to support a decent standard of life'. It was also critical of the growing divide within, and polarization of, our society: 'Wherever we went we saw increasing riches and poverty side by side. It is wrong, in such prosperous times as ours, for men and women to be deprived for long periods of the chance to earn their living'.

The report contained a large number of positive proposals. Some of the most important ones were:

- decent pay rates, underpinned by a minimum wage;
- pay restraint at the upper end of the earnings scale to limit polarization;
- statutory regulation of adequate working conditions;
- equal opportunities policies monitored by a commission.

'Welfare to work'

There are positive signs that the unemployment situation is improving. The concept of 'downsizing' appears to be falling out of favour with some multinational companies. The European Union has introduced a number of positive initiatives specifically focused on alleviating long-term and youth unemployment, and the Labour Government has set in motion its 'Welfare-to-work' provisions as well as giving the 'Low Pay Commission' the task of recommending a minimum wage level. Opponents of the introduction of a fixed minimum wage fear that it will result in a higher rate of redundancies, but experience from America, where it has existed for some time, contradicts this view.

'Welfare-to-work' contains three different programmes. The most expensive programme, utilizing £3.15 billion, is aimed at providing a quarter of a million 18- to 24-year-olds who have been out of work for more than 6 months with a way into work. These young people are to be offered four options, all of which include the equivalent of a day a week of training:

- a job with a private sector employer;
- a job with a voluntary organization;
- work with the public sector 'environment taskforce';
- full-time education or training for up to 1 year for those who lack basic skills.

A second programme costing £350 million is directed at long-term unemployed people. Employers are offered a subsidy of £75 per week to take on individuals who have been unemployed for 2 years or more.

The third programme, costing £200 million, is directed at the 1 million lone parents who are on benefits. The government has estimated that 90 per cent of them want to work, and has recognized that better child-care facilities are essential to allow them to do so. No lone parent is to be compelled to work or penalized if they wish to stay at home. Those who are interested are invited to a 'Job-search interview' when their youngest child reaches the second term of full-time education. Part of this programme has been allocated to provide 'child-care assistant' training for up to 50 000 unemployed young people.

'Welfare-to-work' has its critics, but has been generally well received and has encouraged a mood of optimism. Carey Oppenheim says of it, 'Welfare-to-work represents an important change in social policy; it is about improving the skills and work experience of claimants. It shifts spending from cash benefits to active labour market measures' (*Community Care*, 31 July 1997, p.15).

Unemployment is one of the most serious ills that characterizes modern society. As we have seen, it has a destructive effect on an individual's self-regard, it limits their community participation and it reduces their quality of life.

As a society, we must not accept the fatalism that holds mass unemployment to be unavoidable and permanent. Unemployment has been allowed to affect too many individuals, families and communities for too long. As Michael Ignatieff says: 'What we haven't got used to, and shouldn't get used to, is the injustice of the "market" – which still allocates good jobs to some and bad or no jobs to many' (*20/20*, BBC Radio 4, June 1997).

The consequence of the unfair distribution of work is that the UK is now polarized to the extent that:

- 34 per cent of UK households have no wage-earners;
- 31 per cent have one earner;
- 29 per cent have two earners;
- 6 per cent have more than two earners.

There can be no doubt that many of the people who have sought support from health services, social work and the probation service, and many of those who have become offenders, have experienced the damaging consequences of unemployment, either directly themselves or through another family member.

EXERCISES

1. A close friend comes to stay

A friend is coming to stay with you for the weekend. This friend is 'non-disabled'. Plan the weekend activities for the two of you. Now plan the weekend for yourself and your friend who is either:

- severely visually impaired;
- severely hearing impaired; or
- uses a wheelchair.

Consider the differences in the plans you make in each circumstance.

2. Project on a minority group

Select a minority group that has not been dealt with in this book and produce a detailed project which gives information about the group and focuses on how its members are marginalized and excluded by society. For example, you may choose to examine the social situation of people who are addicted to drugs, people with alcohol-related problems, transsexuals, transvestites, or people with specific medical conditions such as myalgic encephalomyelitis (ME) or sickle cell disease.

3. Choices

You have arrived at work or at college at the beginning of an average working day. This will mean that you have already made a number of choices. On a sheet of paper make a list of all the personal choices you have made so far. These might include what you have decided to wear, whether or not you chose to have breakfast, or how you travelled to work or college.

After making a full list, imagine that you are a service-user living in any *one* of the following settings and make a list relevant to your situation:

- a small group home for people with a learning disability;
- a day centre or resource centre for people with a learning disability;
- the family home of a person with a learning disability;
- an open ward for people with a mental health problem;
- a care home or nursing home for older people;
- a detention centre for asylum-seekers;
- the home of someone who is being cared for by a friend or relative;
- the home of an adult carer who is supporting a disabled person.

4. Media representation of minority groups

With regard to one or more of any of the minority groups covered in this chapter, carry out a media survey on any one day or over a period of a week. Obtain copies of a number of newspapers and magazines and make sure that you include at least one broadsheet newspaper, one tabloid newspaper, a local newspaper and a sample from the ethnic press. Examine these papers for news, features and articles on your chosen group. In addition, you may broaden your study by monitoring television or radio programmes over the same period. Consider the following questions.

(a) Does the group have a high profile or do you feel its interests are marginalized or ignored?
(b) Are members of this group depicted positively or negatively, seriously or disrespectfully?
(c) To what extent have minority group members themselves been involved in the representation of the material produced by the media?

What conclusions do you draw about the media representation of your chosen minority group?

5. Not in my back yard (NIMBY)

You have the task of informing a community about a proposed residential provision which is to be sited within the neighbourhood for one of the following groups of service users:

- travellers;
- people with a mental health problem;
- people with learning disabilities;
- ex-offenders;
- women and children.

At this stage you anticipate an adverse reaction from local residents, and you want to present the group's interests as favourably and honestly as possible. It is important not to gloss over potential difficulties which you think might occur. Draft a letter to local residents outlining what the practical consequence of the proposal might be. This situation could be taken further, as a group discussion or role play, where the individual roles of officials and local residents might be allocated.

6. Reply to the letter

This letter appeared in the newspaper after the Government announced its policy to encourage lone parents into paid work and off welfare benefits. Write a reply to the author of the letter.

Sir: May I, in connection with the row about restricting payments to single parents, make an outrageous suggestion? I think single parents should be split into two categories: the deserving and the not so deserving. Single parents who are so because their partners have died or left them (after committing themselves in the first place to shared parenthood, either by marriage or otherwise) should receive state support sufficient to let them decide whether they want to work or stay at home to look after their children. Single parents who are so through choice or carelessness should be expected to work provided (and this is a big 'but') the government can set up a nation-wide, properly funded and organized system of child-care. I am very willing to have my taxes used to support the first category, who are single parents through no choice of their own. But why should I support women who decide to have babies without the means or the partners to support them?

(Lynne Reid-Banks *Independent*, 27 October 1997, p.20).

7. Mental health quiz

All figures are approximate and relate to the UK, unless otherwise specified.

1. Which group is more likely to experience a mental health problem? **(a)** women; **(b)** children; **(c)** men.
2. In the course of their lifetime, what percentage of people will develop a severe mental health problem? **(a)** 3 per cent; **(b)** 12 per cent; **(c)** 20 per cent.
3. What is the most common adult mental health problem? **(a)** manic-depression; **(b)** schizophrenia; **(c)** anxiety mixed with depression.
4. How many prescriptions are issued every year for tranquillizers and antidepressants? **(a)** 50 000; **(b)** 2 million; **(c)** 6 million.
5. How many people are admitted to psychiatric hospitals each year? **(a)** 80 000; **(b)** 200 000; **(c)** 800 000.
6. Are the majority of people who are admitted to hospitals: **(a)** voluntary patients; **(b)** compulsorily held patients?
7. How many children under 16 years of age are estimated to have a severe mental health problem? **(a)** 30 000; **(b)** 80 000; **(c)** 250 000.
8. How many adults are alcohol-dependent? **(a)** 1 in 20; **(b)** 1 in 200; **(c)** 1 in 1000.
9. About 100 000 ECT treatments are administered each year. What percentage of these are received by women? **(a)** 30 per cent; **(b)** 50 per cent; **(c)** 70 per cent.
10. How many people in England alone take their lives each year? **(a)** 2000; **(b)** 5000; **(c)** 12,000.

Answers on page 263.

QUESTIONS FOR ESSAYS OR DISCUSSION

1. Only heterosexual parents can ever give children a balanced upbringing because they provide appropriate role models.

2. Travellers represent such a threat to 'settled' society that society needs to erect many barriers and blocks in order effectively to stop them living their chosen life-style.

3. Carers have a duty to look after a close friend or relative. The alternative would be for them to be cared for by strangers, and this is never satisfactory.

4. The majority of people who seek asylum in the UK are drawn more strongly by the expected benefits of living in an advanced and prosperous country, than they are repelled by the conditions of danger and abuse that supposedly exist in their country of origin.

5. Ageism experienced by older people is the same phenomenon as that experienced by young people.

6. Every single parent would like to have a partner and substitute parent for their child.

7. It is society that disables a person, not their impairment.

8. Prison should be a more positive experience and aim towards the rehabilitation of an individual. At present prisons merely damage inmates, their families and, ultimately, society.

9. All a carer working with people with HIV can do is to tend to their immediate needs and prepare and counsel them for death.

10. You arrive at a closed swing-door at the same time as a person in a wheelchair. Do you automatically open the door for them? Give reasons for your answer.

11. Paid work is the best form of welfare and the most effective antidote to social exclusion.

12. 'Rights' for people with a mental health condition, without the resources to support them, effectively mean the 'right to complain' and little else.

13. All people with a learning disability should have an independent advocate.

FURTHER READING

Academic sources

Balchin, P. 1995: *Housing policy: an introduction.* London: Routledge. A comprehensive study of housing policy and homelessness in the UK.

Blytheway, B. 1995: *Ageism.* Buckingham: Open University Press. A very engaging and readable exploration of the meaning of old age and the phenomenon of ageism.

Brown, H. 1997: *Social work and sexuality. Working with lesbians and gay men.* London: Macmillan. A clear, introductory account of some of the key practical and theoretical issues raised by homo-sexuality in the context of social work.

Burningham, S. 1989: *Not on your own. The MIND guide to mental health.* Harmondsworth: Penguin. An accessible guide to mental health problems and the professional help that is available. It includes a section on self-help and sources of advice and information.

Council of Churches for Britain and Ireland 1997: *The Churches' enquiry into unemployment and the future of work.* London: CCBI Publications. The report of a Working Party which challenges the defeatism of those who believe that good jobs for all are a thing of the past.

Craft A. 1994: *Practice issues in sexuality and learning disabilities.* London: Routledge. A clear exploration of the need for people with learning disabilities to express their sexuality in ways which are valued by other members of society.

Drakeford, M. and Vanstone, M. (eds) 1996: *Beyond offending behaviour.* Aldershot: Arena. A book that insists that without a concerted effort to address the social circumstances of offenders, attempts to divert them from offending will not succeed.

Hicks C. 1990: *Who cares: looking after people at home.* London: Virago. An in-depth study of the practicality of caring for a friend or relative at home. The book examines the physical and emotional demands made on carers.

Lilley, M. 1996: *Successful single parenting.* Plymouth: How To Books. A positive look at lone parenting with some practical ideas on how to overcome some of the difficulties.

Marr, J. and Kershaw, B. 1998: *Caring for older people: developing specialist practice.* London: Arnold. A collection of contributions from a variety of nursing professionals, including lecturers and practitioners. The book is very informative and accessible and deals comprehensively with the special care needs of older people in the community, residential care and in nursing homes.

Okely, J. 1983: *The traveller-gypsies.* Cambridge: Cambridge University Press. A study of gypsies and other travellers which includes historical aspects, family patterns and life-styles.

Oppenheimer, J. 1997: *Acting on AIDS: sex, drugs and politics.* London: Serpent's Tail. A detailed look at the discrimination experienced by people with HIV infection in this country and throughout Europe.

Shutter, S. 1997: *JCWI immigration, nationality and refugee law handbook.* London: Joint Council for the Welfare of Immigrants. An easy-to-read, comprehensive and detailed source of information about refugee and immigration issues.

Stern, V. 1993: *Bricks of shame,* 2nd edn. Harmondsworth: Penguin. A critical view of the state of British prisons, which questions why an unnecessarily high number of offenders receive costly custodial sentences.

Stopford, V. 1998: *Understanding disability: causes, characteristics and coping,* 2nd edn. London: Arnold. A short, useful handbook which provides a good deal of information and insight into a wide range of impairments. This second edition includes a new section on emotional impairments.

Other literary sources

Atkinson, D. and Williams, F. (eds) 1990: *Know me as I am: an anthology of prose, poetry, and art by people with learning difficulties.* London: Hodder & Stoughton in association with Open University Press.

Boyle, J. 1984: *The pain of confinement: prison diaries.* Edinburgh: Canongate.

Dominique Bauby, J. 1998: *The diving bell and the butterfly.* London: Fourth Estate.

Doty, M. 1996: *Heaven's coast.* London: Jonathan Cape.

Dunn S., Morrison, B. and Roberts, M. (eds) 1996: *Mind readings – writers' journeys through mental states.* London: Minerva.

Dupoy, D. 1988: *Dare to dream. The story of the famous people players.* Toronto: Key Porter Books.

Ignatieff, M. 1994: *Scar tissue.* London: Vintage.

Ireland, T. 1988: *Who lies inside.* Swaffham: GMP Publishers Ltd.

Sarton, M. 1983: *As we are now.* London: The Women's Press.

Shannon, T. and Morgan, C. 1996: *Invisible crying tree.* London: Doubleday.

Swindells, R. 1993: *Stone cold.* London: Hamish Hamilton Ltd.

Wurtzel, E. 1995: *Prozac nation.* London: Quartet Books.

Yates, R. 1992: *If it weren't for the alligators.* Manchester Lifeline Project Ltd.

Films or plays

Oldman, G. 1997: *Nil by Mouth.* UK.

Boyle, D. 1996: *Trainspotting.* UK.

Jarman, D. 1993: *Blue.* UK.

Bogart, P. 1988: *Torch Song Triology.* USA.

6

Caring, policy and social change

SOCIAL CHANGE

Health and social care does not take place within a vacuum. It is therefore important that carers are informed in their work by an understanding of wider social and political issues. Whether a carer is tending to the needs of a friend or relative, or is employed as a paid carer by a statutory, voluntary 'not-for-profit' or private organization, she or he needs to be aware of the relationship between the service user and society in general. In addition, carers need to acknowledge their own relationship with wider society and the dynamic relationship between themselves and those for whom they care, so that their own positions and that of their clients can be seen within the same social context (Fig. 6.1).

Most people who choose to enter the field of health and social care may do so for two main reasons. Primarily they may be motivated by a sense of compassion, which may spring from deep-seated spiritual, moral or cultural grounds, or may simply be an expression of their desire to 'work with people' or 'to do something worthwhile'. The other main concern felt by many entrants to the field of health and social care is to be able to become

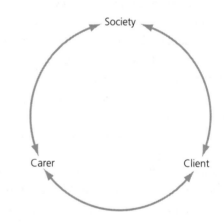

Fig. 6.1

involved in purposeful social change and to be able to help to create a more just society.

Change occurs within society all the time, some of these changes being gradual, while others take place more quickly. The effect of some changes is minimal, but others have a huge and lasting impact. Social carers, by the very nature of their work, are inextricably involved in the process of social change.

Consider, for example, a situation where a carer is preparing a man with a physical impairment for bed. By attending to his physical needs and ensuring that his cultural needs are met and that the client's dignity and self-respect are maintained, the carer automatically becomes involved, however minimally, in the process of purposeful social change. The intervention itself has an immediate effect on the client's well-being, not least because his physical comfort may now allow him to obtain the rest his body needs. If care has been carried out positively, it may well have the effect of increasing the client's confidence and independence, and may contribute to reducing his reliance on other people. The carer's involvement with the service user may thus affect the lives of other people – perhaps those neighbours, relatives or other carers who would otherwise be responsible for the man's care.

Similarly, but on a larger scale – the impact of – for example, the introduction of a group living scheme in a residential care home for older people which gives residents more autonomy, and opportunities to take risks, make decisions and do more things for themselves, can be seen as a clearer and more dramatic example of social change. The ramifications of such a move may spread beyond the walls of the home. The ensuing increased interaction and the greater satisfaction felt by residents who are significantly more involved in their own lives may coincide with an increase in staff morale and a growing sense of purpose within the establishment. Furthermore, the effects of this might be felt by all visitors to the establishment and also by those who share the lives of the workers in the home.

Greater social change clearly occurs following the introduction of new legislation and social policy (or amendments to existing legislation or social policy). Whilst these changes are formally introduced by the government, instigation for change may well have occurred outside. Agitation by service users, practitioners, professional associations and trade unions, and the success of good practice and research, can all directly affect changes in policy.

A carer's understanding of wider society needs to go beyond the general impression created by much of the media and official organizations. The image projected is often one of a stable, balanced society that rewards best those who are talented or hard-working, and ascribes failure either to individual pathology or to misfortune. In other words, the individual is considered to be responsible for his or her circumstances. It is rarely admitted that hardship is often structurally determined. Instead, the impression of social justice is fostered and notions of equality of opportunity and equal rights are taken for granted and considered to be the very basis upon which our society operates.

Anything other than a superficial examination of society will show this picture to be a false one. Throughout this book we have looked at the divisions within society and at the structural inequalities which affect people's lives and their ability to fulfil themselves. In particular, we have noted the damaging effects of oppression, prejudice, discrimination and bias delivered by individuals and organizations from a position of power.

SOCIAL INEQUALITY

The symbol at the core of our unequal society is the unrepresentative political system that excludes the oppressed sectors of society which we have identified. As we have seen, following the 1997 general election, the number of women MPs rose to a record 120, and black membership increased to nine MPs. Furthermore, in the same year there were four MPs who declared themselves to be gay, and a further two MPs who had a physical impairment. We have already noted that this indicates some movement towards a truer reflection of society: 'What with a handful of openly gay MPs, someone in a wheelchair, a few more black faces, Parliament is getting nearer to representing a cross-section of the population' (Suzanne Moore, *Independent*, 9 May 1997, p.21). However, the overwhelming traditional bias remains. The House of Lords and the democratically elected House of Commons are still predominantly the preserve of white, middle-aged, middle-class, assumed heterosexual, non-disabled men. This pattern of representation is repeated throughout the nation states of Europe, except in Sweden, where women form 40 per cent of parliament. Furthermore, the composition of the British Parliament is replicated throughout society's other organizations, although breakthroughs – overcoming the 'glass ceiling', the 'white ceiling' and other discriminatory barriers – continue to occur. Consequently, social change is only gradual, and the influence of structural disadvantage remains powerful.

STRUCTURAL INEQUALITY

> There is a vicious circle of marginalization, with the dice loaded against these people and their families.
>
> ('It Does Not Get Any Better' *The Times*, 15 July 1997, p.10)

There is ample evidence that structural inequality, as shown by levels of poverty, is firmly entrenched within the UK, and that in this respect Britain compares unfavourably with other European countries. It is estimated that as many as one in five of all EC residents in poverty lives in the UK.

Health inequality

There are indications that the divisions between rich and poor actually widened during the 1980s and early 1990s. *Health inequality* broadened:

- between 1982–1986 and 1987–1991, life expectancy among men in social classes IV and V (semi-skilled and unskilled occupations, respectively) fell from 69.8 to 69.7 years;
- among social classes I and II (professional/managerial and technological occupations, respectively) life expectancy for men in 1987–1991 was 74.9 years, more than 5 years higher than that for men in classes IV and V (Whitehead, 1997).

Poorer people tend to experience higher rates of chronic sickness compared to those who are better off, and their children have lower birth-weights, shorter stature and general health which is not so favourable.

There is now also considerable evidence that unemployment causes a deterioration in mental health for many people who experience it.

Income

> First and foremost, I pay my bills and next I see that food is on the table for myself, then for anything else – say underwear or shoe repairs – I have to pick my times. I try saving, but there's always something crops up that I really need it for and I have to delve into it. Its always been like that for me.
>
> (Widowed state pensioner quoted in 'Circle of Life at the Bottom', *Guardian*, 22 October 1997, p.6)

- In 1979 only 7 per cent of families were living on income of less than half the national average (regarded as the best proxy for an official poverty line).
- By 1990–1991 the proportion had risen to 20 per cent, falling to 16 per cent in 1995–1996, towards the end of the long period of Conservative government.
- During this same period, average real income, excluding the self-employed and after housing costs, increased by 38 per cent. The tenth of the population with the highest income enjoyed a 61 per cent rise; the tenth with the lowest suffered a 4 per cent cut (*Guardian*, 17 October 1997, p.5).

So much for the much-heralded 'trickle-down theory', which purported that success at the top would filter through to benefit all.

Paul Sussman, writing for the *Big Issue*, spent some time with politically disaffected young people in Glasgow, and revealed a sense of despair. 'Ironically the saddest thing about Lisa is that she herself is not sad. She accepts her graffitied tenement, absent parents and druggie neighbours as though they were the lot of a normal child. She has no real hopes or expectations, no sense that her situation will get any better. She belongs to a world in which there never has been, and never will be, any feel-good factor' (*Big Issue*, 22 July 1997, p.18). He added that others have lost all sense of their own power to influence events: 'They are a generation for whom the concept of citizenship has ossified' (*Big Issue*, 22 July 1997, p.18).

Education

There is a well-established link between poverty and educational under-achievement, which may stem from lack of stimulation and resources, under-nourishment, absence of support and encouragement, or low teacher expectation. It is also recognized, that the 'handicap' of poor educational attainment has consequences for the rest of a person's life. According to the report *It Doesn't Get Any Better,* produced by the Basic Skills Agency, the effects of low levels of literacy and numeracy were seen in 'unemployment, family breakdown, low incomes, depression and social inactivity'. The report added, 'Poor readers were twice as likely to be on a low wage and four times as likely to live in a household where neither parent worked' (*The Times*, 15 July 1997, p.10).

Alan Wells, director of the Basic Skills Agency, warns about 'the dangers we face in developing an underclass of excluded people; out of work, increasingly depressed and often labelled by themselves as failures' (*The Times*, 15 July 1997, p.10).

The situation is not entirely new. Alan Wells added, 'it is not just that 20 per cent have been getting nothing out of education in the last five years. The long tail of under-achievement is something we have always had. It is still with us. In 1996 almost half of 11 year olds left school without reaching the expected level of English and mathematics' (*The Times*, 15 July 1997, p.10).

Poor, working-class people themselves have developed their own strategies against poverty when they have acted together to form credit unions and food co-operatives and developed community services to meet local need. However, much more commitment is required from Central Government, which needs to be directed at the underlying structural causes of deprivation. In 1997 the Labour Government pledged itself towards the creation of a more inclusive society, beginning with a more egalitarian and effective education system that promises to focus on the attainment of all children. The Government has since set up a 'Social Exclusion Unit' in order to develop policies to counter existing marginalization and prevent its expansion.

Social class

There are those who believe that the nomenclature 'social class' has become insignificant, even as an analytical tool. They regard it as archaic and more difficult to categorize and apply because the traditional boundaries between the classes have become blurred, making distinctions irrelevant. Furthermore, the prominence over the past 20 years of the more easily identifiable factors of gender and race, has tended to obscure the importance of social class. In addition, major changes in technology, the economy and the labour market have profoundly affected class membership.

It is true that some of the indicators of social class have altered and the composition of groups has fluctuated, but the fundamental character of social class is still relevant. Social class remains an essential way of understanding society and its structure, particularly for academics and social policy-makers, despite major changes in technology, the economy and the labour market.

Research by John Galilee of the University of Lancaster has shown social class to be an enduring influence: 'research, which I am currently conducting into the daily lived experiences of middle-class young men in their 20s, has shown that this category is still experiencing the same privileges they have had for generations' (*Guardian*, 31 December 1997, p.16). Similarly, a recently published study of class entitled *A Class Act – the Myth of Britain's Classless Society* (Adonis and Pollard, 1997) found the class system to be very much alive and well.

The government itself has acknowledged the influence of social class, and the existence of an 'underclass' who are excluded from society's mainstream. It now specifically aims to ameliorate social disadvantage and to offer opportunities for people who are structurally underprivileged.

Ethnic minorities

It is now over 20 years since the Race Relations Act 1976 and the establishment of the Commission for Racial Equality (CRE), which continues in its fight to eliminate racial discrimination and to promote equality of opportunity and good race relations. As we have seen, much has been done to combat individual racism, and attempts have been made to do battle against the more hidden aspects of institutional racism. Ethnic monitoring and equal opportunities policies have been implemented by a wide range of industries and service organizations as the value of good race relations has been recognized. Detractors will point to the disparity between the declarations written into equal opportunity policy documents and actual practice. 'Even in social services departments with a strong commitment to recruiting black workers, once you get to the second and third tier there are few black faces' (*Community Care*, 6-12 June 1996, p.21). They may also cynically refer to the reduced significance given to the black perspective by some organizations in the 1990s, particularly in comparison to the 1980s when anti-racism strategies were developed.

Forty-seven per cent of Britain's ethnic minority population was born in this country, 75 per cent of whom are UK nationals (Commission for Racial Equality, 1997c). However, some people have difficulty acknowledging this fact. Gary Younge, writing in the *Guardian* about the contrasting way in which black people are received and accepted in America and the UK, described a 'typical conversation' back home in England:

> Where are you from?
> London.
> Well, where were you born?
> London.
> Well, before then?
> There was no before then.
> Well, where are your parents from?
> Barbados.
> Oh, so you are from Barbados.
> No I'm from London!
>
> (*Guardian*, 11 October 1996, p.19)

Irish people form the largest single ethnic minority by immigration into the UK today and, like their black and Asian counterparts, are concentrated in the most deprived social classes and have lower than average rates of upward social mobility. For instance, with regard to car ownership – an overall measure of standard of living – Irish-headed households were well below the average level in the 1991 census, close to that of the black Caribbean population (*Irish in Britain*, Commission for Racial Equality, 1997b). Irish people in Britain also experience discrimination in education, training and the workplace as well as socially, as do other members of ethnic minorities. 'Of course, being Irish and white, I don't experience discrimination until I open my mouth' (Mary Canty, College Lecturer, 1995).

As we have already seen, people from ethnic minorities, particularly black and Asian groups, experience deprivation on a large scale and they continue to face discrimination in all aspects of their lives – in the community, in school and in the workplace. Prejudice may be expressed as innuendo, harassment or even physical violence. At the same time, thanks to the efforts of the Commission for Racial Equality, black and Asian community groups, the work of black writers and professionals and the contribution of ordinary black people, there is a greater appreciation of the value of living in a multiracial society. More children, particularly in urban areas, are growing up in mixed communities, going to school and forming friendships with children from families with different cultural backgrounds. They have a first-hand opportunity to learn and value differences. There are instances, too, where black and Asian adults have managed to break through the 'white ceiling' into new occupations and make a mark outside the traditional spheres of sport, fashion and entertainment. The rise and growing influence of a distinct black British culture has also been recognized.

However, as Yasmin Ali Brown has pointed out, 'the forces of progress and regression co-exist' (*Independent*, 31 May 1996, p.18). Despite achievements, too many of the lives of ethnic minority people continue to be diminished by the effects of racism. She continues, 'We are faced today with the rage and disappointment of so many black and Asian Britons who still cannot claim a place in this country. It is tragic that whites and blacks with influence have abdicated their responsibility to turn Britain into a standard bearer for racial equality in Europe' (*Independent*, 31 May 1996, p.18).

Women

Women continue to break new ground in all sectors of society. We have seen how many individual women have symbolically broken through the 'glass ceiling' of invisible, entrenched attitudes, procedures and discrimination to obtain positions of authority in hitherto male-dominated spheres. For instance, in 1996 the ordination of women in the Anglican Church represented a major change that had been contested by the majority of the clergy for a very long time. After the first Church of England ordination of a woman in Wales took place in Bangor, North Wales, in January 1997, the Rev. Barry Morgan told the congregation, 'Amidst all the joy there has also to be space for penitence and healing for the long years in which we have wounded these women as individuals and deprived the church of God of their gifts of ministry' (*Sunday Times*, 12 January 1997).

More prosaically, women have made headway in the world of sport. 1996 saw the first Football Association match officiated entirely by women. The following year on 27 August, Wendy Toms became the first woman to 'run the line' in a Premiership football match. Women now make up over 30 per cent of Premiership attendances. The Football Association have altered their rules to accommodate women. A 'linesman' is a thing of the past and has been replaced by 'referee's assistant' and players cautioned under Law 12(1) are guilty of 'unsporting behaviour', which replaced the 100-year-old term 'ungentlemanly conduct'.

More women participate in sport now. An estimated 21 000 women play soccer, which is a threefold increase over the last 10 years; 8000 women play rugby and there are 60 women's registered cricket clubs. Women have now been accepted by the Amateur Boxing Board and are permitted to fight inside the ring with one another.

England's women cricketers were world champions in 1996. However, that is not so widely known because men's sport, even in defeat, still dominates television and newspapers, although women's sport is slowly getting more air-space and media attention. British international women players in many sports may have to lose a day's pay in order to take time to represent their country, whereas their male counterparts may receive thousands of pounds, and fame as well, for doing so.

Despite these landmarks, women remain oppressed. Many institutions are still male dominated and women, particularly working-class and black women, continue to be discriminated against in education and in the world of work. However, the nub of their disadvantage lies in the absence of universal, family-centred policies which could free women from their imposed responsibility of caring for the family at home. Natasha Walker says, 'Until there's a better child-care strategy in this country, women won't have equality' adding that 'the great bedrock of inequality lies in the struggle women experience in combining work and the home' (*Observer*, 27 April 1997, p.25).

As can be seen from Table 6.1, the UK's child-care provision is among the poorest in Europe.

Not only is public child-care provision in short supply, it is also restricted to targeted children who are assessed as being in need. Less than 1 per cent of 0- to 3-year-olds are offered a local authority day-nursery place. Between 1990 and 1993 the number of public day-centre places decreased by 5000, although there has been a continued rise in the number of private nursery places available. The majority of families in the UK care for their own small children, and unregistered childminders are the main source of outside support used. Most other European countries have family-based policies such as: generous statutory maternity leave, statutory paternity or maternal support leave, and leave for family reasons. These policies provide the mother with more initial support and can enable the father, or the child's carer, an opportunity for early and sustained involvement. 'Most member states offer a statutory right to some form of parental leave, or, in the case of Belgium, a universal system of 6–12 months 'career breaks' per worker, subject to employer agreement, available for any reason including care of young children. However, Ireland, Luxembourg and the UK offer nothing' (*A Review of Services for Young Children*, European Commission Network on Childcare, 1996, p.20).

Within the UK there are enormous variations in income and use of child care among families with working mothers. These differences reflect

Table 6.1 Care of pre-school-age children

	Nursery/kindergarten provisions[*]	Infants and very young children: how targeted	Regulation of family day care
Denmark	High	Extensive, universal	Yes
Finland	High	Extensive, universal	Yes
Sweden	High	Extensive, universal	Yes
Italy	High	Variable, to support parents	Yes
France	High	Extensive, working parents	Yes
Norway	Medium	Growing, universal	No
Belgium	High	Limited, at home preferred	Yes
Austria	Medium	Limited, at home preferred	Yes
Germany[†]	Medium	Limited, at home preferred	Yes
Greece	Medium	Limited, at home preferred	No
Luxembourg	Low	Limited, at home preferred	No
The Netherlands	Low	Limited, at home preferred	No
Spain	Medium	Limited, at risk	No
Portugal	Low	Limited, at risk	No[‡]
Ireland	Low	Limited, at risk	No[§]
UK	Low	Limited, at risk	Yes

[*] High, over 80% coverage; medium 50–80%; low, below 50%.

[†] Very different in the old and new Länder.

[‡] Private care is not regulated, but organized day care schemes are.

[§] Some regulation to be introduced under the 1991 Child Care Act.

Source: Miller, J. and Warman, A. 1996: *Family obligations in Europe*. London: Family Policy Studies Centre, p. 30.

the increasing polarization of our society during the 1980s and 1990s. Families with qualified parents in work are more likely to pay for formal child care than families with lower incomes who rely more on family members and friends. There is a growing gap between children's access to good-quality services, and this is dependent upon their parents' income (Table 6.2). For employed mothers of pre-school children:

- 18 per cent of professionals' children are cared for by a grandparent;
- 44 per cent of manual workers' children are cared for by a grandparent.

Other oppressed groups

Public attitudes

As we have seen in Chapter 5, other minority groups continue to be oppressed and excluded from full participation in society. However, for some groups there is now generally a greater degree of public acceptance and support, and this has helped to reduce the stigma they face. For other groups, public attitudes have hardened and public hostility has increased, and they have been pushed further towards the margins of society.

According to consumer research carried out by British Social Attitudes, there is now more public acceptance of gay people. For instance:

- the percentage who said it is acceptable for a homosexual person to be a teacher in a school rose from 41 per cent in 1983 to 55 per cent in 1993;
- the percentage who said it is acceptable for a homosexual person to hold a responsible position in public life rose from 53 per cent in 1983 to 63 per cent in 1993 (Stonewall, 1997b).

These figures reveal the sometimes slow nature of social change.

Attitudes towards single parents have softened in recent years following the vilification that this family form received during the 1970s and 1980s. This is partly due to the increased number of people who have experienced life in a single-parent household, either as a child or as a parent, and a greater appreciation of its strengths and weaknesses, particularly when viewed against a dysfunctional two-parent family.

In the same way that prominent gay men and lesbians have promoted a greater respect for homosexuality, a number of high-profile personalities who have either been single parents themselves or have been brought up by one have improved the social standing of single parents.

The public attitude towards people with HIV and

Table 6.2 Differences in parental income and child-care use

Work-rich families	Work-poor families
Qualified mother	Unqualified mother
Higher than average wages	Low wages
Older mother (over 30 years of age)	Younger mother
In a couple	Lone parent
Partner in work	Partner (if any) out of work
Likely to work full-time	Likely to work part-time
Secure work with sick pay and holiday pay	Insecure work without sick pay and holiday pay
Not dependent on benefits	Likely to depend on benefits
Uses formal child care (nursery, childminder, nanny)	Likely to use informal child care (partner, family, friends, or no child care)

Source: Daycare Trust 1997: *Child care now – making it happen*. Briefing Paper 1. London: Daycare Trust.

AIDS has become more enlightened, now that many of the original myths and fears about the condition have been dispelled. Similarly, there is more understanding of the difficulties faced by unemployed people and an appreciation of the struggle experienced by those who are homeless. Self-help initiatives, such as selling the *Big Issue* magazine, have enhanced the profile of homeless people.

Attitudes towards other minority groups, such as offenders, refugees, gypsies and travellers, have become less sympathetic in recent years. For instance, in 1997, when the National Lottery proposed to give a series of small grants to organizations helping refugees, the MP Ian Bruce urged the National Lottery's Charities Board to consider the so-called 'rattling-tin test' before making awards. In other words, he wanted to ensure that grants were not made to those who he considered were unpopular causes. Another sign of intolerance towards refugees and gypsies is the continuing rise throughout the UK and Europe of extreme right-wing political organizations, many of which promote racism and violence.

A substantial increase in the prison population over the past 10 years has been matched by more severe institutional regimes that reflect a more punitive public and political attitude towards offenders and prisoners. Although there is more sympathy and understanding felt towards people with mental health problems and their families, their public image is still a threatening one. Undue media attention has been focused on a very small number of instances of violence, even murder, carried out by people with severe mental health problems who were living in the community. This distorted concentration on uncontextualized, sensational events has served to damage the public's perception of the policy of 'care in the community'.

Political action and user involvement

Any improvement in the public perception of minority groups is due in part to the contribution of individuals and groups who have expressed their needs and demanded their rights. Foremost among political activists have been disabled people, who have on occasion been prepared to carry out direct action. Demonstrations have taken place at several locations, for instance:

- outside television studios in London, in protest against the patronizing nature of the 'Telethon' appeal;
- at the Blackpool Pleasure Beach, in front of the 'Pepsi-Max' ride, in protest against the fact that disabled people were not allowed access during normal daytime hours;
- in a number of towns and cities throughout the country, where activists have chained themselves to vehicles in protest against the lack of access they have to public transport;
- outside the gates of Downing Street, in Whitehall, where a number of individuals poured red paint over themselves, the road and the gates, in protest at proposed cuts in disabled peoples' benefits.

According to Andy Dick, a disabled college lecturer, 'For many disabled people, direct action is a process of politicization, because it creates the opportunity for them to reclaim their political identity. When disabled people smeared red paint at the gates of Downing Street at the end of 1997, it was more than a publicity stunt. It was disabled people reclaiming the ability to be political' (Dick, A., personal communication, 5 March 1998).

Within the field of health and social care, politicization has mainly taken the form of self-advocacy. Service users have increasingly made themselves heard by supporting one another in stating their individual and collective needs. 'People First' is one of a number of self-advocacy organizations of people with learning disabilities that aims to promote service-user interests. The organization encourages and trains individual service-users to argue their case effectively. It represents the point of view of people with learning difficulties on policy panels, and directly contributes towards training programmes for prospective health and social care workers.

Policies against discrimination

Political or direct action by members of minority groups is not in itself enough. In order to improve the quality of life of oppressed groups effectively, rigorous anti-discrimination legislation is still needed. Twenty years after the introduction of major anti-discrimination legislation concerning women and ethnic minorities, the Disability Discrimination Act (DDA) was passed. This 1995 Act was regarded as insubstantial, however, and it disappointed both disabled people and those who work with them. It is now hoped that the government will fulfil its promise to strengthen the legislation and to introduce full, enforceable civil rights.

It is still permissible to discriminate against people on grounds of age. For example, a recruiting employer may stipulate the age group of prospective workers. The government declined to introduce anti-ageist legislation in 1997, preferring instead to recommend strongly that employers adhere to a code of good practice. Other oppressed groups such as gypsies and travellers, gay people, refugees and people with HIV continue to be denied full civil rights.

Many individuals and groups have turned to the European Courts in the hope of obtaining equality. In 1997, Euan Sutherland successfully challenged as discriminatory the legal age of consent for gay men in the UK, which is 18 years, and out of line with the rest of Europe. However, Jill Percey and Lisa Grant were initially unsuccessful, in February 1998, in outlawing homophobic discrimination in the workplace. They had appealed to be treated in the same way as heterosexual couples with regard to a partner's travel concessions.

All oppressed groups are hopeful that the prevailing social conditions throughout most of the rest of Europe will eventually influence circumstances in the UK. For instance, there are more flexible and generous child-care and parental leave arrangements and family-based working practices in many European countries. The European Union is perceived as being more forward-thinking and less hidebound than Britain. It is also seen as being more committed to social justice.

RESTRUCTURING THE WELFARE STATE

Silly statements abound. . . . One of the silliest is 'We can't afford the Welfare State.'. . . .The reality is that now and in the next century, the question is not 'Can we afford it?' but 'Do we *want* to spend money in this way?' Economics may constrain choice somewhat, but the question is primarily an ethical and political one.

(Andrew Dilnot, Director of the Institute for Fiscal Studies, *Observer*, 30 March 1997, p.7)

On 5 July 1998 the National Health Service celebrated its fiftieth anniversary. Now all that we think of as constituting the 'Welfare State' is at least half a century old. Debate about the affordability of the Welfare State has taken place since its inception at the end of the Second World War. The Conservative governments of the 1980s and 1990s strove to 'roll back the frontiers of the State' in order to make individuals and families more responsible for their own welfare. Whether they actually achieved this remains the subject of controversy.

On coming to power in 1997, the Labour Government energetically set about a radical review of welfare services. This included an examination of the tax and benefits system, unemployment policy, and health and social care services.

The new administration insisted that the Welfare State could not remain static, but rather that as society changes – as old needs disappear and new ones emerge – welfare services should evolve and adapt. A vision of a 'new Welfare State' was the centrepiece of Gordon Brown's first budget as Chancellor of the Exchequer. He introduced the 'Welfare to Work' programme, which aimed to get people off benefits and into paid employment.

On 8 December 1997 the Prime Minister,

Tony Blair, launched the '*Social Exclusion Unit,*' which he said would 'be at the heart of the government, with the remit of co-ordinating our assault on poverty and social exclusion.' He went on to stress that marginalization is not only a matter of poverty: 'social exclusion is about more than just financial deprivation. It is about the damage done by poor housing, ill health, poor education, lack of decent transport but above all the lack of work' (*Independent,* 8 December 1997, p.1). The 12 members of the Unit include representatives from the voluntary sector, the police and probation services and Social Services

Departments. It is set in the Cabinet Office and is directly responsible to the Prime Minister. Some people expressed regret that a more positive title, such as the *Social Inclusion Unit,* had not been used.

Some Labour ministers referred to the Beveridge Report of 1942 and to the *Five Giants* that Beveridge identified as major social problems which the Welfare State was intended to alleviate. The Minister of Public Health, Tessa Jowell, identified the government's social policy in relation to each of the five giants:

- *want* – the introduction of a national minimum wage;
- *idleness* – the 'Welfare to Work' measures;
- *squalor* – a new house-building programme including a return of public or council housing;
- *ignorance* – education policies designed to reduce infant and junior class sizes;
- *disease* – the appointment of a new minister, of 'Public Health' and new measures to control environmental pollution.

THIRTY YEARS ON FROM 'SEEBOHM'

> I would argue for the personal social services to develop in two directions which were explicit in the Seebohm Report. First, for services which are acceptable to the populace at large. . . . Second, a concentration of community social work in deprived areas.
>
> (Bob Holman, *Community Care*, 4 April 1996, p.25)

The Seebohm Committee's report was published in 1968. It had been appointed to review 'the organization of the local authority personal social services ... to ensure an effective family service.' The committee recommended the establishment of all-embracing social services departments, bringing together the children's, welfare, and mental health departments. Specialization gave way to genericism, and smaller agencies to one large agency. A single social worker would now visit and cater for an individual's or family's needs in place of different carers

---

The eight principles

Tony Blair has ordered eight guiding principles to rule Labour's reform of the Welfare State:

- The new Welfare State should help and encourage people of working age to get a job where they are capable of doing so.
- Public and private sectors should work together to ensure that, wherever possible, people are insured against foreseeable risks and make provision for their retirement.
- The new Welfare State should provide public services of high quality to the whole community as well as cash benefits.
- Disabled people should get the support they need to lead a fulfilling life with dignity.
- The system should support families and children as well as tackling the scourge of child poverty.
- There should be specific action to attack social exclusion and help those in poverty.
- The system should encourage openness and honesty and the gateways to benefit should be clear and enforceable.
- The system of delivering modern welfare should be flexible, efficient and easy for people to use.

Fig. 6.2 The eight guiding principles formulated by Tony Blair to rule Labour's reform of the Welfare State. (*Source: The Mirror*, 27 March 1998, p.7. Reproduced with permission.)

from separate organizations. Thirty years after the Seebohm Report, we are witnessing a return to specialisms and a turning away from generic care.

The 30 years since 1968 have been characterized by great uncertainty, change and upheaval. In the 1970s there were major reorganizations in both local authorities, and the NHS. The next decade saw the start of year-on-year financial cutbacks in local authorities and the encouragement of the independent sector in health and social care at the expense of the statutory sector. The 1990s have seen another major re-organization in health and social care, following community care legislation that profoundly affected both the structure and the financing of services. Health and social care professionals could be forgiven for feeling 'punch-drunk' from the many changes that have occurred – they have had to adapt to working within a new internal market and some of them have had to adapt to becoming purchasers as well as, or instead of, providers of care.

CONTINUAL CHANGE IN HEALTH AND SOCIAL CARE

A change of government usually heralds policy changes and new developments. At present, there are as many as eight reviews of health and social care organization, funding and policies that have now been completed or will shortly reach the report stage. They are as follows.

1. A major joint review by the Social Services Inspectorate (SSI) and the Audit Commission, into the role and organization of Social Services Departments. Also under scrutiny is the relationship between health and social care services. The Health Secretary, Frank Dobson, has said that he wants the role of SSDs to be 'more clearly defined' and 'the effectiveness of services costed and tested' (*Community Care*, 6–12 November 1997, p.2).

2. The Burgner report on the 'Inspection and Regulation' functions of SSDs, most importantly in respect of residential homes for older people. Following the publication of the report, the government will issue a White Paper in 1998. In referring to speculation about the recommendations of the review, Frank Dobson has said that 'it was a fair assumption' that the local authorities would lose their regulation function (*Community Care*, 6–12 November 1997, p.2).

3. A 'Royal Commission on the Long-Term Care of the Elderly' was set up on 4 December 1997, and has to report within 1 year. The main focus will be on how the cost of care should be shared between public funds and individuals. However, social care organizations in both the statutory and voluntary sectors have urged the 11 commissioners to take a wider view, and to take in issues such as the type of work-force required for the care of older people, how this work-force is trained, the role of carers, and the kind of caring interventions that should be used. In a separate but related development, a 'Charter on Long-Term Care' has been commissioned by the government.

4. In November 1997, the Utting Report entitled 'People Like Us' (Utting, 1997) was published. Sir William Utting headed a team which had been asked to review the 'safeguards for children living away from home'. The report was damning in its main finding, that children in care were still at risk of abuse because the safeguards contained in the Children Act 1989 were not being fully and effectively implemented. It also concluded that foster care should be more closely regulated and should be managed by local authorities. The report concluded, 'More than regulation is needed … a vigorous rehabilitation of residential care, the modernizing of foster care … [and] the elevation of all boarding schools to the high standards of the best' was required (*Community Care*, 27 November–3 December 1997, p.5).

5. A review of the 'care in the community' policy for people with mental health problems is taking place. This was set up following concern that too many psychiatric hospital places had been lost, with some severely disturbed people being

released prematurely into the community without adequate support.

6. The roles of the probation and prison services and their working relationship are the subject of another review. The actual terms of the review are 'to identify and assess options for closer and more integrated working between the Prison service and the Probation service of England and Wales including any implications for the structure, organization, management, working practices, human resources, funding and legislation governing the functioning of those services'. The setting up of this review has caused grave fears within the Probation Service because it believes its independence is under threat.

7. A 2-month-long review of social work training has concluded that the Central Council for Education and Training in Social Work (CCETSW), set up in 1971, is to be wound up and subsumed within a new organization, which is to be called a 'General Social Care Council' (GSCC). The details of this were the subject of a 1998 government White Paper. The Council will have a wider remit than the CCETSW, for as well as training it will have regulatory powers over the social care work-force. With regard to pre-service and in-service training in social care, GNVQs and NVQs/SVQs are also under scrutiny.

8. Finally, a review of the tax and benefits system is taking place, and already some cuts in or amendments to benefits for single parents and disabled people have been announced.

THE HEALTH AND SOCIAL CARE WORKFORCE

Social work and social care

About 1 015 000 people constitute the UK work-force in social care and social work. This figure has doubled since 1982. It is arguably larger than any other industrial or commercial sector in this country. Within the 'mixed economy of care' there has been considerable movement of workers from one sector to another. The figures are as follows:

- the *private sector* has seen considerable growth since 1980, and is now by far the largest, with 550 000 workers;
- the *statutory sector* has seen a substantial reduction in staff, and the number is currently 315 000;
- the *voluntary sector* has also seen a reduction, although not such a dramatic one, to a current figure of 150 000.

A major 4-year work-force survey conducted by the National Institute for Social Work (NISW) was published at the end of 1997. Among its findings it revealed that about 83 per cent of the social care work-force are women, and that they remain under-represented in management, especially in senior posts.

The work-force as a whole is a stable one, the report revealing an annual turnover of only 9 per cent. On average, staff stay in a job for 10 years. The single most common reason for changing jobs is reorganization. Stress levels are high for most staff, but particularly for managers and social workers. Much concern was expressed by staff about sex and racial discrimination at work. The black staff

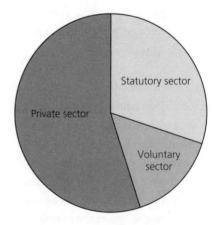

Fig. 6.3 The relative size of the work-forces of the three major sectors which make up the 'mixed economy of care'.

interviewed were 2.5 times more likely to have experienced discrimination than the white staff. Racism from colleagues and managers was reported by 27 per cent of all black staff.

The overall impression of this survey, entitled *The Social Services Work-force in Transition* (Balloch *et al.*, 1997), is of a dedicated work-force under considerable and increasing strain. Obviously the past few years of reorganization and constant change have been the main contributor to this situation. However, other developments in the world of work have played a part. The 'casualization' of work has seen a reduction in secure, permanent posts and an increase in short-term, fixed-contract jobs. There has been a substantial growth in agencies employing staff on a 'casual' short-term basis. Many of these workers will be used in the private sector. Bob Cervi expresses many people's concern: 'It is these "casual" staff that come and go according to demand – not very well-trained and certainly low paid – who help sustain the comparatively low costs of the private sector' (*Community Care*, 20-6 February 1997, p.19).

Health care (figures for England only)

Non-medical staff

In 1996, approximately 940 000 people were employed in the NHS hospital and community health services, of whom 67 per cent were direct care staff and 33 per cent were management and support staff. Just under 80 per cent of the non-medical work-force were women, and over 5 per cent were from ethnic minorities (Fig. 6.4).

Medical and dental staff

The number of hospital, public health medicine and community health service medical and dental staff has grown by 21 per cent since 1986 to 68 010 in 1996. The number of hospital medical staff has increased by 30 per cent over the same period. Hospital medical staff are predominantly male, but more women are now obtaining posts, mainly in junior grades. However, between 1986 and 1996, the proportion of female consultants increased from 14 per cent to 19 per cent. Ethnic minority doctors are

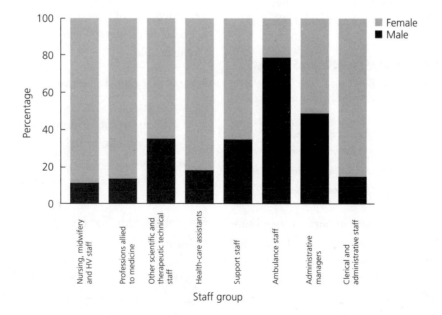

Fig. 6.4 Non-medical staff, categorized by sex for selected staff groups. (*Source: Department of Health Statistical Bulletin*, May 1997, p.4. Crown copyright is reproduced with the permission of the Controller of Her Majesty's Stationery Office.)

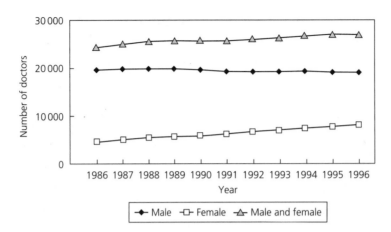

Fig. 6.5 Number of doctors, categorized by sex, October 1986 to October 1996. (*Source*: *Department of Health Statistical Bulletin*, May 1997, p.4. Crown copyright is reproduced with the permission of the Controller of Her Majesty's Stationery Office.)

more likely to be employed at house officer level (21 per cent) than as consultants (11 per cent).

General practitioners (GPs)

Between 1986 and 1996, the number of GPs rose by 9 per cent from 26 529 to 28 937. In 1986, 22 per cent of GPs were female, whereas 10 years later they represented 32 per cent of the total. Furthermore, over 50 per cent of all GP trainees are now female (Fig. 6.5).

SOCIAL SERVICES DEPARTMENTS – AN UNCERTAIN FUTURE?

> privately some social services directors believe their departments will not exist in ten years time.
>
> (Rachel Downey, *Community Care*, 13–19 November 1997, p.10)

Over 20 per cent of all local authority expenditure goes on Social Services Departments, which employ a total of about 234 000 people. Since their creation in 1971, and until the Conservative Government's introduction of 'community care', they were the main providers of social care. This situation has now radically changed. Privatization, the introduction of the 'internal market', 'care management' and the 'contract culture' have transformed Social Services

Departments largely into *purchasers* of services – purchased from the 'independent sector'. The private sector has moved in to run an increasing number of nursing and residential care homes and domiciliary and day care services. Central government's insistence on Social Services Departments shedding their assets has led to many residential homes moving to become 'not-for-profit' trusts. At the same time, the expanded use of foster care has led to a marked decrease in residential care homes for children and young people.

Residential care for older people

> In 1995 in the UK, there were 440 000 residential care beds provided by the independent sector, compared to just 70 000 local authority beds.
>
> (*Community Care*, 20-26 February 1997, p.19)

Residential care for children and young people

> 'More children and young people are placed in foster care than in residential care – two out of three placements are now with foster carers. Residential care costs seven times as much as foster care.
>
> (*Community Care*, 27 November–3 December 1997, p.5)

Fieldwork

As well as residential work, fieldwork has also undergone a thorough transformation, mainly as a result of changes brought about by the National Health Service and Community Care Act 1990 and the Children Act 1989. The traditional role has become fragmented as new roles of 'community care assessment' and 'care management' have taken centre stage. Following the Seebohm recommendations of 1968, 'field social work' was seen to embody the pinnacle of 'professional practice', and field social workers enjoyed a high status. Since then it has been argued that the role has been deprofessionalized, and that it has been supplanted by a routine of needs assessment, drawing up of 'packages of care' and 'care management' responsibilities. In an editorial article in *The Lancet* entitled 'Care management: a disastrous mistake', the view was expressed that

'Highly valued therapeutic skills have been taken away from social workers and replaced by information-gathering best suited to bureaucrats untrammelled by specialist knowledge' (Anon., 1995).

New corporate structures

The actual day-to-day jobs that people do in social care and social work are changing, but so too are management and organizational structures. As we have mentioned, since the beginning of the 1980s the statutory sector has shrunk and local authorities have experienced cut-backs both in responsibilities and in resources. The resulting re-organization has taken a variety of forms. Sometimes social services has been drawn into the same directorate within the local authority as housing, e.g. the London Borough of Richmond (see Fig. 6.6), or it has been merged

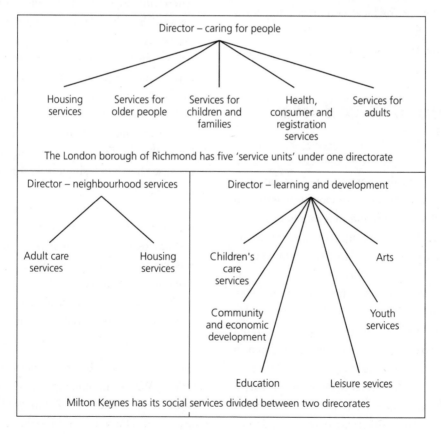

Fig. 6.6 New corporate structures (*Source: Community Care*, 27 November–3 December 1997, p.4).

with education, e.g. Kirklees. In other authorities Social Services Departments' responsibilities have been divided between separate directorates, e.g. Milton Keynes (see Fig. 6.6). In 1990, Kirklees became the first council to develop a 'joint council committee' in place of the traditional social services committee, with social services being linked to education.

New titles for these local authority corporate structures are being introduced, to replace the term 'Social Services Department'. The London Borough of Richmond has adopted the title 'Caring for People', while North Tyneside Council is using 'Care in the Community' which is separated into 'Children's Services' and 'Adult Services'. The next few years are bound to see an increase in such diversity.

There is some pessimism concerning the future of local authority social work. This is epitomized by Daloni Carlisle, who wrote: 'By 2001, social workers will no longer work for local authorities, but for a whole range of charities, trusts and private agencies' (*Community Care*, 15–21 August 1996, p.14).

HEALTH AND SOCIAL CARE – JOINT WORKING

More positively, health services and social care organizations are working more closely together in a range of different ways and in a number of geographical areas. Joint working was encouraged by the NHS and Community Care Act 1990, and by the Children Act 1989. Phrases such as 'multidisciplinary', 'multi-agency' and 'cross-functional' working have become commonplace and reflect this constructive innovation. 'Integration' and 'integrated working' are expected to develop and strengthen in the immediate future, following the completion of the joint review of the Social Services Inspectorate and the Audit Commission. It is clear that many health and social care workers wish to see the demolition of the so-called 'Berlin Wall' which they feel separates their respective disciplines.

Integration is not easy. It has resource implications, and there are often clashes between different agency structures and professional cultures. Professional rivalry and competition are also likely to occur. Nevertheless, some interesting innovations have taken place, and have been deemed to be successful. Two examples will be given here.

1. In Shipley, West Yorkshire, Social Services Department care managers were placed in four GP surgeries for 18 months. They remained under the supervision of their Social Services Department managers, but the public clearly perceived them as being part of the primary health care team. Structural problems arose because the care managers did not have equal power, in terms of commissioning and purchasing, to the GPs. However, there were still some positive aspects to the working relationship. These included the following: communication between health and social care workers improved; assessment of clients' needs became more holistic, as the GP or district nurse assessed health care needs at the same time as the care manager assessed social care needs; a climate of trust and co-operation developed as the two cultures underwent mutual change, the main beneficiaries being the service users, especially older people, because they had a single access point for health and social care.

2. A similar experiment was started in 1992 in Runcorn, Cheshire, in relation to patients of a GP practice who were over 65 years old. Again it was considered a success. Referrals and admissions to hospital were reduced, lengths of stay in hospital were shortened, and both of these improvements occurred without an increase in the workload of GPs or community nurses.

The Government has encouraged joint working practices. When announcing the setting up of 10 'Health Action Zones' (HAZs) in 1997, Health Secretary Frank Dobson said, 'the aim of these zones is to help health service organizations, local authorities, community groups, charities and local businesses to forge innovative new partnerships to improve health and modernise services' (*Community Care*, 23–29 October 1997, p.19).

Health and local authorities can bid to be designated as an HAZ, but in order to be successful they must prove that they have already been working co-operatively together. By the deadline in February 1998, 41 bids had been received by the Department of Health. The introduction of the zones was generally welcomed, but some fear that they may be large and overly bureaucratic.

TRAINING FOR WORK IN THE CARING SERVICES

It is time to stop talking about the value of training. How many more reports, how many complaints before we really take training seriously?

(Frank Dobson, Health Secretary, *Community Care*, 6–12 November 1997, p.2)

Two significant announcements which affected training for social work were made in 1996, at about the same time. First, the London School of Economics (LSE) stated that it was closing its social work courses. This was especially poignant because it was the LSE that had pioneered professional social work training (for probation officers) in the 1920s. In addition, other universities have made plans to offer alternative courses to the Diploma in Social Work (DipSW). This represents a departure from a universal social work qualification. The second announcement, made by the Open University (OU), was that from February 1998 its newly developed 'open learning' package leading to the Diploma in Social Work would receive its first intake of students. Barbara Kahan was one of the people who had developed the course and she spoke enthusiastically about it: 'It's giving everybody access to a DipSW – there is no need to go away to College for two years. Such flexibility means that people can tailor it to their individual requirements in terms of time and geography. That is very important' (*Community Care*, 30 October–5 November 1997, p.30).

Training for social care and social work has always been piecemeal. Of the 1 015 000 members of the UK social work and social care labour force, only a small percentage are professionally qualified. The state of training has been variously described as 'a mess' or 'in crisis'. Several different bodies awarded qualifications at different levels and stages (including pre-vocational, vocational, professional and post-qualifying). The national co-ordinating body, the Central Council for Education and Training in Social Work (CCETSW), met with mounting criticism both from within and outside social care and social work. Eventually it was considered to be weak and ineffective, and its demise was announced in December 1997. As we have stated earlier, it is to be subsumed within a General Social Care Council.

The 'crisis' in professional social work training has been multifaceted.

- Cutbacks in local authority expenditure have meant that many training sections have been reduced in size or closed down, and Social Services Departments have concentrated their resources on direct services.
- The reduction in training funds has resulted in a drastic fall in the number of staff seconded on to DipSW courses.
- In 1995, the Home Office announced that the probation service would withdraw from social work training.
- The DipSW has always been beset by a shortage of suitable practice placements.

It is hoped that the establishment of the General Social Care Council will bring new energy and impetus to training for the caring services. The suggestion of joint pre-qualifying training for health and social care staff has been welcomed, and the need to strengthen anti-discriminatory and anti-oppressive practice elements within all levels of training has also been acknowledged. Finally, there has been a call for the needs of those staff working with children, particularly in a residential setting, to be better catered for. Proposals for improved training in child development, handling difficult behaviour and children's specific health and educational needs will help to improve the status of this sector and to ease the problem of staff retention.

ENHANCED SERVICE-USER INVOLVEMENT

> I would like services that enable me to be independent and empower me to do what I want to do. For example, as a blind person I find it very difficult to go shopping on my own, so I need someone to help me, but to do that at the moment I have to pay somebody or ask a volunteer for help, and that can sometimes be difficult.
>
> (A disabled person from Coventry, speaking to the Citizens' Commission on the Future of the Welfare State, *Community Care*, 12–18 June 1997, p.19)

Service users' voices, their views about services and their ideas for improvement in service delivery are heard much more frequently and more clearly today than in the past. They are now rightly regarded as the experts. People with communication difficulties are being encouraged to comment on service delivery. Pictorial representations, such as those shown in Fig. 6.7, are increasingly being used in order to facilitate the expression of service users' views and their ideas for improvement.

The joint review of social services mentioned earlier has taken a service user or citizen perspective. The Project Director of the review, Andrew Webster, recently wrote: 'Quality is to be judged from the point of view of those who receive and pay for services, not from the views (however professional) of those who provide them' (*Community Care*, 27 November–3 December, 1997, p.6).

If 'empowerment' is to be more than just a word or a paper exercise, then not only must service users' views be heard, but they must also be involved in

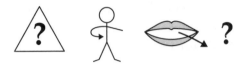

Q. How do I complain?

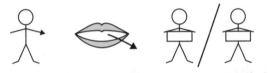

A. You can talk to the Community Access Co-ordinator *Arif* who will try to sort things out with you. If you don't feel things are any better or if you want to complain about the Community Access Co-ordinator, then you can speak to the Community Support Manager *Hannah*

Fig. 6.7 This illustration, part of a sequence of related drawings, may be used by a support worker working alongside a service user in order to convey the complaints procedure. Some service users will be able to glean the information themselves, using the combination of pictures and words. (*Source*: Owl Housing Ltd, *Link project complaints procedure*.)

planning and delivering services. 'Mission Statements' and 'Citizen Charters' are laudable, but alone they are not enough. Unless they are enacted and seen to have a practical reality, they may suffer the same fate as many 'equal opportunity' policies – that is, people will become disillusioned with them and cynicism will set in.

The Citizens' Commission on the Future of the Welfare State, quoted above, published its report *It's our Welfare* in 1997 (Beresford and Turner, 1997). It described its task as a large-scale 'listening exercise'. The report, which covered the whole of the country, relayed how users of welfare services felt about those services. Some of its main findings were as follows:

- that service users want to be as independent as possible, and do not want to be 'trapped in welfare';
- that they would rather be in paid work than in receipt of benefits;
- that they believed education and training was the best route out of welfare and into decent jobs;
- that there is a lack of reliable information about welfare benefits and services;

- that many perceived welfare state services as often being insensitive, unresponsive and unaccountable to them (the benefits system came out worst on this);
- that existing provision for complaints and redress in both benefits and services was inadequate;
- that being in receipt of welfare, particularly benefits, carries with it an increasing stigma today. Service users feel that both the public and the media have a part to play in the creation of stigma.

As we have already mentioned, listening on its own is not enough. However, there is a growing number of encouraging initiatives by the service providers themselves to involve users more fully.

- In places as far apart as Surrey, Wiltshire and Sheffield, local Social Services Departments are encouraging the involvement of user groups.
- Some Social Services Departments have actively encouraged children and young people to be involved in the recruitment and selection of staff for residential care homes. Some children and young people have taken part in interviewing panels.
- A user-led project called 'Shaping Our Lives' is currently in progress under the auspices of the National Institute for Social Work, and is funded for 2 years by the Department of Health. Part of the project's brief is to look at ways in which users can be practically involved in community care initiatives.

There is a growing number of examples of service-users' groups themselves acting on their own initiative. The range of activity is very wide. People with mental health problems have formed self-support groups which act independently of any service providers. A growing number of these represent black people with mental health problems. As we have seen, both disabled people and people with learning disabilities have developed self-advocacy and other support groups. Some service users have also been involved in 'direct action' protests.

Protester Brenda Green justified her participation in direct action in order to avoid her worst fear, 'that we will be back where we used to be when disabled people were stuck in their own homes or bussed to day centres, and were totally dependent on social services' (*Guardian*, 23 December 1997, p.4).

User involvement is recognized as being an essential component of quality assurance. After all, service users are in the best position to comment on existing services and to suggest improvements (Fig. 6.8).

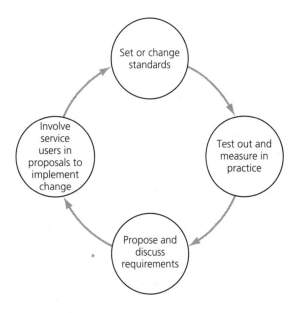

Fig. 6.8 Quality assurance cycle.

CARE IN A EUROPEAN CONTEXT

The social integration of all citizens goes to the heart of all existing welfare state policies. Areas that need to be looked at include the fight against poverty, youth opportunities, the elderly, equal treatment of third country nationals, disabled people, the fight against racism and xenophobia and the problems of rural populations.

(European Commission, 1993, p.3)

Europe may still seem remote to many people, including those of us who are involved in health, social care and social work. However, our social, political and economic links with the 14 other countries that, together with the UK, make up the European Union (EU) are becoming increasingly important. For instance, none of us could travel very far from our home before finding a project which had received funds from the EU.

The European Union contains 371 million people, of whom about 58 million live in the UK. The Union is managed by five bodies.

1. The democratically elected *European Parliament* contains 626 members (MEPs), of whom UK voters elect 87 members. It meets in Strasbourg, France, and it has an office in London. Elections take place every 5 years.
2. The *Council of Ministers* consists of national government Ministers from each of the 15 member states. This is the main decision-making body. The participating ministers vary according to the topic under discussion. The headquarters secretariat is based in Brussels, Belgium.
3. The *European Commission* (EC) is responsible for preparing and implementing European law. It consists of 20 Commissioners who are appointed by national governments for 5 years. The UK has two commissioners. The EC is based in Brussels, and has offices in England, Scotland, Wales and Northern Ireland.
4. The *European Court of Justice* (ECJ) consists of 13 judges assisted by six Advocates-General. It rules on the interpretation and application of EC law. It has no power to overturn the decisions of UK courts. It assists our courts in applying EC law by answering questions from UK judges. It sits in Luxembourg.
5. The *Court of Auditors* monitors the budget and financial activities. It is located in Luxembourg.

The original impetus for the formation of the EU came after the Second World War. It was intended to prevent such a tragedy from ever happening again, and also to improve the member states' economies

by working together. The first countries came together in 1951 when six of them (France, Germany, Italy, Belgium, The Netherlands and Luxembourg) signed an economic agreement for the production of coal and steel. In 1957 a treaty creating the European Economic Community (EEC), also known simply as the European Community (EC), was signed in Rome. It is now referred to as the European Union (EU). More countries joined later, including the UK in 1973, and 13 others have recently applied to become members. The official symbol of the EU is the blue flag with a circle of 12 yellow stars (Fig. 6.9). The number of stars will always remain the same even when new countries join the Union.

On 7 February 1992 at Maastricht in The Netherlands, the Treaty on European Union was signed. This agreed on a number of important issues:

• It established *citizenship* of the EU. Every person who holds the nationality of a member state is a citizen of the Union, which enables them to vote and to stand as a candidate in European elections.
• It decided that a 'single currency' would be introduced by the beginning of 1999.
• Most relevant to those of us who work in health and social care will be the *Social Chapter* contained in the Maastricht Treaty. This was annexed to the Treaty, and the UK government of the time refused to sign it. However, the present government has pledged to do so. Its full title is the *Agreement on Social Policy*. It contains the principles set out originally in the *Community Charter*

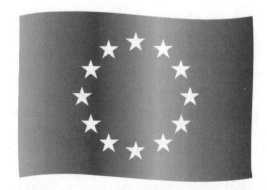

Fig. 6.9 The flag of the European Union.

of *Fundamental Social Rights of Workers*, which had been drawn up and adopted in Strasbourg, France, in December 1989.

The Social Chapter's 12 principles include:

- the right to vocational training;
- the right of women and men to equal treatment;
- the right to health protection and safety at work;
- a decent standard of living for older people;
- improved social and professional integration for disabled people.

As members of the European Union, health and social carers and social workers have the same freedom of movement as any other worker. There are a number of reciprocal 'exchange' or 'secondment' arrangements whereby workers in this country can spend time abroad in the caring services, and foreign nationals can gain experience in the UK.

A few years ago attempts were made to bring this country's professional social work training courses into line with those in many other European countries, by extending the length of courses from 2 to 3 years. The government refused to make this change. It is to be hoped that a newly created 'General Social Care Council' will attempt to have this proposal accepted. Another small indication of our close links with the EU was announced in January 1998, when it was reported that the University of Portsmouth and Sheffield Hallam University had obtained funding in order to develop the first MA degree in European social work. Colleges in Denmark, Finland, Norway, Sweden and The Netherlands are to follow suit.

CONCLUSION

Some (government) Ministers believe social work and probation have failed. In fact, both have been starved of resources.

(Harry Fletcher, Assistant General Secretary of The National Association of Probation Officers, *Observer*, 14 September 1997, p.4)

In November 1997, 'Group 4' – a private security company that had been running prisons in this country – announced that it wanted to appoint three social workers, who would wear the company's corporate uniforms, to work in its new private prison, Altcourse, in Liverpool. An advertisement in the *Liverpool Echo* stated that Group 4 were looking for 'experienced social work professionals to work in a uniformed capacity, assisting custody staff' (*Liverpool Echo*, 20 November 1997, p.6). Many people expressed anger and disbelief at the development, finding the idea of social workers/probation officers in uniform to be anathema. The assistant general secretary of the National Association of Probation Officers (NAPO) thought that it was a 'bizarre development'. He asked, 'Who are these social workers to be accountable to, their prisoner clients, the public or to shareholders with a vested interest in high rates of incarceration?' (*Observer*, 23 November 1997, p.6).

This incident illustrates the fact that social work is constantly changing, and that its work-force is always faced with new challenges. This has been true at all times since the publication of the Seebohm Report 30 years ago. In 1980, Colin Brewer and June Lait published a book called *Can Social Work Survive?* (Brewer and Lait, 1980) At the time, neither of them was working as a social worker – Brewer was a consultant psychiatrist and Lait was a university lecturer. They wrote 'social work … in general and casework in particular are usually without any specific effect and frequently without any measurable effect at all' (Brewer and Lait, 1980, p.165). They went on to warn, 'Without major and painful changes social work may well have to struggle not merely for funds but for its very survival' (Brewer and Lait, 1980, p.188).

Social work as an activity may be secure, but we are once again in a time of great uncertainty for the statutory agencies that employ social workers and probation officers. Social Services Departments and Probation Services are still experiencing financial cuts, and these are expected to continue. There are even fears for the survival of social services and the probation service as independent entities. Both are currently under review, and the present government has at least considered the possibility of creating new community care authorities to replace Social Services Departments and merging the probation service with the prison service.

Alongside fears for the future there have been a number of positive developments and reasons for optimism. Some of these have already been mentioned:

- the creation of a General Social Care Council (GSCC). This should strengthen the central leadership of social care, raise its profile and improve the public perception of caring. It should also create improved training opportunities in the caring services;
- improved multidisciplinary and co-operative working practices between health and social care. The White Paper on the NHS entitled *The New NHS: Modern, Dependable*, published in December 1997 (Department of Health, 1997b), further encourages joint working;
- the continued development of the service-user movement. Agencies that provide care are also increasingly committed to listening to users and involving them more fully in practical ways;
- the Labour Government is committed to bringing about 'one nation' – an *inclusive* society. To this

end the Government set up the Social Exclusion Unit.

By 1997 it was clear that polarization had become extreme. In 1979, some 1.2 million households in the UK had no adult member in paid work. In 1995 this figure had risen to 3 million households, so that one in five households in the UK had no wage earner. At the same time, the salaries of top professionals had never been higher – a Judge received £76 000 a year, an accountant £190 000 per annum, a barrister received £350 000 and a City financier anything from £400 000 to more than £1 million a year.

The present government will require the assistance of social workers and probation officers in attempting to bring *social exclusion* to an end. It is encouraging, therefore, that both disciplines are represented among the 12 members of the Social Exclusion Unit. However, more resources are urgently needed. Ultimately, budgets affect the quality of care provided. Financial rewards and conditions of service also determine the morale of those providing it.

At a time of considerable upheaval and change in the caring services, those who make up the workforce need to be careful that they do not become despondent. There are plenty of discouraging developments, but there are also many refreshing and challenging innovations.

EXERCISES

1. Joint working – health and social care

Outline the advantages to individuals and organizations brought about by working collaboratively. What barriers exist that prevent agencies from working together, and how can they be overcome?

2. Inspecting for good practice

An inspector from the local authority Social Services Department is planning an 'announced' inspection of a care home for older people. The inspector will need to ensure that certain regulations are met, but how will he or she be able to establish that a high quality of care is being provided? What are the indicators that an inspector might view as significant:

(a) through *observation*?

(b) through *talking to management and staff*?

(c) through *talking with residents*?

3. Maintaining health, safety and security

Below are nine Performance Criteria taken from Unit U4 of NVQ level 3. You have put yourself forward for assessment on these nine criteria. Provide written explanations of what you would do for each.

(a) What would be the appropriate form of dress, approach and hygiene to comply with good health and safety practice?

(b) How would you explain to a client, for example, the need to wear rubber gloves or other protective clothing?

(c) What should you do immediately before and after contact with others, equipment or instruments – and why?

(d) If a person has open cuts or fresh abrasions, what action should be taken?

(e) What are notifiable diseases and to whom should they be reported?

(f) If you are lifting, how should this be done?

(g) When you are not immediately accessible, e.g. while taking a client shopping, what information should be passed on and to whom?

(h) How would you minimize the risk of personal danger?

(i) To whom would you report an accident and how would it be recorded?

4. Equal opportunities policies

You work in a care organization. What systems would you establish to ensure that equal opportunities policies are met with regard to the following criteria?

(a) culture.

(b) gender.

(c) race.

(d) social class.

(e) disability.

(f) sexual orientation.

(g) age.

(h) marital status.

5. Anti-oppressive practice

The purpose of this exercise is to reveal the extremes of bad practice in order to emphasize the value of anti-oppressive practice. In small groups, design a 'racist', 'sexist' or 'disablist' residential care home that would discriminate against older people either directly or indirectly. Consider all aspects of residential care provision, including staffing, selection procedures, decor, materials, food, rules and regulations.

QUESTIONS FOR ESSAYS OR DISCUSSION

1. With regard to the Welfare State, the question is not 'can we afford it?' but rather 'do we want it?'.

2. Beveridge's 'Five Giants' are as prominent today as they were in 1942.

3. The private sector can provide better and more efficient health and social care services than the statutory or voluntary sectors ever could.

4. Why shouldn't social workers and probation officers wear a uniform?

5. Local Authority Social Services Departments and Health Authorities should merge, and the sooner this happens the more efficient the service offered will become.

6. Less money should be invested in maintaining large-scale service organizations, and more should be provided to communities, so that local people can decide upon and create the services that they require.

FURTHER READING

Academic Sources

Ackers, L. and Abbott, P. 1996: *Social policy for nurses and the caring professions*. Buckingham: Open University Press. A social policy text specifically geared to those working in health and social care. It covers the development of welfare and different ideological approaches and examines current provision.

Adams, R. 1996: *The personal social services*. Harlow: Longman, A comprehensive review of the history and organization of the personal social services, as well as much detail about the services that they offer.

Allott, M. and Robb, M. 1998: *Understanding health and social care – an introductory reader*. London: Sage. Covering both health and social care, this collection of readings discusses the political context of caring, as well as the various settings in which care takes place.

Hantrais, L. 1995: *Social policy in the European Union*. London: Macmillan. This book examines the development of social policy in Europe, including those measures taken to eradicate social exclusion. It also discusses the relationship between European and national policy-making.

Holman, B. 1993: *A new deal for social welfare*. Oxford: Lion Publishing. A critique of right-wing approaches to the welfare state and 'contract culture'. It suggests new alternatives to bring about a less unequal society.

Timmins, N. 1996: *The Five Giants – A biography of the Welfare State*. London: Fontana. A very detailed history of the Welfare State, with an analysis of progress to date on eradicating Beveridge's 'Five Giants'.

Other literary sources

Armitage, S. 1989: *Zoom*. Newcastle upon Tyne: Bloodaxe Books.

Dickens, M. 1980: *The listeners*. Harmondsworth: Penguin.

England, H. 1986: *Social work as art: making sense for good practice*. London: George Allen & Unwin.

Konrad, G. 1975: *The case worker*. London: Hutchinson.

Laken, B. 1984: *More than a friend*. Oxford: Lion Publishing.

Sayer, P. 1993: *The absolution game*. London: Sceptre.

7

Towards positive practice

> Perhaps by the Millennium the rhetoric of anti-discriminatory practice empowerment and partnership can become a reality.
>
> (Phyllida Parsloe, *Community Care*,
> 4–10 April 1996, p.24)

In order to develop positive practice it is necessary for carers to identify with, and more fully understand, the needs of those people for whom they care. There is a requirement for carers to have a good working knowledge of the effects of discrimination, oppression and social exclusion. Throughout this book we have seen how various groups of people are structurally disadvantaged within society, and how prejudicial attitudes and discriminatory practices combine to impoverish their lives, so that they do not participate as fully in society as they otherwise might. An acknowledgment of the structural disadvantage experienced by the majority of service users helps the carer, social worker or health worker to resist the temptation to blame the person or people for whom they care. Seeing the service user in his or her social setting rather than in isolation is one step towards obtaining a more rounded perspective. In pursuing positive practice we should be aiming to reduce the gap which often exists between social carers and their clients.

We have seen from our examination of social class and the 'underclass' that many members of our society are deprived of full citizenship and suffer a range of deprivations. The same is true for many women, black people and members of other minority groups such as gay men, refugees and homeless people. We must attack the oppression which prevents all of these groups from participating fully in our society, and we must aim for *full citizenship* for all.

QUALITIES OF A CARER

In order to achieve full citizenship for all we need, as far as possible, to aim to see the world through the eyes of those for whom we care – as the saying goes, 'To walk a mile in another person's moccasins'. As Harper Lee writes in *To Kill a Mockingbird*, 'You never really understand a person until you consider things from his point of view – until you climb into his skin and walk around in it' (Lee, 1960, p.35).

We need, therefore, to develop an empathy for others regardless of any differences in social class, gender, racial origin, culture, sexual orientation, age or life-style. We should note that we are not capable of absolute empathy because our experience will never fully correspond to that of another person. However, we should always aspire to be as sensitive to others as possible.

A number of essential qualities are needed in an effective carer in addition to empathy. These include personal qualities such as sensitivity, assertiveness, honesty, love and compassion, and a predilection to

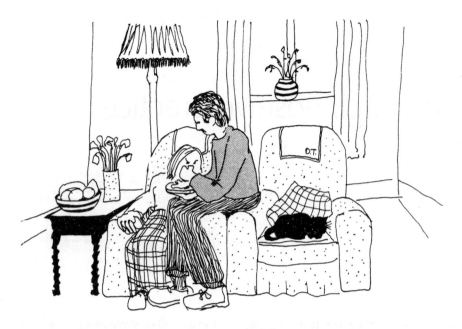

Knowledge and communication are an integral part of practical social care.

demonstrate the basic courtesies of politeness and respect. Also needed are communication and interpersonal skills, including the ability to listen, and the ability to like people and show warmth, friendliness and cheerfulness.

In addition, it is important that carers can demonstrate practical abilities in order to instil confidence in those for whom they care, such as the ability to lift and assist with mobility and to apply basic nursing skills, including emergency first aid. Certain attitudes are also essential, such as patience, tolerance and acceptance. Of course knowledge must precede all good practice. This might be academic knowledge, an awareness of the role and function of caring and other organizations, an insight into the needs of minority ethnic cultures, an ability to draw on personal life-experience and a commitment to increasing self-knowledge, or a developed political awareness.

(*Note:* These qualities are more fully explained in Chapter 8 of *Inside the Caring Services* (Tossell and Webb, 1994.)

CHANGE AND THE AGENCIES IN WHICH WE WORK

Some of us who are engaged in social care, health care and social work will be working in large, often bureaucratic organizations. It is very tempting to feel overwhelmed and 'swamped' as an individual in such a large set-up. Frequently this feeling is accompanied by pessimism about our agency's ability to change or develop in a positive way. Large bureaucracies can seem to have a life of their own, and one which is resistant to change. We need to acknowledge that many caring organizations, in common with other institutions and establishments, have a vested interest in maintaining the *status quo*. Senior and middle management is still, in the main, dominated by white, middle-class, middle-aged males.

BURNOUT

It is possible to be overwhelmed by the nature and volume of responsibility that is sometimes placed

Table 7.1 The jobs that take the strain; the jobs listed have been identified by Professor Cary Cooper, of the University of Manchester Institute of Science and Technology, as carrying a risk of 'high stress'

- Medicine – both doctors and nurses
- Teaching – especially in the primary sector
- Jobs in the construction industry
- Middle managers, whose numbers have been severely depleted as part of the 'downsizing' process during the recession
- Police
- Ambulance staff
- Social workers
- Journalists
- Staff in newly privatized organizations and public servants in some areas

Source: Independent, 17 November 1994.

upon an individual within a care organization, be they at basic grade or managerial grade. This is manifested in high staff turnover rates and the high levels of stress-related illness found in health and care occupations. A number of workers have succumbed to the pressure of daily workloads.

In 1994, Northumberland County Council were held liable for a social worker's nervous breakdown. Mr Walker, a senior social worker, maintained that the breakdown he suffered was caused by a huge increase in child abuse cases, and he was awarded substantial damages.

SELF-AWARENESS AND SELF-DEVELOPMENT

It is important not to become despondent about the inherent resistance of bureaucracies, because this can only be disabling. Instead, we need to be more positive and remember that we *can* control what we do – and own our behaviour and practice. Doing this in small, immeasurable ways contributes to change around us and eventually to change in wider society,

although we will not always be conscious of this process.

The most important resource that we bring to health and social care is ourselves. This is not a static entity, but a resource which is undergoing constant change and development. In order to retain a high standard of personal practice, we need to examine our attitudes, behaviour and approach continually, and to develop our own personal strategies for effective care.

TAKING RISKS AND BEING ASSERTIVE

In addition to monitoring our own personal practice, we also have a responsibility to challenge the practice of others as well as the policies of the employing organization when we feel that these are having a detrimental effect on the lives of service users. However, this will often involve taking risks, because our challenges may offend those we work with and may, in the extreme, actually damage working relationships or even career advancement. We need to overcome this fear and confront bad practice in an assertive manner. Compromise and, worse still, collusion with poor standards of practice are never acceptable.

For example, a carer may be tempted to tolerate racist comments made by a white resident of a care or nursing home towards a black member of staff or a fellow resident. The carer may compromise by only making a tentative objection, or he or she may collude, by ignoring its occurrence, in order not to offend the white resident. Neither option is satisfactory. It is all too easy to patronize and make excuses for someone's age or cultural background. Our behaviour and that of others should be consistent at all times and in all settings.

LANGUAGE AND ANTI-DISCRIMINATORY AND ANTI-OPPRESSIVE PRACTICE

As we have said, our health and social care practice should be aimed at counteracting the exclusion of any individual in our society, whether on grounds of class, gender, race or culture, age, disability, sexual orientation or life-style. In this regard, we should be continually vigilant in examining ourselves and our language and attitudes. In order to aid this process we can read, think, observe and discuss relevant issues with family, friends, colleagues and clients. One of the most important factors to check is our own *language*, because how we speak or write is usually how we think, and it reflects our attitudes and beliefs. The words we use will convey to others how we see them. Certain words and phrases will carry negative and possibly harmful connotations, while others will communicate dignity and respect.

Language is constantly evolving – more rapidly now, due to the increased awareness of its importance. Service users have contributed to this process not least by stating how they wish to be referred to.

Early this century, people who today would be described as having mental health problems were still being variously labelled as 'lunatics' and 'imbeciles'. Similarly, people with learning disabilities were formerly described as 'defective' or 'retarded', and were universally referred to as being 'mentally handicapped' until relatively recently. In 1989, the Campaign for Mental Handicap (CMH) changed its name to Values Into Action (VIA) because its members considered that they could not 'continue much longer with a name which includes a term – "mental handicap" – which is confusing and offensive' (*CMH Newsletter 56*, Spring 1989, p.1).

Within schools, the category 'educationally subnormal' (ESN), officially in use until well into the 1980s, was both stigmatizing and degrading to young people and their families. The term 'special needs' was introduced as a more respectful way of highlighting a young person's learning difficulty and the need for specialist educational provision.

In fairness, many of the outmoded words and terms that were originally used to categorize people were neutral descriptions of a condition. Some of them have only acquired a negative connotation over time. For instance, the word 'spastic' relates to the clinical condition of spasticity that affects an individual's control and movement. In 1994, the Spastics Society also changed its name to 'SCOPE', with the intention of projecting a modern, positive image.

However, client groups today are still commonly lumped together by the media and individuals solely in terms of their 'limitations' when they are referred to as *the* homeless, *the* elderly or *the* unemployed.

The growing interest in consumerism and empowerment during the 1990s, and the established rights of service users to have access to certain records, have meant that health and social careworkers have had to develop and use a more sensitive and respectful language.

Proposed changes to accepted language may meet with resistance. For instance, the charge of 'political correctness' (or 'PC', as it is also known) is often levied by detractors at any attempts to challenge existing, taken-for-granted, oppressive language. The statement 'You are only being PC' is used to 'put down' innovation. The phrase 'being politically correct' developed a bad name, mainly due to its media-led association with ludicrous or petty superficial changes. Today it is still used to denigrate change – yet to be opposite, to be politically incorrect, would be to damage people and continue to act with discrimination towards them, and this is unacceptable.

CHALLENGING RACISM

There has been an increasing recognition of the central need for anti-racist practice. Social care organizations have provided their own Codes of Practice. The Social Care Association produced a short *Action Checklist* (Social Care Association, 1990) for practitioners and managers in order to promote good practice. According to this booklet, anti-racist practice:

- is the responsibility of all practitioners;
- challenges racism in all practice settings;
- takes steps to remedy the shortcomings of provision for black people;
- is active in seeking out racism;
- consciously highlights the multiracial nature of our society.

The Social Care Association's 'strategy' for putting this check-list into operation is also extremely useful.

- *Think* about your racism together with that of your colleagues.
- *Accept* that the problems exist.
- *Plan* for action.
- *Challenge* racism, including the racism inside yourself.
- *Review* progress and decide on further action.

The check-list also provides more details and encourages us to aim for personal goals, which may include the ability:

> to actively seek awareness and understanding of your own racism and that of others; to examine how your attitudes and behaviour contribute to racism . . . to seek to avoid cultural and racial stereotyping; to openly disagree with any racist joke or action; and to promote a positive image of black people within social care settings.
>
> (Social Care Association, 1990)

An important part of our anti-racist strategy is to support our colleagues who work for changes in practice. We must oppose policies which collude with the oppression of black people. It is important to be clear that anti-racism is not about preferential treatment – it is aimed at redressing inequality and establishing social justice. It is there-

fore something in which we must all be involved. Frequently a single black person can be made a scapegoat, or labelled as 'difficult' or a 'trouble-maker', by colleagues who simply disagree with him or her. We should also avoid a situation in which we contribute to one black person in a team being pressurized into being the so-called 'expert' on race issues or racism. Instead we need to ask questions directly of policy-makers, administrators and managers.

We need to update our practice continually in order to remain in touch with social change. One way in which we can do this is to participate in anti-racist training and encourage others to take part as well, in order to share what we have learned and to try to apply it to the work setting. It is important to discuss the issues involved in an open and honest way.

Other ways in which we could be anti-racist would be, for example, to introduce positive images and experiences of black people, to share their history and life-stories, to celebrate their customs and festivals, to have their food prepared in traditional ways, and to enjoy culturally appropriate music, dance, games and pastimes. Decisions relating to any or all of these may depend upon management policies. However, we each have a responsibility to press for their introduction.

If we work with many people from different cultures (for example, Greek, Chinese, Punjabi or Polish), and a large number of the members of that community do not speak English, we may need to learn the language in order to improve communication. The least we can do is to learn the most common 100–200 words and some regularly used phrases, and thus help to break down barriers.

NON-SEXIST PRACTICE

Men must examine the sexism within themselves and not tolerate it or collude with it in other men, regardless of age. Often sexism will be subtle or

...ous – as when, for example, when a man ...over' women in a team meeting. It may not be ... y for a man even to realize that he is doing this. However, men need to monitor their behaviour in this respect, perhaps by talking to others. It should be pointed out that it is not only women who are 'talked over' – the same thing happens to some men. Not everyone is comfortable expressing themselves in public, and we need to recognize that all of us have a valid contribution to make, whatever our style. What we can do to facilitate this is to make space and provide encouragement for others, so that every individual has a full opportunity to be heard.

All clients, but particularly women, should have the right to choose a carer of their own gender. This is important in situations where physical care is being provided and intimate matters are under discussion, for example in counselling. Similarly, all women should have the opportunity to choose to be supervised by another woman, whether they are paid social carers, volunteers, or students on training courses or placements. They may find this arrangement less threatening and more conducive to learning and self-disclosure.

NON-DISABLIST PRACTICE

Disabled people are commonly patronized, pitied or ignored. All of these unhelpful responses contribute to the exclusion of disabled people or people with learning difficulties. Treating disabled people in this way prevents them from living as fully integrated and fulfilled individuals. The very word 'disability' is in itself disparaging. This point was confirmed by the Wagner Report, which stated, 'The commonly applied label "disabled" emphasizes disability at the expense of ability and, without discussion, assumes dependency. Which one of us would wish to be characterized by what we are unable to do?' (National Institute for Social Work, 1988a, p.103).

Not only do disabled people have to come to terms with their particular physical or mental impairment, but they also have to cope with society's disablist attitudes when they want to be seen as ordinary people with ordinary human emotions who are capable of making a valuable contribution to society. The way in which they are dealt with and depicted affects their self-image and self-belief. As Ann MacFarlane says, 'It can be difficult, almost impossible, to have a good self-image and confidence if you are being "cared for" as a disabled person in a way which leads you to perceive yourself as a "burden" or "helpless"' (*Arthritis News,* February 1990).

EQUAL OPPORTUNITIES

Many people feel that their employers' equal opportunities policies are merely statements of good intent but are not translated into effective practice, and there is some evidence that this is indeed the case: 'There are institutions where dozens get printed, left on shelves and ignored' (*Community Care,* 6–12 June 1996, p.21).

One way of ensuring their relevance and application is for all of us to familiarize ourselves with what has been laid down by our employer. In order to keep the issues alive, we need to share our understanding of equal opportunities with other people and continually monitor its application, and in order to reflect our changing society it should be kept under review. A standardized equal opportunities statement is likely to be taken for granted or ignored, and will run the risk of being merely 'tokenistic'.

For many years now organizations and professional bodies have declared their commitment to equal opportunities. For instance, they are incorporated in the British Association of Social Workers *12 Principles of Social Work Practice* outlined in Table 7.2.

EMPOWERMENT

Empowerment may be viewed as a particular form and style of positive action. In 1992, the Bishops'

Table 7.2 The 12 principles of social work practice

- Knowledge, skills and experience used positively for the benefit of all sections of the community and individuals
- Respect for clients as individuals, and safeguarding their dignity and rights
- No prejudice in self, nor tolerance of prejudice in others, on the grounds of origin, race, status, sex, sexual orientation, age, disability, beliefs or contribution to society
- Empowerment of clients and their participation in decisions and defining services
- Sustained concern for clients, even when unable to help them or where self-protection is necessary
- Professional responsibility takes precedence over personal interest
- Responsibility for standards of service and for continuing education and training
- Collaboration with others in the interests of clients
- Clarity in public as to whether acting in a personal or organizational capacity
- Promotion of appropriate ethnic and cultural diversity of services
- Confidentiality of information and divulgence only by consent or, exceptionally, in evidence of serious danger
- Pursuit of conditions of employment which enables these obligations to be respected

Source: British Association of Social Workers.

Committee for Community Relations published a pamphlet entitled *From Charity to Empowerment: The Church's Mission Alongside Poor and Marginalized People.* This pamphlet explored different approaches to empowerment:

> Some approaches stress being with and listening to the poor and marginalized. Some stress the creation of a space where people can meet, exchange views, acquire skills, experiment and become involved. Other approaches focus on the need for an organization controlled by people themselves which they can use as a base of power to address society. Some centre around funding. None the less, all these approaches have in common an emphasis on standing with people in their struggle rather than doing things for them
>
> (Bishop's Committee for Community relations, 1992)

The principle of *empowerment* in social care has been around for some time in different guises, although the word itself has only relatively recently come into common parlance. Even now the word is open to a range of varying interpretations, but it fundamentally concerns issues of authority, power and control, and how these affect service users' lives.

It is more useful to consider empowerment as a continuum, rather than in absolute terms. It would be extremely difficult to find situations of either complete empowerment or its total absence – most practice will lie somewhere in between.

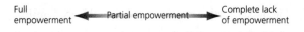

Full empowerment ← Partial empowerment → Complete lack of empowerment

Fig. 7.1

Some people object to the concept of empowerment because they do not believe that permanent power can ever be *given* to another person or group. If it were possible to give it, it could just as easily be possible for it to be taken away. Furthermore, they feel that power can only truly be seized. Others would see this as representing a rather extreme philosophical objection that denies the power inherent in the caring role. Such people feel that any intervention which is aimed at enabling clients, by definition automatically makes a contribution to their empowerment. For example, the creation of a safe environment in which a client is able to express him- or herself freely, or the creation of structures in which clients make more decisions for themselves, is part of the process.

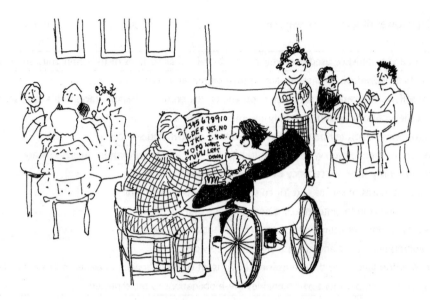

The use of an alphabet board enables a person with cerebral palsy to express exactly how he likes his food. By pointing to individual letters with his tongue, he indicates to his friend or carer his precise requirements. This is an example of empowerment.

ADVOCACY AND SELF-ADVOCACY

The idea of advocacy is an old one. We are familiar with someone acting on behalf of another who may not be able to speak for him- or herself. They speak for that person and in so doing represent his or her best interests. A daily example can be found in the criminal courts, where solicitors or barristers act as advocates for those they represent.

McKenzie person

Less formally, the support of a friend in the role of a 'Mckenzie person' is relied upon by people at a tribunal hearing. They obtain moral support from their McKenzie person who may, if required, speak on the person's behalf. Alternatively, the person her- or himself may deal with the questioning, having gained the necessary strength and support from their friend.

More recently, the term has been introduced into social care and social work to describe such occa-sions when, for example, a social worker represents the interests of his or her client at a tribunal, a community psychiatric nurse attends his or her client's job interview, or when a probation officer supports his or her client at the housing department in an attempt to secure accommodation.

However, advocacy can be seen to be patronizing because the social carer or social worker, who is in a position of authority, mediates or negotiates on behalf of the client, who is relatively powerless. Of course it is very often this power differential that makes advocacy essential – it defends the weak against the strong. Malcolm Payne describes the essential nature of advocacy as 'arguing for change where power has created an existing decision or pre-disposition against the client' (Payne, 1986, p.118).

Self-advocacy

The negative implications of the patronizing nature of advocacy have led to the development of self-advocacy and a growing number of self-advocacy projects. It is seen that a social carer may actually 'disable' a client by acting 'for' them, and may prevent them from acting assertively. Instead, self-advocacy aims to enable clients to act on their own in their own and best interests – to speak for themselves. It is therefore central to the concept of empowerment, as it is about making decisions and choices for oneself and being assertive.

Frequently a self-advocacy project will develop from a collective or group activity in which common problems are shared – for example, with a social welfare agency or housing department. Different ways of tackling the problem may be explored and, at a later stage, rehearsals, simulations or role-plays may take the participants further. All are designed to lead to a point where the client feels reasonably safe and sufficiently confident to make contact or intervene on their own behalf. This does not, of course, rule out the possibility of the group remaining in existence as a background support.

POSITIVE PRACTICE TODAY

Positive practice in social care should involve affirming some or all of the following, both as policy and as practical action.

Rights

This involves insisting that clients' *citizen, legal* and *welfare rights* are upheld and respected at all times. This is clearly a very important part of full social citizenship. It also requires all carers to gain as much reliable, up-to-date information as possible about any rights which may improve the quality of life of those for whom they care.

User or citizen involvement

This is another term, currently very much in vogue, which needs to be translated into practice in order to avoid becoming mere rhetoric. Clients can be involved at all stages – in planning service, deciding how they are to be delivered most effectively, and in running their own services as much as possible and budgeting for those services. Except in exceptional circumstances, all clients should be present and involved in their own reviews, care programme meetings or 'case conferences'.

Legislation such as the Children Act 1989, and the National Health Service and Community Care Act 1990, has enshrined the principle of user involvement wherever this is possible. Service users are now consulted, or more actively involved, at every stage of the assessment and care-planning process. In some instances, service users may hold their own care budget and purchase their own care.

For many years Peter Beresford and Suzy Croft have been studying user involvement in services which, in their own words, are 'more democratic and appropriate'. However, as they point out, there are pitfalls – for example, when social care agencies merely want user involvement to help deliver a cheaper, more cost-effective service. However, if it is done well, the clients involved can gain more confidence and learn new skills and abilities. At best, they say, 'where empowerment is the aim, people decide the agenda for themselves.... This model comes closest to realizing the idea of self-advocacy in social services' *(Community Care Supplement,* 27 April 1989).

Access to records

Health and social care agencies hold a great deal of information about clients, much of which is of an extremely personal nature. Since the Data Protection Act 1984, the Access to Personal Files Act 1987 and the Access to Medical Records Act 1988, patients and service users have had access to certain records about themselves. This has meant that practitioners have needed to be more mindful of what they have recorded about service users. Records need to be factual and opinion has to be identified and substantiated.

Information technology, which was barely visible in social services 10 years ago, has been introduced and harnessed with varying degrees of success by different health and social care agencies. Now all local authorities have large network systems for record-keeping. However, according to Professor Jan Pahl, 'Social services are still behind the times,' because 'few social services departments use 'E-mail' and the Internet, unlike the health service' (*Community Care*, 19–24 June 1997, p.21). He adds that this is partly due to the resistance of some workers to technology because 'Social work is a very face-to-face culture' (*Community Care*, 19–24 June 1997, p.21).

Computers can benefit Social Services Departments in four main ways, namely for record-keeping, service planning, communication and information research. Individuals will have to acknowledge the usefulness and increasing presence of information technology in all care settings. Carers now need to develop and maintain computer skills in order to be able to utilize technology to the ultimate benefit of service users.

There are instances where residents of care homes are communicating with the outside world through the Internet, and software programs have been designed in order to facilitate communication with people with learning disabilities. Information technology is here to stay, and skill development and familiarization are becoming a vital aspect of care.

Complaints and redress

Following the NHS and Community Care Act 1990, all local authorities have been obliged to produce clear complaints procedures. Other health and social care organizations have also published their own complaint procedures. In addition, a number of charters exist, including the Patients' Charter, the Mental Services Patients' Charter and the Local Authority Community Care Charters.

Local Authorities and Health Authorities are also required to produce combined annual community care plans. These joint community care plans out-

Table 7.3 A typical local area Community Care Charter setting out the key principles and standards to which authorities are committed

The core commitments state that the Social Services Department will:
- respond to users' and carers' needs;
- ensure that services are accessible;
- communicate clearly;
- respect confidentiality;
- involve carers and users;
- be competent;
- be polite and courteous;
- comply with health and safety standards;
- set standards for all services and monitor them;
- take comments and complaints seriously.

line services and describe the rights of patients and service users. In many ways patients and service users may now be more aware of their rights, and we should welcome this situation. We should encourage and honour their complaints because they may lead towards an improvement in the service.

Get to know your community

In following the aim of seeing service users in their social setting and not in isolation, we need to acquaint ourselves with their immediate physical environment and local neighbourhood. Getting to know the patch where you work, whatever its setting – residential, day care, domiciliary or field – will involve a knowledge of all the resources in the community including shops, clubs, pubs, groups and any specialist facility, e.g. for disabled people or for a particular ethnic minority group.

A good up-to-date knowledge of the community in which we work can be especially helpful for breaking down barriers in a residential setting which may seem rather cut off from the neighbourhood life around it. We always need to be aware that residential provision is an integral part of community care.

Find support

Whether we are paid social carers, carers for a friend or relative at home, or volunteers, most of us need and benefit from the support of others. Where a form of support – possibly a group – already exists we should think of joining it to make our own unique contribution. If no form of support exists, we should think about starting one because there are usually others who feel isolated and who will benefit from contact.

The value of a support group for carers or volunteers is that it gives them the opportunity to express themselves, to share their problems and to learn from other carers. For some, the group can be a great source of confidence and support. In particular, Nick Fielding outlined the special value of an all black carers' group, one of several black, Asian or Chinese carers' groups that have been set up throughout the country.

> The group gives an opportunity for its members to discuss their problems and to share them – realizing that someone else has to deal with similar issues can often be uplifting. It also allows the members to socialize, share recipes and discuss issues relating to the black community or home background which they might feel constrained to mention in a predominantly white group.
>
> Sometimes it's just important to talk in our own 'Patois'.
>
> (*Community Care*, 11 January 1990, p.15)

CONCLUSION – THE PERSONAL AND THE POLITICAL

Political and social policy issues, such as poverty, poor housing, or a lack of child-care provision or community facilities, cannot be separated from personal circumstances – each affects the other. As a reflection of this, individual positive practice in social care often needs to be accompanied by action for political change for a more humane, kinder, less unequal and less unjust society. There are a number of ways in which we, as social carers, can combine the personal and the political in a meaningful, life-enhancing way.

If we join with either staff or clients to press for a new facility – for example, play space or the installation of a crèche, or the provision of a regular meeting room in our local area – this *collective experience* can energize us, galvanize others into action and give us a valuable experience of shared assertiveness. Such an experience can help us, as carers and clients, to break out of our individualism and eradicate feelings of isolation. It can also help us to politicize ourselves and others, and raise our awareness of how much fuller life could be in our community. Empowerment would result, and it would help us to move away from what Bill Jordan described as the 'totally privatized, commercialized world of individual and household self-sufficiency and self-interest' (*Community Care*, 19 April 1990, p.28).

Thankfully, the old social-care world of 'us' working for 'them' is disappearing. Power-sharing, partnership and democratic ways of working in the social-care world of human need are far more appropriate. As Terry Bamford states, 'The old paternalism will not do. Client self-determination and a deliberate attempt to widen the opportunities for choice available to clients should be at the core of future services' (*Social Work Today*, 4 January 1990).

Good work practice has always been essentially about enabling clients to achieve more control over their own lives. Increased awareness of the detrimental effect of the marginalization process on certain groups in society, the growth of the consumer voice in social care and enhanced user involvement have all contributed to the creation of conditions that are more favourable to the enabling process. Any client-centred social care practice that fully acknowledges the importance of the clients' social setting will help to translate the theories and policies of heath and social care, and so move towards a more caring community.

1. Examining our behaviour in positive practice

Most of the time we behave in one of the four ways described below:

- non-assertive or passive – 'I will withdraw or retreat from the situation';
- aggressive – 'I will win at all costs';
- manipulative – 'I will use any method at my disposal';
- assertive – 'I will speak my mind, but will also take into account how others feel or think'.

Usually, as carers, we might assume that being assertive is the most appropriate way to act. However, at times one of the other three approaches might be more suitable. Think of examples of situations in which each of the four behaviours might be most appropriate.

2. What would you do?

(a) Colleague's behaviour
You work in a care home for people with learning disabilities. You notice that your colleague, Rose Horrocks, brings her own cup to work and insists on drinking from this. She will not use the cups provided and shared by the other staff and residents. When she uses cutlery from the home she elaborately ensures that it is clean, sometimes re-washing the item. The home has a dish-washer and, so far as you are concerned, operates good, safe hygiene practices. However, all of the staff and residents have free access to the kitchen and there is no guarantee that every item that is in the drawers and cupboards has been through the dish-washer.

What is your responsibility in this matter? Should you take any action as:

(a) a colleague?
(b) as her supervisor?

(b) Supervision
Although you recognize that your supervisor, Beryl Chyut, is trying to be accommodating towards you, particularly during supervision, you do not feel at ease with her. You regard her as being brash, anxious and unyielding. Outside supervision she is sometimes short with you, for instance when you recently asked for help with the computer, she typically showed irritability, by rolling her eyes to the ceiling, before she reluctantly assisted you, but not in an enabling way. You sit in close proximity to each other, on either side of the computer that you share, so you can overhear each other very easily when speaking on the telephone. You find her loud voice off-putting and are somewhat intimidated by her presence when making calls of your own. Eventually, in a formal feedback session, you learn from her that she is not satisfied with the number of visits and reports that you are producing, but she is unclear about the number she would expect you to complete. When you tell her that you have seven reports outstanding, she tells you quite earnestly, but in an offhand way. 'Well, you could do those in a day'. This is quite unrealistic so far as you are concerned, and conflicts both with what you regard as being feasible, and with your perception of the work rate of your colleagues. Her remark is consistent with an earlier, unhelpful claim that she could 'knock off reports in 10 minutes'.

You feel undermined and oppressed by Beryl, rather than being supported and properly guided.

(a) What implications does a poor relationship between any two members have for the rest of the team?
(b) Outline the steps that an individual would need to take if they were unhappy with the quality of supervision and guidance they were receiving.
(c) As Beryl, how would you feel about receiving this feedback from the person you supervise? What would be your response?
(d) As Henry, the section manager for both parties, what measures or actions could you take to help to resolve the grievances raised by the supervisee?

3. Carers' handbook

You are employed by a local branch of a national voluntary organization working with people with disabilities, and have been given responsibility for preparing a booklet for those who care for people in their own home. Include information on financial benefits, community resources, places of interest to visit, free entertainments, leisure facilities, statutory help, relevant organizations, local support networks and the availability of aids and adaptations.

4. Integration or special provision?

You are a social worker working with the family of a 13-year-old child who has a moderate learning disability and is also physically disabled and a wheelchair user. The girl, Marva James, has been offered the opportunity to attend a mainstream school full-time, and whilst her father would support such a move, her mother is against it, primarily because she feels that Marva is too vulnerable and would 'only experience failure'. To date Marva has been attending the same special school since she was 4 years old. The school was purpose-built and is constructed on one level; it has wide corridors and hand-rails throughout the building. The care within the school is of a very high standard, and teaching takes place in small groups with a low staff-student ratio. The facilities are good and pupils can receive physiotherapy and hydrotherapy on the school premises. The academic emphasis is mainly on developing basic reading and writing skills. Marva likes school *and has achieved a great deal.*

Over the past 12 months Marva has also been attending a mainstream comprehensive, initially 1 day per week during the first term, and finally for 3 days of the week during the third term. The school is not fully adapted for wheelchair use, but it is mainly on one level. Marva has been provided with her own word-processor and is eligible for additional individual teacher support with lessons under the conditions of her educational special needs statement. In other words, she is entitled to the exclusive support of an additional teacher in the classroom. However, this facility has not yet been arranged by the local education authority.

Marva likes her new school and no longer wants to go to the special school. She does not see herself as having the same problems as other children with learning

difficulties, and would regard a permanent move to a mainstream school as an achievement in itself. She wants to take up the chance of repeating the second year and to start full-time in September.

Mrs James, Marva's mother, is concerned that Marva will now be exposed to the possibility of ridicule by other children, and fears that she may even be at risk of physical injury in a large mainstream school. More significantly, she worries that Marva will 'only experience failure'. Marva would have to study for GCSEs, in which both her mother and father fear she will not do well. 'I want her to be able to read and write. . .but because of the National Curriculum she has to do French. What good will that do her?'

Despite the reservations of her mother, Marva's father would like to see his daughter experience mainstream full-time education in order that she may encounter some of the difficulties presented by the outside world as early as possible in her life. He argues that the younger she is when she is exposed to the reactions of 'able-bodied' people, the better adjusted she will be by the time she reaches adulthood. Mrs James is concerned that her daughter's already low self-image will be further damaged when she spends time away from the protective and supportive surroundings of the special school. How would you go about helping the parents to make a decision about Marva's full-time education?

5. Community care cases

You are the *duty social worker* for the team working with older people. Consider what action you would take in the following circumstances.

(a) *Bernard Gillespie*

Your senior approaches you with a referral of an older man, Bernard Gillespie, whom a neighbour says is neglecting himself. He has no food in the house. It is late in the day and she asks you to undertake an emergency visit. She gives you a £10 note from petty cash in case you have to buy him a hot meal. When you arrive at the man's house, in a rural part of the community, you get no reply so you go to the home of a neighbour, Mrs Erica Davidson and she returns to his house with you. You then see Mr

Gillespie making his way towards you from the side-door of the house. As he turns to go into the house you notice his shirt tail hanging out of his trousers – it is stained with what appears to be faeces. He leads you through the dark kitchen past the table, on which there stands a bag of groceries. The house is poorly lit, the carpet is smooth with ingrained dirt and you are loath to sit down in the vacant armchair. By the side of Bernard's chair is a bucket, three-quarters full of pale brown liquid. He explains that this is 'slops' to give to the chickens he keeps in the back garden. He says that he is perfectly well, and gets all the help he needs from his other neighbour (the one who made the referral), and from his sister who visits once a week to take his washing and bring him some groceries. Bernard does not want any help and thanks you for your concern. After you have left Mr Gillespie's home, Mrs Davidson tells you that, in her opinion, he has deteriorated since the recent loss of his brother with whom he lived for many years. She would like to do more for him but he has not allowed her to because he does not like women (except his sister). Instead he unrealistically relies on his other neighbour who, Erica informs you, is no longer able to help because he has a job outside the home and is caring for his own sick mother. You are satisfied that Bernard is safe for the evening, but you feel that he needs support. What do you recommend and how do you produce a value-free report of his circumstances?

(b) Doreen Burns

You receive a telephone call from the angry son of Doreen Burns, a woman who is living in sheltered housing. Recently she fell during the night and the assistant warden attended to her. Mrs Burns had cut her head badly. Mr Burns thinks that his mother is not safe in her fourth-floor flat, and he would like her to be transferred to residential care. He says that he is, at the moment of talking to you, holding the blood-stained towel that was used to soak up the blood from his mother's head wound. If you do not agree to meet with him and his wife he will complain to the director and go to the newspapers. Mr Burns and his wife have complained in the past. The last duty social worker they dealt with was, according to Mr Burns, 'absolutely hopeless'. You contact the warden, who says that although Mrs Burn's wound bled profusely she had been well attended and had not been in any danger. Her fall was an isolated occurrence. The warden feels that Mrs Burns is happily placed in her flat and has no desire to be transferred to residential care, and that the family are trying to use the accident as a lever to get her transferred so that they will feel better themselves.

Your senior asks you to arrange an initial meeting as a matter of urgency.

Role play the initial meeting. Decide who you think should be present and where the meeting should be held.

(c) Roy Fletcher

Mr Fletcher is 65 years old and been living in warden-controlled accommodation following a stroke 2 years earlier. He is normally able to get about by himself, and regularly goes to the pub for his lunch, but he is suffering from gout at present which makes it difficult for him to walk. He has taken to staying in bed each morning and has asked the warden, Meg Morris, to make him bacon and eggs. As a favour she has made his breakfast on a couple of occasions, but she really does not have time to do this regularly. He also has a home carer to help him to get washed and dressed for half an hour each morning. Meg is requesting that the carer's time be extended to an hour each morning so that she can prepare breakfast for Mr Fletcher. He has had meals-on-wheels in the past but refused to eat them. Mrs Morris would like to have the additional daily care for a period of 2 weeks, by which time she hopes that his gout may be controlled medically, and that he will then be able to bear weight on his foot and resume his normal routine.

QUESTIONS FOR ESSAYS OR DISCUSSION

1. Discrimination-awareness training introduces new terms and language, but drives prejudice and discrimination underground.

2. There has been severe criticism of the standard of residential and nursing home care for older people. In what ways can you improve the service offered to older people who are residents in a care or nursing home, so that they may be more fulfilled and more independent?

3. The idea of 'full citizenship' is not attainable in an unequal society like our own.

4. Empowerment and its application with regard to user involvement is flawed because the power involved is granted rather than taken.

5. Organizational efficiency, keyboard proficiency and a high case-turnover rate are important skills for modern social workers and health professionals. They override such traditional qualities as empathy, compassion and client-centredness.

6. Individual positive social care practice is divorced from wider social change.

FURTHER READING

Academic sources

Ahmed, A. 1990: *Practice with care.* London: Racial Equality Unit. A very detailed code of practice aimed at those working with black communities within the social services context. It highlights the relevance of the Race Relations Act to other aspects of social work legislation, and provides examples of good practice.

Bell, L. 1993: *Carefully – a guide for home care assistants.* London: Ace Books. A useful handbook for home carers that promotes good practice and independence. Accessible material.

Carmichael, K. 1992: *Ceremony of innocence tears: power and protest.* London: Macmillan. A book that looks at the feelings engendered by caring, and more particularly the role, purpose and value of tears. Very readable, compassionate and uplifting.

Centre for Policy on Ageing. 1996: *A better home life.* London: Centre for Policy on Ageing. An update of the very popular *Home life: a code of practice for residential care*, which was written as a guide for care-home owners established under the Regis-

tered Homes Act 1984. This book is as readable and resourceful in its recommendations of good practice as its predecessor.

Harvey, C. and Philpot, T. (eds) 1994: *Practising social work.* London: Routledge. An outline and explanation of some of the wide range of social work techniques used today. Very clear, with contributions from a number of current practitioners.

Tossell, D. and Webb, R. 1994: *Inside the caring services*, 2nd edn. London: Edward Arnold. An accessible, simple and comprehensive overview of the caring services, including both statutory and voluntary sectors. The book also highlights ways of performing social care and social work, and the basic qualities of a carer.

Other literary sources

Axline, V. M. 1990: *Dibs – in search of self.* Harmondsworth: Penguin.

Bach, R. 1973: *Jonathan Livingston Seagull.* London: Pan.

Fournier, A. 1966: *Le grand meaulnes.* Harmondsworth: Penguin.

Fynn. 1977: *Mister God this is Anna.* London: Fount/Collins.

Jefferies, R. 1968: *The story of my heart.* London: Macmillan.

Morrison, B. 1994: *And when did you last see your father?* London: Granta Publications.

ANSWERS TO MENTAL HEALTH QUIZ
(P.219)

1. (a)
2. (a)
3. (c)
4. (b)
5. (b)
6. (a) – approximately 95 per cent are voluntary patients
7. (a)
8. (a)
9. (c)
10. (b)

References

Acton, T. 1974: *Gypsy politics and social change.* London: Routledge and Kegan Paul.

Adonis, A. and Pollard, S. 1997: *A class act – the myth of Britain's classless society.* London: Hamish Hamilton.

Age Concern. 1996: *Older people in the UK. Some basic facts.* London: Age Concern.

Alcorn, K. and Browning, P. 1998: *National Aids manual.* London: NAM Publications.

Anderson, I. and Morgan, J. 1997: *Social housing for single people? A study of local policy and practice.* York: Joseph Rowntree Foundation.

Anon. 1995: Care management: a disastrous mistake. *Lancet* **345**, 399–401.

Archbishops' Commission on Rural Areas. 1990: *Faith in the countryside.* London: Churchman.

Baker, A. and Townsend, P. 1996: Post-divorce parenting: rethinking shared residence. *Child Care and Law Quarterly* **8**, 217–20.

Balchin, P. 1995: *Housing policy – an introduction.* London: Routledge.

Balloch, S., Andrew, T., Davey, B. *et al.* 1997: *The Social Services workforce in transition.* London: National Institute for Social Work.

Bamford, T. 1990: *The future of social work.* London: Macmillan.

Barnes, C. 1991: *Disabled people in Britain and discrimination.* London: Hurst & Co.

Beresford, P. and Turner, M. 1997: *It's our welfare. Report of the Citizen's Commission on the future of the Welfare State.* London: National Institute for Social Work.

Bishops' Committee for Community Relations. 1992: *From charity to empowerment: the Church's mission alongside poor and marginalized people.* London: Bishop's Committee for Community Relations.

Blackstone, T. 1990: *Prisons and penal reform.* London: Chatto and Windus.

Boyson, R. 1987: *The defence of the family. The battle against permissiveness.* Watford: Church Society.

Brackx, A. and Grimshaw, C. (eds) 1989: *Mental health care in crisis.* London: Pluto Press.

Brandon, D. (ed.) 1989: *Mutual respect. Therapeutic approaches to working with people who have learning difficulties.* Surbiton: Good Impressions Publishing.

Brewer, C. and Lait, J. 1980: *Can social work survive?* London: Temple Smith.

Brown, G.W., Brolchan, M.N., and Harris, T. 1975: Social class and psychiatric disturbance among women in an urban population. *Sociology* **9**, 225–54.

Bulmer, M., 1989: *The goals of social policy.* London: Unwin Hyman.

Burgess, A. 1997a: *Fatherhood reclaimed. The making of the modern father.* London: Vermilion.

Burgess, A. 1997b: *Carlton parenting campaign fathers.* London: Institute for Public Policy and Research.

Campling, J. (ed.) 1989: *Learning the hard way. A feminist list.* London: Macmillan.

Carers' National Association. 1997: *Who we are, what we do.* London: Carers' National Association.

Carey-Wood, J. *et al.* 1995: Settlement of refugees in Britain. Home Office Research Study. London: HMSO.

Centrepoint. 1996: *The new picture of youth homelessness.* London: Centrepoint.

Chambers, C. *et al.* 1996: *Celebrating identity – a resource manual for practitioners working with black children and young people, including black children of mixed parentage.* Stoke-on Trent: Trentham Books.

Church Action on Poverty. 1996: *Women and low pay.* Manchester: Church Action on Poverty.

Church Action on Poverty. 1997: *Unemployment and the jobseeker's allowance – the people.* Manchester: Church Action on Poverty.

Cochrane, R., and Stopes-Roe, M. 1981: Women, marriage, employment and mental health. *British Journal of Psychiatry* **139**, 137–45.

Cohen, B. 1988: *Caring for children; service policies for child care and equal opportunities in the UK. Report for the European Commission Child Care Network.* Brussels: Commission of the European Communities.

Commission for Racial Equality. 1989: *From cradle to school – A practical guide to race, equality and childcare.* London: Commission for Racial Equality.

Commission for Racial Equality. 1996: *Roots of the future. Ethnic diversity in the making of modern Britain.* London: Commission for Racial Equality.

Commission for Racial Equality. 1997a: *Ethnic minority women. Fact sheet.* London: Commission for Racial Equality.

Commission for Racial Equality. 1997b: *Irish in Britain.* London: Commission for Racial Equality.

Commission for Racial Equality. 1997c: *Migration and citizenship. Fact sheet.* London: Commission for Racial Equality.

Commission for Racial Equality. 1997d: *No limits visible. Women challenging race and sex discrimination.* London: Commission for Racial Equality.

Commission for Racial Equality. 1997e: *Policing and race in England and Wales. Fact sheet.* London: Commission for Racial Equality.

Commission for Racial Equality. 1997f: *Racial attacks and harassment.* London: Commission for Racial Equality.

Commission for Racial Equality. 1997g: *Racial equality and the Asylum and Immigration Act. 1.* London: Commission for Racial Equality.

Commission for Racial Equality. 1997h: *Refugees and asylum-seekers.* London: Commission for Racial Equality.

Commission for Racial Equality. 1997i: *Criminal justice in England and Wales.* London: Commission for Racial Equality.

Commission for Racial Equality. 1997j: *Employment and unemployment.* London: Commission for Racial Equality.

Cook, S. L. 1994: *Surviving social work education. Black student's handbook.* London: Race Equality Unit.

Council of Relatives to Assist in the Care of Dementia (CRAC Dementia). 1994: *Caring for dementia: early onset dementia. A living bereavement – the wife's story.* London: CRAC Dementia.

Daycare Trust. 1997: *Briefing Paper. Childcare now. Making it happen.* London: Daycare Trust.

Department of Education. 1985: *Swann Report. Education for All – The Report of the Committee of Enquiry into the Education of Children from Ethnic Minority Groups.* London: HMSO.

Department for Education and Employment. 1995: *Report of the UK Delegation on the Fourth UN World Conference on Women.* London: Department for Education and Employment.

Department for Education and Employment. 1996: *Work and the family: ideas and options for childcare. A consultation paper.* London: Department for Education and Employment.

Department of Health. 1995: *Variations in health – what can the Department of Health and the NHS do?* London: Department of Health.

Department of Health. 1997a: *Young carers – Something to think about. Report of four SSI workshops May–June 1995.* London: The Stationery Office.

Department of Health. 1997b: *The new NHS: modern, dependable.* London: The Stationery Office.

Dibblin, J. (ed.) 1991: *Wherever I lay my hat – young women and homelessness.* London: Shelter.

Disability Alliance. 1988: *The financial circumstances of disabled adults living in private households. Briefing paper No. 2.* London: Disability Alliance.

Disraeli, B. 1980 (originally published in 1845): *Sybil, or the two nations*. Harmondsworth: Penguin.

Donnellan, C. (ed.) 1996: *Men, women and equality. Independence. Vol. 18*. Cambridge: Cambridge University Press.

Doty, M. 1996: *Heaven's coast: a memoir*. London: Jonathan Cape.

Doyle, R. 1996: *The woman who walked into doors*. London: Minerva.

Elkington, G. and Harrison, J. 1997: *Caring for someone at home*. London: Carers' National Association.

Equal Opportunities Commission. 1995a: *In pursuit of equality. A national agenda for action. Policy Paper 2*. Manchester: Equal Opportunities Commission.

Equal Opportunities Commission. 1995b: *In pusuit of equality. Policy Paper 5. Media*. Manchester: Equal Opportunities Commission.

European Commission. 1993: *European social policy (background report)*. London: European Commission.

European Commission. 1996: *How is the EU meeting social and regional needs?* London: European Commission.

European Commission Network on Childcare. 1996: *A review of services for young children*. London: European Commission Network on Childcare.

Fernando, S. (ed.) 1995: *Mental health in a multi-ethnic society*. London: Routledge.

Field, F. 1989: *Losing out: the emergence of Britain's underclass*. Oxford: Basil Blackwell.

Ford, C., Shaw, R., and Morris, J. 1997: *Controlling your own personal assistance services*, 2nd edn. Derby: British Council of Organizations of Disabled People.

Formaini, H. 1990: *Men – the darker continent*. London: Mandarin.

Frayne, B. and Muir, J. 1994: *Nowhere to run. Underfunding of women's refuges and the case for reform*. London: London Housing Unit.

Friedli, L. and Scherzer, A. 1996: *Positive steps: mental health and young people*. London: Health Education Authority.

Fryer, P. 1984: *Staying power – the history of black people*. London: Pluto Press.

Giddens, A. 1982: *Sociology – a brief but critical introduction*. London: Macmillan.

Goldthorpe, J. 1980: *Social mobility and class structure in modern Britain*. Oxford: Oxford University Press.

Hanmer, I. and Statham, D. 1988: *Women and social work – towards a woman-centred practice*. London: Macmillan.

Hansard Society. 1990: *Women at the top*. London: Hansard Society.

Hansard Society. 1996: *Women at the top: progress after 5 years. A Follow-Up Report to the Hansard Society Commission on Women at the Top*. London: Hansard Society.

Hantrais, L. 1995: *Social policy in the European Union*. London: Macmillan.

Health Education Council. 1987: *The health divide: inequalities in health in the 1980s*. London: Health Education Council.

Heidensohn, F. 1985: *Gender and crime*. London: Macmillan.

Hite, S. 1988: *Women and love*. Harmondsworth: Penguin.

Holman, B. 1992: *Reconstructing the common good. Tawney Lecture*. London: Christian Socialist Movement.

Holman, B. 1997: *Towards equality: a Christian manifesto*. London: SPCK.

Home Affairs Committee. 1986: *Report on racial attacks and harassment*. London: HMSO.

Home Office. 1990: *Crime, justice and protecting the public*. London: HMSO.

House of Lords Select Committee on the European Commission. 1985: *Income taxation and equal treatment for men and women*. London: HMSO.

Hough, M. and Mayhew, P. 1985: *Taking account of crime. Key findings from the 1984 British Crime Survey*. London: HMSO.

Howard League for Penal Reform. 1994: *Fact sheet 4. The Howard League's programme of action for reforming the prison system*. London: Howard League.

Hutton, W. 1997: *The state to come.* London: Vintage.

Inner London Education Authority. 1985: *Race, sex and class. 6. A policy for equality.* London: ILEA.

Jacobs, B. 1988: *Racism in Britain.* Bromley: Helm.

Joint Council for the Welfare of Immigrants. 1997a: *The new asylum and immigration proposals.* London: JCWI.

Joint Council for the Welfare of Immigrants. 1997b: *Immigration and nationality handbook.* London: JCWI.

Joint Council for the Welfare of Immigrants. 1997c: *Annual Report and Policy Review.* London: JCWI.

Jones, C. 1983: *State social work and the working class.* London: Macmillan.

Jordan, B. 1989: *The common good – citizenship, morality and self-interest.* Oxford: Basil Blackwell.

King's Fund. 1995: *Tackling inequalities in health: An agenda for action.* London: King's Fund.

Langan, M. and Lee, P. (eds) 1989: *Radical social work today.* London: Unwin Hyman.

Lee, H. 1960: *To kill a mockingbird.* London: William Heinemann.

Letts, P. 1983: *Double trouble – sex, discrimination and one-parent families.* London: National Council for One-Parent Families.

Littlewood, R. and Lipsedge, M. 1982: *Aliens and alienists.* Harmondsworth: Pelican.

Lobstein, T. 1997: *British lifestyles, 1994.* London: National Food Alliance.

Luthura, M. 1997: *Britain's black population. Social change, public policy and agenda.* Aldershot: Arena.

McNeil-Taylor, E. 1985: *Bringing up children on your own.* London: Fontana.

Mack, J. and Lansley, S. 1985: *Poor Britain.* London: Allen and Unwin.

Mallinson, I. 1988: *The social care task.* Surbiton: Social Care Association.

Mama, A. 1989: *The hidden struggle – statutory and voluntary sector responses to violence against black women in the home.* London: Race and Housing Research Initiative.

Marshall, G., Newby, R. and Rose, D. 1988: *Social class in modern Britain.* London: Hutchinson.

Marx, K. and Engels, F. 1975: *Manifesto of the Communist party.* Harrow: Foreign Languages Press.

Mental Health Foundation. 1996: *Improving services for Asian people with learning difficulties.* London: Mental Health Foundation.

Ministry of Housing and Local Government and the Welsh Office. 1967: *Gypsies and other travellers.* London: HMSO.

Morris, J. 1990: *Our homes, our rights.* London: Shelter.

Murray, C. 1984: *Losing ground: American social policy 1950–1980.* New York: Basic Books.

Myrdal, G. 1962: *Challenge to affluence.* New York: Pantheon.

National Association for the Care and Resettlement of Offenders. 1995: *Criminal justice digest.* London: NACRO.

National Association for the Care and Resettlement of Offenders. 1997: *Getting serious about youth crime.* London: NACRO.

National Association of Probation Officers. 1989: *Working with lesbians and gay men as clients of the service – good practice guidelines.* London: National Association of Probation Officers.

National Council For One-Parent Families. 1988: *70th Anniversary Annual Report (NCOPF).* London: National Council For One-Parent Families.

National Council For One-Parent Families. 1990: *Key facts.* London: National Council For One-Parent Families.

National Institute for Social Work. 1988a: *Wagner Report. Residential care – a positive choice.* London: National Institute for Social Work.

National Institute for Social Work. 1988b: *Wagner Report. Residential care – the research reviewed.* London: National Institute for Social Work.

National Institute for Social Work. 1996: *Creating a home from home – a guide to standards. Residential forum.* London: National Institute for Social Work.

Norman, A. 1985: *Triple jeopardy: growing old in a second homeland.* London: Centre for Policy on Ageing.

O'Dwyer, C. 1994: *Homelessness – what's the problem?* London: Shelter.

Office of Population Censuses and Surveys. 1988: *The financial circumstances of disabled adults living in private households. Surveys of disability in Great Britain. No. 2.* London: HMSO.

Okely, J. 1983: *The traveller-gypsies.* Cambridge: Cambridge University Press.

Oliver, M. 1990: *The politics of disablement.* Basingstoke: Macmillan Education.

Oppenheimer, J. and Reckitt. 1997: *Acting on Aids: sex, drugs and politics.* London: Serpent's Tail.

Orbach, S. 1978: *Fat is a feminist issue.* London: Hamlyn.

Paterson, J. 1997: *Disability rights handbook*, 22nd edn. London: Disability Alliance Educational and Research Association.

Payne, M. 1986: *Social care in the community.* Birmingham: British Association of Social Workers.

Perry, A. (ed.) 1996: *Sociology: insights in health care.* London: Arnold.

Philo, G., Henderson, L., McLaughlin, G. *et al.* 1993: *Mass media representation of mental health/illness: report for Health Education Board for Scotland.* Glasgow: Glasgow University Media Group.

Raynor, P., Smith, D., Vanstone, M. 1994: *Effective probation practice.* Basingstoke: BASW/ Macmillan.

Rosen, M. (ed.) 1991: *Give me shelter.* London: Shelter.

Rowlands, O. 1998: *Informal carers.* London: HMSO.

Roy, A. 1997: *The God of small things.* London: Flamingo.

Royal College of Psychiatrists. 1997: *Every family in the land.* London: Royal College of Psychiatrists.

Ryan, W. 1976: *Blaming the victim.* London: Vintage.

Sarton, M. 1992: *As we are now.* London: The Women's Press.

Sayce, E. 1997: *Respect – time to end discrimination on mental health grounds.* London: MIND Publications.

Sheffield Gypsy and Traveller Support Group. 1992: *Response to the Consultation Paper 18–8–92 'Reform of the Caravan Sites Act 1968'.*

Sickle Cell Society. 1997: *A brief guide to sickle cell disorders.* London: Sickle Cell Society.

Simons, K. 1995: *My home, my life: innovative approaches to housing and support for people with learning difficulties.* Bristol: Values into Action/Nora Fry Research Centre.

Smith, P. 1985: *Language, the sexes and society.* Oxford: Basil Blackwell.

Social Care Association. 1990: *Code of practice.* Birmingham: British Association of Social Workers.

Stewart, G. and Stewart, J. 1993: *Social work and housing.* Basingstoke: BASW/Macmillan.

Stonewall. 1997a: *Same-sex couples and the law. Fact sheet.* London: Stonewall.

Stonewall. 1997b: *Public opinion on lesbian and gay rights. Fact sheet.* London: Stonewall.

Tossell, D. and Webb, R. 1994: *Inside the caring services*, 2nd edn. London: Edward Arnold.

Twitchin, J. 1988: *The black and white media book. Handbook for the study of racism and television.* Stoke-on-Trent: Trentham Books Ltd.

UNISON. 1997: *Sexual harassment – some guidelines for UNISON branches. Women in UNISON.* London: UNISON.

University of Warwick, 1994: *Labour Market Structure and Prospects for Women.* Warwick University, p. 57.

Utting, W. 1997: *People like us: the Report of the Review of the Safeguards for Children Living Away from Home.* London: HMSO.

Walker, A. 1994: *Half a century of promises – the failures to realise 'community care' for older people.* London: Counsel and Care.

Ward, S. 1986: Power, politics and poverty. In Golding, P. (ed.), *Excluding the poor.* CPAG.

Whitehead, M. 1997: *Health inequalities.* London: HMSO.

Wilson, M. and Francis, J. 1997: *Raised voices – African-Caribbean and African users' views of mental health services in England and Wales.* London: MIND Publications.

Women in Mind. 1990: *Finding our own solutions – women's experiences of mental health care.* London: Women in Mind.

Index